NEURAL CORRELATES OF CONSCIOUSNESS

NEURAL CORRELATES OF CONSCIOUSNESS
Empirical and Conceptual Questions

edited by Thomas Metzinger

A Bradford Book
The MIT Press
Cambridge, Massachusetts
London, England

Second printing, 2002

© 2000 Massachusetts Institute of Technology

This book was set in Times New Roman on '3B2' by
Asco Typesetters, Hong Kong and was printed and
bound in the United States of America.

Library of Congress Cataloging-in-Publication Data

Neural correlates of consciousness : empirical and conceptual questions / edited by Thomas Metzinger.
 p.   cm.
 Includes bibliographical references and index.
 ISBN 0-262-13370-9 (hardcover : alk. paper)
 1. Consciousness. 2. Neuropsychology. I. Metzinger,
Thomas, 1958–
QP411.N48   2000
612.8′2—dc21   99-087947

Contents

Preface

This volume tries to make a bold step forward. For the first time ever, it unites a number of highly renowned neuroscientists and philosophers, from all over the world, who are together investigating the way in which the content of subjective experience is correlated with events in the brain. The current collection grew out of the conference "Neural Correlates of Consciousness: Empirical and Conceptual Questions," which took place June 19–22, 1998, in Bremen, Germany. I had the honor to act as the principal organizer for this conference, and I am now very pleased to be able to present a small selection of the many excellent contributions that were made there.

The 1998 Bremen meeting was a special event for the consciousness research community for several reasons. One was that it was organized and supported by two newly founded and particularly dynamic academic institutions: the Association for the Scientific Study of Consciousness (ASSC) and the Hanse-Wissenschaftskolleg in Delmenhorst. I am deeply indebted to both organizations, and want to take the opportunity to thank some of the people who have helped me. First, the members of the ASSC conference committee: Bill Banks, David Chalmers, Christof Koch, Antti Revonsuo, and Patrick Wilken. They assured the scientific quality of the meeting, and in doing so indirectly made it possible for this volume to come into existence. Second, I wish to thank all those who have supported me on the level of local organization. Professor Dr. Dr. Gerhard Roth, as director of the hosting institution, financially secured the enterprise and, with continuous enthusiasm, backed it up on many levels. Ingeborg Mehser, Diana Garde, Martin Meier, Beatrice Riewe, and Marion Wachholz-Logemann mastered a number of unforeseeable difficulties and took countless burdens off my back. I could not have done without the continuous support from the superb team in the Hanse-Wissenschaftskolleg. The same is true, in particular, of my wife, Anja. She is my continuous source of strength and inspiration. In a way, however, I am most proud of the student team led by John-Dylan Haynes, Harald Schmidt, and Sven Schütt: Jakob Bösenberg, Christina Egger, Christine Häßler, Martin Haindorff, Jürgen Hanken, Alexander Hillmann, Stefan Huth, Tobias Gronau, Ulrich Kühne, Heide Müller-Leiendecker, Marcus Naumer, Anett Noster, and Andreas Wawrzinek. Some of them may not yet know it, but they are the consciousness researchers of the future.

San Diego, July 1999

NEURAL CORRELATES OF CONSCIOUSNESS

Introduction: Consciousness Research at the End of the Twentieth Century

From False Intuitions to Psychophysical Correlations

In 1989 the philosopher Colin McGinn asked the following question: "How can technicolor phenomenology arise from soggy gray matter?" (1989: 349). Since then many authors in the field of consciousness research have quoted this question over and over, like a slogan that in a nutshell conveys a deep and important theoretical problem. It seems that almost none of them discovered the subtle trap inherent in this question. The brain is not gray. The brain is colorless.

Obviously, the fundamental methodological problem faced by any rigorous research program on consciousness is the subjectivity of the target phenomenon. It consists in the simple fact that conscious experience, under standard conditions, is always tied to an individual, first-person perspective. The subjective qualities inherent in a phenomenal color experience are a paradigm example of something that is accessible from a first-person perspective only. Color consciousness—regardless whether in gray or in Technicolor—is a *subjective* phenomenon. However, the precise nature of the relationship of such first-person phenomena to elements within the domain of objectively describable events is unclear. From an objective, third-person perspective all we find in the world are electromagnetic radiation and the reflectance properties of middle-sized objects, wavelength mixtures and metamers, retinal input vectors and activation patterns in the visual system. None of these, so far, map nicely and systematically onto the chromatic primitives of subjective, visual experience. It is just as our physics teacher in high school always told us: From a strictly objective perspective, no such things as colors exist in the world. Therefore, the pivotal question is *not* How do we get from gray to Technicolor?

The core question is if at all—and if so, in what sense—physical states of the human nervous system, under a certain description, can be successfully mapped onto the content of conscious experience. This content can be a simple qualitative feature like "grayness" or "sogginess." There are also complex, nested forms of conscious content like "the self in the act of knowing" (see, e.g., chapters 7 and 20 in this volume) or high-level phenomenal properties like "coherence" or "holism" (e.g., chapters 8 and 9 in this volume). But what, precisely, does it mean that conscious experience has a "content"? Is this an entity open to empirical research programs and interdisciplinary cooperation? And what would it mean to map this content onto physical states "under a certain description"? In other words: What kinds of relations *are* psychophysical correlations? Do we have a workable conception of the isomorphism we are obviously assuming? If one is seriously interested in getting away from the naïveté of popular discussions concerning consciousness, the first thing one has to understand is that we know the world only under representations. For philosophers this is a point of great triviality, but since the large majority of contributors in this volume address empirical issues, a few short remarks may be in order. Let me explain.

Theoretical and Phenomenal Models of Reality

One way to know the world (and ourselves) is under *theoretical* representations. For instance, we can use descriptions of the brain generated by empirical research in the cognitive neurosciences. Neurophysiological descriptions of certain brain areas or neural algorithms describing their computational properties are typical and well-known examples. We can also gain further knowledge under conceptual interpretations of such descriptions generated by analytical philosophers of mind. For instance, philosophers might speak about the way in which a certain abstract property, such as a causal role, is "realized" by a certain concrete state in the brain. Both types of descriptions are linguistic representations, and their content is propositional.

Another way to know the world (and ourselves) is under a *phenomenal* representation. For instance, to come back to our initial example, we can use the content of conscious experience generated by our own brain in the act of visually perceiving another brain in order to gain knowledge about the world. "Grayness," for instance, is one important aspect of the content of a phenomenal representation. The subjectively experienced colors of a rainbow or those of a movie in Technicolor are further examples. The format of phenomenal representations is something for which we currently possess no precise terminology, but it is obviously not of a syntactically structured, linguistic kind, and their content is only very rarely of a conceptual or propositional nature. You don't need language to be conscious—a nonlinguistic creature could certainly have the subjective experience of "grayness."[1] Again, there are also conceptual interpretations of the content of conscious representations itself (for instance, generated by phenomenologically oriented philosophers of mind), and in some cases such descriptions constitute a valuable source of information.

At the end of the twentieth century we have some good ideas about what it could mean for an empirical theory (the first type of representation) to possess "content." However, it is unclear what it means, precisely, to claim that states of consciousness (the second type of representation) have "content." I am not going to answer this question here. But let me frame it in a simplified way that may serve to illustrate an important aspect of the underlying issue. The problem may consist in the fact that phenomenal representations are special in having *two* kinds of content. Philosophers sometimes speak of the *intentional content* and of the *phenomenal content* of mental representations. Consider the following example: While visiting one of the new underground laboratories for experimental philosophy of mind, which are mushrooming all over the world, you suddenly find yourself holding a freshly excised human brain in your hand and, looking at it, you

have the phenomenal experience of "grayness" and "sogginess." The next night, after awaking from a nightmare in which you subjectively relived exactly the same scene, including precisely the same visual and tactile qualities, you realize that you have just had a complex hallucination. This time, fortunately, it was all a dream.

What was the difference between the two episodes? In a first and very rough approximation one might say the following: In the initial case your relevant mental state had intentional *and* phenomenal content. The intentional content consisted in the fact that this mental state actually referred to something in the external world; there really *was* a brain in your hand. The phenomenal content consisted, for example, in the subjectively experienced qualities of "grayness" and "sogginess." In the second case, however, there was *only* phenomenal content, because no such thing as a brain existed in your present environment—your hand was paralyzed and your visual system was decoupled from external input (regarding dreams as a model system for phenomenal experience, see chapter 4 in this volume). If you remove the external component, you seem to get very close to the pure experiential content (on the neural correlates of spontaneous visual hallucinations and on bistable phenomena, see chapters 14 and 15 in this volume).

It is probably safe to say that a majority of experts in the relevant areas of philosophy would, while wholeheartedly disagreeing about the nature of intentional content, at least subscribe to the thesis that phenomenal content, in a strong sense, supervenes on properties of the brain.[2] That is, as soon as all internal and contemporaneous properties of your brain are fixed, all properties of your conscious experience are fully determined as well. What is determined is how being in these states *feels* to you, not if these states are what philosophers would call "epistemic states"—states that actually carry knowledge by relating you to the world in a meaningful way. In the short introductions written for the parts of this volume, I will use the concept of "phenomenal content" in accordance with this loose, nontechnical definition: The phenomenal content of your mental representations is that aspect which, being independent of their veridicality, is available for conscious experience from the first-person perspective while simultaneously being determined by inclusively internal properties of your brain.

What is the upshot of this first conceptual clarification? Consciously experienced colors or the tactile experience of "sogginess" are parts of a *phenomenal* model of reality. The content of global conscious states like waking or dreaming is the content of phenomenal models of reality, episodically activated by the brain of an individual human being. Wavelength mixtures and the like are theoretical entities in *scientific* models of reality. Scientific models of reality are generated by socially interacting groups of human beings. This point is important in order to prevent a second possible form of popular naïveté lurking in the background. The reality of the brain as well as the reality of consciousness as described by science are, strictly speaking, not "the" objective domain. They are the result of *intersubjective* cooperation within scientific communities. If readers will permit the use of a connectionist metaphor: A theoretical model is more like a distributed and coherent pattern in a social network, dynamically unfolding its informational content while subtly changing the internal landscape of the overall system. It is also interesting to note that, in parallel with the renaissance of systematic research programs on conscious experience, we are starting to discover the neural correlates of social cognition as well (see chapter 22 in this volume).

If individual human beings, maybe as observers of a neurosurgical operation or, while in the basement of a pathology institute as witnesses of the dissection of a corpse, consciously look at the exposed brain of a fellow human being, then they will, under standard conditions, experience this brain as having the color gray. *Their* brains

activate individual phenomenal models of reality, including the visually perceived brain. From an objective point of view, however, both brains involved in this perceptual relation are absolutely colorless. There are no colors in the external world. Matter never was gray. So what is it that generates those false intuitions often leading us astray? It is the fact that theoretical reality-modeling is anchored in phenomenal reality-modeling, and that phenomenal reality-modeling is characterized by an all-pervading naive realism.

From a strictly subjective point of view there is only one brain, and in all its concrete sogginess and grayness it is certainly not perceived by another brain, but by a self-conscious *person*. This person enjoys what Revonsuo (see chapter 4 in this volume) has called an "out-of-the-brain-experience": a very robust sense of presence in and the immersion into a seemingly real world outside the brain. Yet many theoretical considerations and a flood of empirical data now strongly point to the conclusion that in all its ultimate realism, this form of experiential content is itself entirely dependent on the internal workings of an individual brain. And trying to understand this nexus between the virtuality of an external existence and the internal dynamics of biological information-processing certainly is more exciting than any popular debate could ever be. While the Mysterian's trap is just a rhetorical bogeyman, we are actually faced with much deeper theoretical issues and an extremely interesting set of empirical challenges. This book is about these challenges. How could genuine first-person phenomenal experience emerge in a self-organizing physical universe?

The NCC: Correlating Phenomenal Content with Properties of the Brain

Given this context, what does it mean to look for the "neural correlates of consciousness" (NCC)? The idea of an NCC has been around in discussions since about 1980, and was probably first used in print by Francis Crick and Christof Koch (1990). In some cases it will mean looking for correlations between certain events in the brain—under a certain representation, as described on a certain neurobiological level of analysis—and for certain events in the ongoing dynamics of phenomenal experience—under a certain representation, as described by the attending, cognizing subject, usually in the everyday terminology of "folk phenomenology." In other cases it will mean looking for correlations between the occurrence of events of the first kind—again, as neuroscientifically described—and the occurrence of events of the second kind—as only *indicated* in a nonlinguistic manner by the subject, such as in pushing a button. Generally speaking, the epistemic goal—what we really want to *know*—in the type of correlation studies relevant to consciousness research consists in isolating the *minimally sufficient neural correlate* for specific kinds of phenomenal content (see chapter 2 in this volume). Such a correlate, however, will always be relative to a certain class of systems and to internal as well as external conditions. In this empirical context it will be the minimal set of properties, described on an appropriate level of neuroscientific analysis, that is sufficient to activate a certain conscious content in the mind of the organism.

However, mapping does not mean reduction. Correlation does not mean explanation. Once strict, fine-grained correlations between brain states and conscious states have been established, a number of theoretical options are still open. Additional constraints therefore will eventually be needed. Important questions are What is the true nature of these psychophysical correlations? Are we justified in interpreting them as *causal* relations? What additional constraints would have to be introduced in order to speak of *lawlike correlations* (see chapter 3 in this volume)? Is a fully reductive account, or even an eliminativist strategy, possible? (See, e.g., P. M.

Churchland 1985, 1986, 1988; P. S. Churchland 1986.)

Assume that we find a strict and systematic correlation between a certain brain property or type of neural event N and the subjectively experienced phenomenal property of "sogginess" S. This is entirely compatible with Cartesian dualism: The underlying relation could indeed be a causal one, namely causal *interaction* between events in two ontologically distinct domains. If the ideas of Descartes or those of Popper and Eccles (see Popper and Eccles; Popper 1996) were correct, then we would certainly find neural correlates of consciousness. However, it could also be the case that we have only a unidirectional arrow pointing from N to S, a causal one-way street leading upward from the brain into the conscious mind. If *epiphenomenalism* were true, phenomenal experience as such would be causally inefficacious.[3] Certainly most neuroscientists today would rather be epiphenomenalists than dualists. The problem is this: Empirical correlation data do not help us to decide between those two positions. A third possibility is that there may be no direct causal relationship between N and S at all; they could both be dependent on a single event in the past or upon repeated singular events, constantly reestablishing the observed correlation. The classical position for the first type of interpretation is the Leibnizian concept of prestabilized harmony, the second model is historically represented by "occasionalist" philosophers like Arnold Geulincx and Malebranche, who thought that God would, *ad occasionem*, actively correlate the minds of all human beings with their body whenever necessary. The methodological problem in the background is that of *screening off* N and S from more distant, alternative causes (see chapter 17 in this volume). One typical example of the absence of direct causal relationships between highly correlated sets of events is clocks: Usually large numbers of clocks and watches in our environment all show the same time, though they do not possess direct causal links in any interesting sense.

If we find strict, fine-grained, and systematic correlations between neural and phenomenal types of events, this does not rule out a fourth possibility. There may be *no* causal relationship between events like N and S at all, neither direct nor indirect, because both of them are just different aspects of one underlying reality. *Double-aspect theories* would assume that scientifically describing N and phenomenally experiencing S are just two different ways of accessing one and the same underlying reality. Spinoza is a beautiful classical example of this philosophical intuition, as is Herbert Feigl with his "neutral monism" version of the early identity theory.[4] Identity theorists frequently thought that the relation between types of mental and physical events was simply that of *contingent identity*. Just as concepts like "morning star" and "evening star" turned out to be coextensive (referring to the same part of reality, the planet Venus), so, they thought, as science advances, mental and physical concepts would in the same way eventually turn out to be referring to one and the same part of reality (see, e.g. Place 1956, 1988). Identity theories are maximally parsimonious and do justice to the principle of the causal closure of the physical world, and as such they seem ideally suited as an underlying research heuristic for the cognitive neurosciences. However, they have their own logical intricacies and difficulties, none of which I am going to discuss here.[5]

What this brief look at some possible ontological interpretations of empirical correlations between mind and brain illustrates is that a full-blown theory of consciousness will need much more than correlation data alone. Taken by themselves, those data simply underdetermine the shape any comprehensive theory will have to take. On the other hand, the work presented in this volume certainly is an impressive beginning. We clearly see a new phase of consciousness research, which is now definitely expanding from the realm of more abstract and speculative models into the field of gathering "harder" and more domain-specific data. And in the end it may even turn out that as we gain new insights about what all those difficult concepts like "first-person perspective," "subjective access," and "introspective individuation of conscious states by their phenomenal content" might actually refer to in terms of their necessary neuro-computational underpinnings, some of our theoretical intuitions about what is really needed to successfully bridge the explanatory gap (see Levine 1983, 1993) will shift as well.

Being a philosopher, I will not attempt to develop a general introduction into what the problem of consciousness amounts to for the cognitive neurosciences.[6] I have given a somewhat more comprehensive introduction into the philosophical issues associated with conscious experience elsewhere (see Metzinger 1995a), and will not repeat myself here.[7] However, let me briefly point to a third possible form of naïveté, which has to be avoided if we want to achieve genuine progress on consciousness.

In order to get away from the shallowness and the constant misunderstandings inherent in many popular discussions of conscious experience, one has to first understand that reduction is a relationship between *theories*, and not between phenomena. A primitive scientistic ideology would be just as bad as succumbing to Mysterianism. Neither serious empirical researcher nor philosopher wants to "reduce consciousness." All that can be reduced is one *theory* about how the contents of conscious experience come into existence to another *theory* about how the contents of conscious experience come into existence. Our theories about the phenomena change. The phenomena stay the same. A beautiful rainbow remains a beautiful rainbow even after an explanation in terms of electromagnetic radiation has become available. Of course, if one takes a second look, it is here where one discovers yet another danger of naïveté lurking in the background: One factor that makes consciousness such a very special target for scientific research is that our own beliefs about it can subtly *change* the contents and the functional profile of subjective experience itself. Consciousness—as well as science—is a culturally embedded phenomenon (see chapter 8 in this volume).

Soft Issues: The Wider Context of Consciousness Research at the Turn of the Millennium

In the closing section of this general introduction I will briefly draw attention to a number of "soft" issues associated with the search for the NCC. I know that many of my readers will not be interested in these aspects of the problem. They may safely skip the remaining part of this introduction and continue reading in chapter 2. I am also aware that this is a risky enterprise, since there is a rising suspicion about the value of philosophical contributions in consciousness research in general and since a large variety of potential misunderstandings exist. On the other hand, I am convinced that there is an important set of more general and *normative* issues associated with the kind of research now expanding so forcefully. For the twenty-first century's mind sciences, these issues will definitely become more pressing and relevant. They certainly deserve attention. For the scientific community it is vital to keep an eye on these issues from the very beginning, because they will eventually shape our image of ourselves and the cultural foundations of our societies. There is a large normative vacuum emerging, and it is important for it not to be filled by popular irrationalism and by people who are just promoting their own interests and pet ideologies. Those of us who are seriously interested in the growth of knowledge as a good in itself must also face the consequences of this growth. We have to see to it that the ensuing issues in the wider context eventually are resolved with the same degree of professional attention, rationality, and rigorousness which goes

into searching for the neural correlates of consciousness. Let me briefly highlight three aspects.

Anthropology Assessment

There is a new image of man emerging, an image that will dramatically contradict almost all traditional images man has made of himself in the course of his cultural history. For instance, to start with a rather trivial point, it will be strictly incompatible with the Christian image of man, as well as with many metaphysical conceptions developed in non-Western religions. Since about 1990 we have learned more about the human brain than in the three preceding centuries. Not only the cognitive neurosciences and consciousness research, but also a growing number of new disciplines like evolutionary psychology, artificial life, and cognitive robotics, are generating a flood of new insights into the foundations of mentality. Implicit in all these new data on the genetic, evolutionary, or neurocomputational roots of conscious human existence is a radically new understanding of what it *means* to be human. Although there is not yet a comprehensive formulation of a new anthropology, the accelerating change in the conception we have of ourselves is becoming more and more obvious. This certainly is an exciting development. As a philosopher, of course, I like to look at it as a new and breathtaking phase in the pursuit of an old philosophical ideal: the ideal of self-knowledge. However, nobody ever said that a deepening of self-knowledge cannot have painful, sobering, or other emotionally unattractive aspects.

Humanity will certainly profit from the current development. But we will also pay a price, and in order to effectively minimize this price, it is important to assess potential consequences of a reductionist neuroanthropology as early as possible. Just as in technology assessment, where one tries to calculate potential dangers, unwanted side-effects and general future consequences of new technologies introduced into society, we need a new kind of anthropology assessment. We have to start thinking about the consequences a cultural implementation of a new image of man might have.

It may be helpful to differentiate between the "emotional price" and the "sociocultural price." The emotional price consists in a certain unease: We feel insecure, because many of our unscrutinized beliefs about ourselves suddenly seem obsolete. What about rationality and free will—is it really true that our own actions are to a much larger extent determined by "subpersonal" and unconscious events in the brain than we have always liked to assume? If the minimally sufficient neural cause for an overt action and the minimally sufficient neural correlate of the phenomenal experience of *myself now deciding* to carry out this action actually diverge, does this mean that my subjective experience of initiating my own action is some kind of internal confabulation? Is the experience of agency an illusion, a fragile mental construct (see chapter 21 in this volume)? Is conscious thought just a phenomenal echo of the zombie within me talking to itself (see chapter 6 in this volume)? And is there really no such thing as a soul? If the property of selfhood, of "being someone," is not a supernatural essence, but basically a biologically anchored *process* (see chapter 20 in this volume), is there any hope for survival after death? From a purely theoretical perspective the finiteness of human existence in itself does not constitute a problem.

Mortality, however, also is an emotional problem, which we cannot simply brush away by some intellectual operation. The desire for individual survival is one of the highest biological imperatives, mercilessly burned into our limbic system by millions of years of evolution. However, we are the first creature on this planet to have an awareness of the fact that eventually all attempts to observe this bioemotional imperative will be futile. This awareness of mortality will be greatly enhanced as we—especially people outside the academic world and in nondeveloped countries—learn more and more about the neural correlates of consciousness. This is only one element of what I have called the "emotional price." Doubts about the extent to which we actually are free and rational agents are further examples.

There will be a sociocultural price for the current development as well. Unfortunately, this aspect is much harder to assess. First of all, the image we have of ourselves in a subtle, yet very effective, way influences how we live our everyday life and how we interact with our fellow human beings. A popularized form of vulgar materialism following on the heels of neuroscience might therefore lead us into another, reduced kind of social reality. If our image of ourselves is a radically demystified image, then we run the risk of losing a lot of the magic and subtlety in our social relationships. Should believing in a soul or in an irreducible core of our personality one day become just as absurd as stubbornly believing that the sun actually revolves around the Earth is today, then the social and emotional pressures on people who, for whatever reason, have chosen to live their lives outside the scientific image of the world will greatly increase. This may well lead to conflicts, to cultural, and conceivably to civil, warfare. Even today presumably more than 80 percent of the people on this planet do not live their lives against the background of the scientific image of man and, in their personal lives, do not accept even the most general standards of rationality. Almost all of them have never heard of the idea of an NCC, and many of them will not even *want* to hear about it. In short: Existing gaps between the rich, educated, and secularized parts of global society and the poor, less informed, and religiously rooted parts may widen in a way that proves to be unbearable or outright dangerous. One last aspect of the potential sociocultural price to be paid consists in unwanted side effects of new technologies, and they must be rationally assessed and minimized as well.

Consciousness Ethics

We are currently witnessing the beginning of a truly revolutionary development: Subjective experience becomes technologically accessible, in a way it has never been in the history of mankind. This is particularly obvious in the thematic context of this book. Once we know the neural correlate of a specific kind of phenomenal content, we can, in principle, selectively switch this content on and off (see chapters 16–19 in this volume). We can start to modulate it, amplify it, and arguably we can even *multiply* it in artificial systems by realizing the same computational function, the same causal role on another kind of physical hardware. Biological psychiatry, neuropharmacology, and medical neurotechnology, as today manifested in new forms of short-term psychotherapy or new generations of mood enhancers, in the transplantation of embryonic nerve cell tissue or the implantation of brain prostheses, are just the tip of the iceberg. Many of the neuro- and information-processing technologies of the future are going to be *consciousness technologies*, because their main goal will be to directly change the phenomenal content of their targets' mental states. In psychiatry and other branches of medicine this will certainly be a blessing for generations of patients to come. But as it becomes possible to influence and manipulate conscious experience in ever more precise and reliable ways, we face a new ethical dimension. Therefore, more than a research ethics for the cognitive neurosciences or an applied ethics for neurotechnology is needed. We may have to go beyond the concept of mental health used in medicine or psychiatry, and start thinking about what states of consciousness are interesting or desirable *in principle*.

Developing a normative theory of conscious states would be a difficult problem in many respects. First, it would mean constructing a theory that offers not normative judgements of actions, but a normative evaluation of *ways of subjectively experiencing the world*. Maybe one could analyze consciousness ethics as a new branch of ethics dealing with actions having the primary goal of deliberately changing the phenomenal content of mental states possessed by the agent or other persons. Of course, many people have long been seeking a convincing theory about what good and desirable states of consciousness actually are. But it is far from clear if searching for such a theory is even a coherent goal. Does it really make sense to speak of a "good" state of consciousness? In everyday life, are there really states of subjective experience that are "better" than others? A general ethics for conscious experience would inevitably have to face all the foundational issues concerning the epistemic status and the universalizability of ethical norms, which any moral philosophy has to confront. Personally, I tend to be rather skeptical with regard to the prospects of such an ethics for consciousness.

However, decisions will have to be made. And it is interesting to note how large the scope of normative considerations in this realm would be. They would range from pedagogics to euthanasia, from animal rights to robotics, and from drug policy to media policy. It is also surprising to see how far concrete questions range; an ethics of consciousness could attempt to answer them in a more systematic way: What states of consciousness do we want to show our children? What state of consciousness do we eventually want to die in? What states of consciousness would we like to be illegal in our societies? What types of conscious experience do we want to foster and integrate into our culture? What states of consciousness are we allowed to force on animals (e.g., when attempting to isolate the NCC)? Should we really try to build conscious machines before we have understood why our own form of subjective experience is accompanied by so much suffering? How can we design media environments so that they do not endanger our mental health, but increase our own autonomy and the quality of our conscious lives? If we have answers to these questions, we may soon be able to achieve practical solutions in a more efficient way—by bringing about the NCC of the desired phenomenal state. We might then move on by seeking answers to questions of a more pragmatic kind: How can scientific research on consciousness help us to realize our normative goals? How can we use this research to further minimize the price we pay as much as possible?

Consciousness Culture

Anthropology assessment and ethical considerations are not enough. The issue is not just how to avoid the adverse side effects of a very special and controversial kind of scientific progress. Rather, the crucial point is that new insights about the structure of mind and the wealth of knowledge generated by empirical research on the phenomenon of conscious experience *themselves* have to be culturally implemented. We have to move away from a purely defensive position (as is currently widespread in the humanities), away from any cheap, counterproductive resentment. Laying the foundations for a consciousness culture means taking a more active attitude, a—nevertheless critical—point of view that allows us to ask positive questions like How would a future culture look that uses the results of consciousness research in a fruitful way? Can a *positive* vision be developed? How to protect the individual from new potentials for manipulation and the dangerous side effects of commercially exploited, newly emerging consciousness technologies is just one half of the challenge we will be facing in the future. The other half consists in using those new insights and technologies to *raise* the degree of individual autonomy, in order to help individual human beings live in the states of consciousness in which they have decided to live. Obviously, one necessary precondition consists in being ready to face the facts. *Ought* implies *can*, and objective knowledge is important for any realistic judgement of the options open to us.

A consciousness culture will have nothing to do with organized religion or a specific political vision. Rather, it has to be a rational and productive strategy to transfer new knowledge and new possibilities for action into a global sociocultural context. New knowledge and new technologies, which doubtless, with ever-accelerating speed, will emerge from research activities in the empirical mind-sciences in the next millennium, have to be integrated into society in a way that gives a maximum of people free access to them. A rational consciousness culture, it seems safe to say, will always have to encourage individuals to take responsibility for their own lives—and make continuous attempts at creating a social context that allows them to actually do so. Our current lack of a genuine consciousness culture can be interpreted as an expression of the fact that the project of enlightenment got stuck. What we need is not faith, but knowledge; what we are lacking is not a new metaphysics, but a new variant of practical rationality. In short, the third bundle of "soft issues" to which I briefly wanted to point at the end of this introduction is constituted by the urgent necessity to *embed* the current technological and the current theoretical development in a sustainable process of cultural evolution that can keep pace with stormy future developments. It has not been my intention to make any positive suggestions here. All I want to do is throw some light on the broader context in which the search for the NCC is taking place at the turn of the millennium.

However, consciousness culture, just like self-knowledge, is an old philosophical project. Cicero (1971; *Tusculanae disputationes*, II 5) conceived of philosophy as *cultura animi*, as taking care of and cultivating the soul—and in this sense I have only advertised a very old concept of philosophy that went out of fashion a long time ago. Maybe defining the love of wisdom as cultivating the soul is a classical motif that could inspire us as we take our first steps in the present situation. One has to admit, though, that the initial conditions for the time-honored project of a consciousness culture have changed slightly since the time of Cicero. It therefore remains an open question whether a convincing new interpretation of this classical motif, in light of our recent discoveries about the neurobiological foundations of consciousness and subjective experience, could actually be achieved.

Notes

1. The important question, which I am deliberately skipping in this short introduction, runs in the opposite direction: Could we coherently conceive of a class of representational systems that *only* knows the world under theoretical propositional representations, never having had any kind of subjective experience? In other words, Could the epistemic projects of science and philosophy, at least in principle, be successfully pursued by an unconscious race of machines? Or are even the meaning and the truth of scientific theories ultimately constituted by the fact that they are generated in groups of *phenomenal subjects*—systems that also know the world (and themselves) under phenomenal representations?

2. In philosophy of mind, the concept of supervenience stands for an attempt to formulate a coherent and *nonreductive* form of materialism, capturing the essential theoretical intuitions behind many previous strategies for solving the mind–body problem. For the concept of supervenience, see Kim 1993. For an excellent and accessible introduction to philosophy of mind, well suited for empirical researchers and other non-philosophers, see Kim 1996.

3. Here the classical position is Thomas Huxley's. For a recent exposition of problems surrounding the notion of epiphenomenalism, see Bieri 1992. Herbert Feigl saw the problem of introducing "nomological danglers," a new class of psychophysical laws "dangling out of" the closed causal network of the physical world, as early as 1960: "These correspondence laws are peculiar in that they may be said to postulate 'effects' (mental states as dependent variables) which by themselves do not function, or at least do not seem to be needed, as 'causes' (independent variables) for any observable behaviour" (Feigl 1960: 37).

4. See Feigl 1958; for a collection of texts regarding early identity theory, see Borst 1970.

5. Regarding formal and semantic difficulties of the identity theory, see Kripke 1971, 1972; for the more influential "multiple realization argument" see Putnam 1975, 1992; for a brief introduction to functionalism Block 1980. A good way to enter the current debate is Kim 1998. Important edited collections are Borst 1970; Heil and Mele 1993; Lycan 1990; Warner and Szubka 1994.

6. See Bock and Marsh 1993; Cohen and Schooler 1997; Davies and Humphreys 1993; Marcel and Bisiach 1988; Milner and Rugg 1992 for edited collections. Examples of important individual contributions are Shallice 1988; Weiskrantz 1997; see also the references to monographs given in the introductions to individual parts of this book.

7. An excellent, recent introduction is Güzeldere 1997. For substantial encyclopedia articles, containing further references, see Diemer 1971; Grauman 1966; Landesman 1967; Lormand 1998; Metzinger and Schumacher 1999; NN 1904.

References

Bieri, P. (1992). Trying out epiphenomenalism. *Erkenntnis* 36: 283–309.

Block, N. (1980). What is functionalism? In Block, N., ed. (1980). *Readings in the Philosophy of Psychology. Vol. 1.* Cambridge, MA: Harvard University Press.

Block, N., Flanagan, O., and Güzeldere, G., eds. (1997). *Consciousness: Philosophical Debates.* Cambridge, MA: MIT Press.

Bock, G. R., and Marsh, J., eds. (1993). *Experimental and Theoretical Studies of Consciousness.* New York: Wiley.

Borst, C. V., ed. (1970). *The Mind/Brain Identity Theory.* London: Macmillan.

Churchland, P. M. (1985). Reduction, qualia, and the direct introspection of brain states. *Journal of Philosophy* 82: 8–28.

Churchland, P. M. (1986). Some reductive strategies in cognitive neurobiology. *Mind* 95: 279–309. Reprinted in *A Neurocomputational Perspective.* Cambridge, MA: MIT Press.

Churchland, P. M. (1988). Reduction and the neurobiological basis of consciousness. In A. Marcel and E. Bisiach, eds., *Consciousness in Contemporary Science.* Oxford: Oxford University Press.

Churchland, P. S. (1986). *Neurophilosophy: Toward a Unified Science of the Mind–Brain.* Cambridge, MA: MIT Press.

Cicero, Marcus Tullius (1971). *Tusculan disputations.* Loeb classical library; Cambridge, Mass.: Harvard University Press.

Cohen, J. D. and Schooler, J. W., eds. (1997). *Scientific Approaches to Consciousness.* Mahwah, NJ: Lawrence Erlbaum Associates.

Crick, F. H. C., and Koch, C. (1990). Towards a neurobiological theory of consciousness. *Seminars in the Neurosciences* 2: 263–275.

Davies, M., and Humphreys, G., eds. (1993). *Consciousness: Psychological and Philosophical Essays.* Oxford: Basil Blackwell.

Diemer, A. (1971). Bewußtsein. In J. Ritter, ed., *Historisches Wörterbuch der Philosophie.* Vol. 1. Basel: Schwabe Verlag.

Feigl, H. (1958). The "Mental" and the "Physical." In H. Feigl, M. Scriven and G. Maxwell, eds., *Minnesota Studies in the Philosophy of Science: Concepts, Theories and the Mind-Body-Problem*, Vol. 2. Minneapolis: University of Minneapolis Press.

Feigl, H. (1960). Mind–body, *not* a Pseudo-Problem. In S. Hook, ed., *Dimensions of Mind.* New York: Collier Macmillan.

Graumann, C.-F. (1966). Bewußtsein und Bewußtheit. Probleme und Befunde der psychologischen Bewußtseinsforschung. In W. Metzger and H. Erke, eds., *Allgemeine Psychologie: Vol. I: Der Aufbau des Erkennens.* vol. 1 of K. Gottschaldt et al., eds., *Handbuch der Psychologie.* Göttingen: Verlag für Psychologie.

Güzeldere, G. (1997). Introduction: The many faces of consciousness: A field guide. In Block et al. 1997.

Heil, J., and Mele, A., eds. (1993). *Mental Causation.* Oxford: Clarendon Press.

Kim, J. (1993). *Supervenience and Mind.* Cambridge: Cambridge University Press.

Kim, J. (1996). *Philosophy of Mind.* Boulder, CO: Westview Press.

Kim, J. (1998). *Mind in a Physical World. An Essay on the Mind–Body Problem and Mental Causation.* Cambridge, MA: MIT Press.

Kripke, S. (1971). Identity and necessity. In M. Munitz, ed., *Identity and Individuation.* New York: New York University Press.

Kripke, S. (1972). Naming and necessity. In D. Davidson and G. Harman, eds., *Semantics of Natural Language.* Dordrecht: Reidel Publishing Company. Revised version as monograph (1980), *Naming and Necessity.* Cambridge, MA: Harvard University Press.

Landesman, C., Jr. (1967). Consciousness. In P. Edwards, ed., *The Encyclopedia of Philosophy.* Vol. 2. New York: Macmillan/Free Press.

Levine, J. (1983). Materialism and qualia: The explanatory gap. *Pacific Philosophical Quarterly*, 64: 354–61.

Levine, J. (1993). On leaving out what it's like. In Davies and Humphreys 1993. Reprinted in Block et al. 1997.

Lormand, E. (1998). Consciousness. In E. Craig and L. Floridi, eds., *Routledge Encyclopedia of Philosophy.* London: Routledge.

Lycan, W. G., ed. (1990). *Mind and Cognition.* Oxford: Basil Blackwell.

Marcel, A., and Bisiach, E., eds. (1988). *Consciousness in Contemporary Science.* Oxford: Oxford University Press.

McGinn, C. (1989). Can we solve the mind–body problem? *Mind* 98: 349–366. Reprinted in Block et al. 1997.

Metzinger, T. (1995a). Introduction: The problem of consciousness. In Metzinger 1995b.

Metzinger, T., ed. (1995b). *Conscious Experience.* Thorverton, UK: Imprint Academic; Paderborn: mentis.

Metzinger, T., and Schumacher, R. (1999). Bewußtsein. In H.-J. Sandkühler, ed., *Enzyklopädie der Philosophie.* Hamburg: Meiner.

Milner, D., and Rugg, M., eds. (1992). *The Neuropsychology of Consciousness.* London: Academic Press.

NN. (1904). Bewußtsein. In R. Eisler, ed., *Wörterbuch der philosophischen Begriffe.* Berlin: Ernst Siegfried Mittler und Sohn.

Place, U. T. (1956). Is consciousness a brain process? *British Journal of Psychology* 47: 44–50. Reprinted in Borst 1970.

Place, U. T. (1988). Thirty years on—Is consciousness still a brain process? *Australasian Journal of Philosophy* 66: 208–219.

Popper, K. R. (1996). *Knowledge and the Body–Mind Problem: In Defence of Interaction.* London: Routledge.

Popper, K. R., and Eccles, J. C. (1977). *The Self and Its Brain: An Argument for Interactionism*. Berlin, Heidelberg, London, New York: Springer.

Putnam, H. (1975). *Mind, Language, and Reality*. Vol. 2 of his *Philosophical Papers*. Cambridge, UK: Cambridge University Press.

Putnam, H. (1992). Why functionalism didn't work. In J. Earman, ed., *Inference, Explanation and Other Frustrations. Essays in the Philosophy of Science*. Berkeley: University of California Press.

Shallice, T. (1988). *From Neuropsychology to Mental Structure*. Cambridge: Cambridge University Press.

Warner, R., and Szubka, T., eds. (1994). *The Mind–Body Problem. A Guide to the Current Debate*. Oxford: Basil Blackwell.

Weiskrantz, L. (1997). *Consciousness Lost and Found: A Neuropsychological Exploration*. Oxford: Oxford University Press.

I FOUNDATIONAL ISSUES AND CONCEPTUAL PROBLEMS

David Chalmers and Ansgar Beckermann, the first two authors in this introductory part of the book, are philosophers. Antti Revonsuo and Gerhard Roth, the two contributors following them, are philosophers who in a later phase of their research career became neuroscientists. Their contributions will guide readers into the three middle sections of this volume. Almost all chapters in this middle part focus on the empirical aspects of the ongoing search for the neural correlates of consciousness. However, as readers will undoubtedly notice, many authors turn out to be deeply sensitive to the more theoretical and metatheoretical issues associated with this newly emerging field of research. The final section of this collection will round off the debate by returning to questions of a philosophical and more speculative kind.

What do we actually mean by the concept of a "neural correlate of consciousness"? David Chalmers offers an introductory analysis of this concept and of some of the more general philosophical and methodological issues associated with it. If a neural correlate of consciousness is taken as a specific system in the brain whose activity directly correlates with states of conscious experience, then two questions immediately follow: What is a "state of consciousness"? And what makes a correlation a "direct correlation"?

Chalmers points out that we will often be interested in the correlates of specific types of *phenomenal content* (see chapter 1). The crucial question, as he puts it, is whether the representational content in the neural system matches up with the representational content in, for instance, visual consciousness. States of consciousness, in this way of thinking about them, are individuated by their experiential content, by *what* is subjectively experienced through them. Does "direct correlation" mean that we are looking for neural systems that are necessary and sufficient for consciousness? Chalmers thinks this is too strong a requirement, since it might turn out that there exists more than one neural correlate of a given conscious state. There might, for example, be two systems M and N such that a certain state of M suffices for being in pain and a certain state of N also suffices for being in pain. If we would want to say that both M and N count as neural correlates of this specific conscious content, then both of them would be sufficient but neither would be necessary.

The interesting concept, however, is not merely that of a sufficient neural correlate of consciousness. We do not want irrelevant brain properties to enter into our description of this correlate. What we should be looking for is a *minimally sufficient neural system*. It is defined by (a) being sufficient to bring about the corresponding state of consciousness and (b) the fact that no proper *part* of it suffices by itself to bring about this corresponding state of consciousness. After this important conceptual tool has been established, Chalmers goes on to investigate the domain, the relevant range of cases and conditions under which such a tool can be applied. He closes by offering a series of methodological outcomes from a philosophical perspective.

Once correlations between neural and phenomenal states have been achieved, we face another deep theoretical problem: the explanatory gap (see Levine 1983, 1993). Since nothing in the physical or functional correlates of a phenomenal state helps us to understand why this state subjectively *feels* in a certain way, a special sort of "intelligibility gap" arises. Why so? Phenomenal states are not fully characterized by the causal role the play (e.g., in the generation of behavior). They also have a distinct qualitative character, and many of us can always imagine that whatever realizes the causal role in the brain can be separated from this qualitative, subjective content. There seems to be no *necessary* connection (e.g., from a certain activation pattern in the visual system to *this* specific shade of indigo I am experiencing now). This intuitive separability is one major root of Cartesian intuitions in the philosophy of mind: Reductive strategies to explain qualia and consciousness seem to leave a gap in the explanation, in that, strictly speaking, such explanations cannot really be *understood*. They do not seem to us to say, in principle, what we want to know. In order to overcome this difficulty, we need a much deeper understanding of the logic behind psychophysical laws; we need an understanding of what it would mean to possess general bridge principles connecting brain states to states of conscious experience.

Ansgar Beckermann in his contribution offers a careful analysis showing how the current theoretical debate is deeply rooted in discussions about the concept of "emergence," which took place at the beginning of the twentieth century.

Could a phenomenal quality—like the one given in the visual experience of a certain shade of indigo—be an *emergent* property in the sense that (a) it is a true law of nature that all brains with a certain microstructure will generate the conscious experience of indigo, while (b) the occurrence of an indigo-experience cannot (not even in principle) be deduced from the most complete knowledge of the properties possessed by all the neural components making up the microstructure, either in isolation or within other arrangements? This was C. D. Broad's definition in his famous book *The Mind and Its Place in Nature*. What are the laws connecting properties of parts to properties of complex wholes? Are they, in the case of phenomenal experience, unique and ultimate laws, which cannot be derived from the general laws of nature? Could a Martian consciousness researcher, who had complete scientific knowledge about the brains of humans but no visual modality, maybe not a even a nervous system, *predict* the occurrence of a sensation of indigo? Or would she be unable even to form a concept of the sensation of indigo before having experienced it at least once? Beckermann offers a clear exposition of the problems we currently face when trying to take the step from empirical correlation studies to fully reductive and genuinely explanatory accounts of phenomenal experience. However, he also remarks that the fact of the non-deducibility of the qualitative character possessed by conscious states

from the current laws of neurobiology may simply be a *historical* fact—reflecting an insufficiently advanced state of the neuroscience of consciousness.

This is the point of departure for Antti Revonsuo. He asks what it would take to finally transform the current state of consciousness studies into a rigorous scientific research program on consciousness. We are presently witnessing what in theory of science would be called a "preparadigmatic stage": There is no one coherent theory of consciousness that could serve as the unified background for criticism and systematically organized further developments. Revonsuo points out that what we should strive for is first and foremost a *biological* theory of consciousness, an empirically based strategy that regards consciousness primarily as a biological phenomenon. However, although the volume of empirical research relevant for understanding phenomenal experience in cognitive neuroscience is so large that it is probably the best starting place for the enterprise in general, the metaphysics of cognitive neuroscience appears to be merely some vague and philosophically outdated version of functionalism.

Revonsuo proceeds to isolate some of the major problems that have to be solved. First of all, the initial assumptions of a scientific research program for consciousness have to be clearly formulated. The ontological assumptions for a theory of consciousness have to be conceptually framed in a manner acceptable for a biological research program. Since the corresponding assumptions in cognitive neuroscience are inappropriate, novel levels of description and explanation have to be introduced. At least one level has to capture the first-person point of view (see chapter 20, this volume). Also, a resolution of the "paradox of isomorphism" is needed: If consciousness, as Revonsuo assumes, resides strictly in the brain, then there must be some level of organization in the brain that quite directly resembles the content of conscious experience. In developing initial answers to these questions, he proposes that, in accordance with what he terms the "standard hierarchical model of the world", a serious research program should reconceptualize consciousness as the phenomenal level of organization in the brain. A complete description of the brain, Revonsuo argues, *necessarily includes* this level of description, which cannot be imported from any other discipline but must be contributed by the science of consciousness itself. In fleshing out his own proposals he then investigates the role of dreams as a model system for consciousness and as a metaphor for subjective experience in general. The conscious brain, in this view, is nature's own virtual reality system that creates an "out-of-the-brain-experience" for the organism, so that the individual can act in a meaningful way in the world. The main task for the research program on consciousness is to describe the phenomenal level systematically, and to capture it through empirical investigations.

The last contribution in this introductory section leads the reader from the philosophy of consciousness into the realm of empirical research. Gerhard Roth draws our attention to the *historical dimension* associated with conscious experience. The human brain can be seen as the result of many millions of years of biological evolution, and it is rational to assume that this is also true of at least major portions of the neural correlates of consciousness embedded in this brain. In short, ontogenetically as well as phylogenetically speaking, conscious experience is an acquired phenomenon. There will be *stages* in which it has naturally developed. If we look across species boundaries and into the evolutionary history of nervous systems on this planet, we will very likely find simple and complex, older and more recent, general and strictly species-specific NCCs as well as types of phenomenal content going along with them. But how are we—foundational issues in philosophy put aside for now—going to find an answer to the question of whether members of other biological species have phenomenal experiences as well?

Roth proposes a number of strategies: (1) to check groups of animals for the presence of those cognitive functions which in humans can be exerted only consciously; (2) to examine which parts of the human brain are necessary for (and active during) the different states of consciousness; (3) to examine which of these centers of the human brain are present (and active) in the brains of those animals which—based on behavioral evidence—show certain states of consciousness; (4) to compare the ontogeny of cognitive functions, including states of consciousness in humans, with the ontogeny of the human brain. In the ideal case, the first appearance of certain states of human consciousness should coincide with the maturation of certain centers in the human brain.

If we look at the project of correlating conscious experience with its physical substrates from this new angle, it becomes obvious that any fine-grained analysis will demonstrate that there are not only many different stages in the development of a hypothetical NCC, but also a wider variety of phenomenal states than many of us may have previously thought. The complexity of the research domain called "conscious experience" is rooted in the complexity of its history and in the structural richness of forms brought about by the evolution of life on our planet.

Further Reading

Beckermann, A. (1992). Supervenience, emergence, and reduction. In A. Beckermann, H. Flohr, and J. Kim, eds., *Emergence or Reduction? Essays on the Prospects of Nonreductive Physicalism.* Berlin: Walter de Gruyter.

Beckermann, A. (1997). Property physicalism, reduction and realization. In M. Carrier and P. Machamer, eds., *Mindscapes: Philosophy, Science, and the Mind.* Konstanz: Universitätsverlag; Pittsburgh: University of Pittsburgh Press.

Block, N., Flanagan, O., and Güzeldere, G., eds. (1997). *Consciousness: Philosophical Debates.* Cambridge, MA: MIT Press.

Broad, C. D. (1925). *The Mind and Its Place In Nature*. London: Kegan Paul, Trench, Turbner, and Co.

Byrne, R. (1996). *The Thinking Ape: Evolutionary Origins of Intelligence*. Oxford: Oxford University Press.

Chalmers, D. J. (1995). Facing up to the problem of consciousness. *Journal of Consciousness* Studies 2: 200–219. Reprinted in S. Hameroff, A. Kaszniak, and A. Scott, eds. (1996). *Toward a Science of Consciousness*, (Cambridge, MA: MIT Press); and in J. Shear, ed. (1997). *Explaining Consciousness: The Hard Problem*. Cambridge, MA: MIT Press.

Chalmers, D. J. (1996). *The Conscious Mind: In Search of a Fundamental Theory*. Oxford: Oxford University Press.

Chalmers, D. J. (1998). On the search for the neural correlate of consciousness. In S. Hameroff, A. Kaszniak, and A. Scott, eds., *Toward a Science of Consciousness II*. Cambridge, MA: MIT Press.

Davies, M., and Humphreys, G., eds. (1993). *Consciousness: Psychological and Philosophical Essays*. Oxford: Basil Blackwell.

Levine, J. (1983). Materialism and qualia: The explanatory gap. *Pacific Philosophical Quarterly* 64: 354–361.

Levine, J. (1993). On leaving out what it's like. In Davies and Humphreys 1993. Reprinted in Block et al. 1997.

Pearce, J. M. (1997). *Animal Learning and Cognition*. 2nd ed. Hove, UK: Psychology Press.

Revonsuo, A. (1994). In search of the science of consciousness. In A. Revonsuo and M. Kamppinen, eds., *Consciousness in Philosophy and Cognitive Neuroscience*. Hillsdale, NJ: Lawrence Erlbaum.

Revonsuo, A. (1995). Consciousness, dreams, and virtual realities. *Philosophical Psychology* 8: 35–58.

Revonsuo, A., Wilenius-Emet, M., Kuusela, J., and Lehto, M. (1997). The neural generation of a unified illusion in human vision. *NeuroReport* 8: 3867–3870.

Roth, G. (1998). *Das Gehirn und seine Wirklichkeit: Kognitive Neurobiologie und ihre philosophischen Konsequenzen*. Frankfurt am Main: Suhrkamp.

Roth, G., and Prinz, W., eds. (1996). *Kopf-Arbeit: Gehirnfunktionen und kognitive Leistungen*. Heidelberg: Spektrum Verlag.

What Is a Neural Correlate of Consciousness?

David J. Chalmers

The search for neural correlates of consciousness (NCCs) is arguably the cornerstone of the recent resurgence of the science of consciousness. The search poses many difficult empirical problems, but it seems to be tractable in principle, and some ingenious studies in recent years have led to considerable progress. A number of proposals have been put forward concerning the nature and location of neural correlates of consciousness.

A few of these include 40-hertz oscillations in the cerebral cortex (Crick and Koch 1990), intralaminar nuclei in the thalamus (Bogen 1995), reentrant loops in thalamocortical systems (Edelman 1989), 40-hertz rhythmic activity in thalamocortical systems (Llinás et al. 1994), extended reticular-thalamic activation system (Newman and Baars 1993), neural assemblies bound by NMDA (Flohr 1995), certain neurochemical levels of activation (Hobson 1997), certain neurons in the inferior temporal cortex (Sheinberg and Logothetis 1997), neurons in the extrastriate visual cortex projecting to prefrontal areas (Crick and Koch 1995), and visual processing within the ventral stream (Milner and Goodale 1995). (A longer list can be found in Chalmers 1998. Review articles on neural correlates of consciousness, especially visual consciousness, can be found in Crick and Koch 1998 and Milner 1995.)

As the full title of this book (*Neural Correlates of Consciousness: Empirical and Conceptual Questions*) suggests, all this activity raises a number of difficult conceptual and foundational issues. I can see at least five sorts of foundational questions: (1) What do we mean by "consciousness"? (2) What do we mean by "neural correlate of consciousness"? (3) How can we find the neural correlate(s) of consciousness? (4) What will a neural correlate of consciousness explain? (5) Is consciousness reducible to its neural correlate(s)?

The first two questions are conceptual questions, the third is an epistemological or methodological question, the fourth is an explanatory question, and the fifth is an ontological question. The first, fourth, and fifth are versions of general questions that philosophers have discussed for a long time (my own view on them is in Chalmers 1995; 1996). The second and third questions are more specific to the NCC investigation. I have discussed the third question in Chalmers (1998). Here I want to focus on the second question.

What does it mean to be a neural correlate of consciousness? At first glance, the answer might seem to be so obvious that the question is hardly worth asking. An NCC is a neural state that directly correlates with a conscious state, or that directly generates consciousness, or something like that. One has a simple image: When your NCC is active, perhaps your consciousness turns on in a corresponding way. But a moment's reflection suggests that the idea is not completely straightforward, and that the concept needs some clarification.

Here, I will attempt a little conceptual spadework in clarifying the concept of an NCC. I don't know that this is the deepest problem in the area, but it seems to me that if we are looking for an NCC, it makes sense to get clear on what we are looking for. On the way I will try to make contact with some of the empirical work in the area, and see what concept of NCC is at play in some of the central work in the field. I will also draw out some consequences for the methodology of empirical work in the search. Most of this is intended as a first step rather than a last word. Much of what I say will need to be refined, but I hope at least to draw attention to some interesting issues in the vicinity.

As a first pass, we can use the definition of a neural correlate of consciousness given in the program of the ASSC conference. This says a neural correlate of consciousness is a "specific system in the brain whose activity correlates directly with states of conscious experience." This yields something like the following:

A neural system N is an NCC if the state of N correlates directly with states of consciousness.

There are at least two things to get clear on here. First, what are the relevant "states of consciousness"? Second, what does it mean for a neural state to "correlate directly" with states of consciousness? I will look into both these things in turn.

States of Consciousness

I will take it that the states of consciousness we are concerned with here are states of subjective experience or, equivalently, states of phenomenal consciousness. But what *sorts* of states are relevant? In the NCC literature, I can see a few different classes of states that are sometimes considered.

Being Conscious

The first option is that the states in question are those of being conscious and of not being conscious. The corresponding notion of an NCC will be that of a neural system whose state directly correlates with whether a subject is conscious or not. If the NCC is in a particular state, the subject will be conscious. If the NCC is not in that state, the subject will not be conscious.

This is perhaps the idea that first comes to mind when we think about an NCC. We might think about it as the "neural correlate of creature consciousness," where creature consciousness is the property a creature has when it is conscious, and lacks when it is not conscious.

Although this is an interesting notion, it does not seem to capture the sort of NCC that most work in the area is aimed at. As we'll see, most current work is aimed at something more specific. There are, however, some ideas that can be

taken as aiming at this notion at least in part. For example, the ideas of Bogen (1995) about the intralaminar nucleus seem to be directed at least in part at this sort of NCC.

Examining current work, it's interesting to note that insofar as there is any consensus at all about the location of this sort of NCC, the dominant view seems to be that it should be in or around the thalamus, or at least that it should involve interactions between the thalamic and cortical systems in a central role. Penfield (1937) argued that "the indispensable substratum of consciousness" lies outside the cerebral cortex, probably in the diencephalon (thalamus, hypothalamus, subthalamus, epithalamus). This theme has been taken up in recent years by Bogen, Newman and Baars (1993), and others.

Background State of Consciousness

A related idea is that of the neural correlate of what we might call the background state of consciousness. A background state is an overall state of consciousness such as being awake, being asleep, dreaming, being under hypnosis, and so on. Exactly what counts as a background state is not entirely clear, since one can divide things up in a number of ways, and with coarser or finer grains; but presumably the class will include a range of normal and of "altered" states.

We can think of this as a slightly finer-grained version of the previous idea. Creature consciousness is the coarsest-grained background state of consciousness: it is just the state of being conscious. Background states will usually be finergrained than this, but they still will not be defined in terms of specific contents or modalities.

A neural correlate of the background state of consciousness, then, will be a neural system N such that the state of N directly correlates with whether a subject is awake, dreaming, under hypnosis, and so on. If N is in state 1, the subject is awake; if N is in state 2, the subject is dreaming; if N is in state 3, the subject is under hypnosis; and so on.

It may well be that some of the thalamocortical proposals discussed above are intended as, or might be extended into, proposals about this sort of NCC. A more direct example is given by Hobson's (1997) ideas about neurochemical levels of activation. Hobson holds that these levels can be grouped into a three-dimensional state-space, and that different regions in this space correspond to different overall states of consciousness: wakefulness, REM sleep, non-REM sleep, and so on. When chemical levels are in a particular region in this space, the subject will be awake; when in they are another region, the subject will be in REM sleep; and so on. On this reading, one might see the neurochemical system as an NCC of the sort characterized above, with the different regions in state-space corresponding to correlates of the various specific background states.

Contents of Consciousness

There is much more to consciousness than the mere state of being conscious, or the background state of consciousness. Arguably the most interesting states of consciousness are *specific* states: the fine-grained states of subjective experience that one is in at any given time. Such states might include the experience of a particular visual image, of a particular sound pattern, of a detailed stream of conscious thought, and so on. A detailed visual experience, for example, might include the experience of certain shapes and colors in one's environment, of specific arrangements of objects, of various relative distances and depths, and so on.

Specific states like these are most often individuated by their *content*. Most conscious states seem to have some sort of specific content representing the world as being one way or another. Much of the specific nature of a visual experience, for example, can be characterized in terms of content. A visual experience typically represents the world as containing various shapes and colors, as containing certain objects standing in

certain spatial relations, and so on. If the experience is veridical, the world will be the way the experience represents it as being. If the experience is an illusion or is otherwise misleading, the world will be other than the experience represents it. But either way, it seems that visual experiences typically have detailed representational content. The same goes for experiences in other sensory modalities, and arguably for many or most nonsensory experiences as well.

Much of the most interesting work on NCCs is concerned with states like these. This is work on the neural correlates of the contents of consciousness. Much work on the neural correlates of visual consciousness has this character, for example. This work is not concerned merely with the neural states that determine that one *has* visual consciousness; it is concerned with the neural states that determine the specific contents of visual consciousness.

A nice example is supplied by the work of Logothetis and colleagues on the NCC of visual consciousness in monkeys (Logothetis and Schall 1989; Leopold and Logothetis 1996; Sheinberg and Logothetis 1997). In this work, a monkey is trained to press various bars when it is confronted with various sorts of images: horizontal and vertical gratings, for example, or gratings drifting left and right, or faces and sunbursts (I will use horizontal and vertical gratings for the purposes of illustration). After training is complete, the monkey is presented with two stimuli at once, one to each eye. In humans, this usually produces binocular rivalry, with alternating periods of experiencing a definite image, and occasional partial overlap. The monkey responds by pressing bars, in effect "telling" the experimenter what it is seeing: a horizontal grating, or a vertical grating, or an interlocking grid.

At the same time, neurons in the monkey's cortex are being monitored by electrodes. It is first established that certain neurons respond to certain stimuli: to horizontal lines, for example, or to flowers. Then these neurons are monitored in the binocular rivalry situation, to see how well they correlate with what the monkey seems to be seeing. It turns out that cells in the primary visual cortex (V1) don't correlate well: When the monkey is stimulated with horizontal and vertical gratings but "sees" horizontal, a large number of "vertical" cells in V1 fire as well. At this point, most cells seem to correlate with retinal stimulus, not with visual percept. But farther into the visual system, the correlation increases, until in the inferior temporal (IT) cortex, there is a very strong correlation. When the monkey is stimulated with horizontal and vertical grating but "sees" horizontal, almost all of the relevant horizontal cells in IT fire, and almost none of the vertical cells do. When the monkey's response switches, indicating that it is now "seeing" vertical, the cell response switches accordingly.

These results naturally lend themselves to speculation about the location of a visual NCC. It seems that V1 is unlikely to be or to involve an NCC, for example, due to the failure of V1 cells to correlate with the contents of consciousness. Of course there are still the possibilities that some small subset of V1 is an NCC, or that V1 is a neural correlate of some aspects of visual consciousness but not of others, but I leave those aside for now. On the other hand, IT seems to be a natural candidate for the location of an NCC, due to the strong correlation of its cells with the content of consciousness. At least it is natural to suppose that IT is a "lower bound" on the location of a visual NCC (due to the failure of strong correlation before then), though the NCC itself may be farther in. None of this evidence is conclusive (and Logothetis and colleagues are appropriately cautious), but it is at least suggestive.

It is clear that this work is concerned with the neural correlates of the *contents* of visual consciousness. We are interested in finding cortical areas whose neural activity correlates with and predicts specific contents of consciousness, such as experiences of horizontal or vertical lines, or of flowers or sunbursts. The ideal is to find a neural system from whose activity we might determine the precise contents of a visual experience, or at least its contents in certain respects (shape, color, and the like).

Interestingly, it seems that in doing this we are crucially concerned with the the representational contents of the neural systems themselves. In the Logothetis work, for example, it is important to determine the receptive fields of the cells (whether they respond to horizontal or vertical gratings, for example), in order to see whether the receptive fields of active cells match up with the apparent contents of visual consciousness. In essence, the receptive field is acting at least as a heuristic way of getting at representational content in the neurons in question. Then the crucial question is whether the representational content in the neural system matches up with the representational content in visual consciousness.

This suggests a natural definition of a neural correlate of the contents of consciousness:

A neural correlate of the contents of consciousness is a neural representational system N such that representation of a content in N directly correlates with representation of that content in consciousness.

Or, more briefly:

A content NCC is a neural representational system N such that the content of N directly correlates with the content of consciousness.

For example, the Logothetis work lends itself to the speculation that IT might contain a content NCC for visual consciousness, since the content of cells in IT seems to correlate directly (at least in these experiments) with the contents of visual consciousness. (Much more investigation is required to see whether this correlation holds across the board, of course.)

This definition requires that we have some way of defining the representational content of a neural system independent of the contents of consciousness. There are various ways to do this. Using a cell's receptive field to define its representational content is probably the simplest. A more refined definition might also give a role to a system's projective field, and to the sort of behavior which activity in that system typically leads to. And there may be still more complex notions of representational content, based on complex correlations with the environment, patterns of behavior, and activity in other cells. But even a crude definition of representational content (e.g., the receptive field definition) is good enough for many purposes, and can yield informative results about the visual NCC.

It is arguable that much work on the visual NCC tacitly invokes this sort of definition. Another example is Milner and Goodale's (1995) work on the two pathways of visual perception. They suggest that the ventral stream is largely for cognitive identification and decision, while the dorsal stream is largely for on-line motor response; and that visual consciousness correlates with activity in the ventral stream.

Much of the support for this work lies with patients who have dissociations between specific contents of conscious perception and the contents involved in motor response. For example, a subject with visual form agnosia (e.g., Milner and Goodale's patient D.F.) cannot consciously identify a vertical slot but can "post" an envelope through it without problem; subjects with optic ataxia (e.g., those with Balint's syndrome) can identify an object but cannot act appropriately toward it. The dissociations here appear to go along with damage to the ventral and dorsal pathways, respectively.

What seems to be going on, on a natural interpretation of these results and of Milner and Goodale's hypothesis, is that for these subjects, there is a dissociation between the contents represented in the ventral pathway and those represented in the dorsal pathway. In these cases, the character of a motor response appears to be determined by the contents represented in the dorsal pathway, but the character of conscious perception appears to be determined by the contents represented in the ventral pathway.

Thus one can see Milner and Goodale's hypothesis as involving the suggestion that the ventral stream contains the neural correlates of the contents of visual consciousness. The hypothesis is quite speculative, of course (though it is interesting to note that IT lies in the ventral stream), but it seems that the content-based analysis provides a natural interpretation of what the hypothesis is implicitly claiming in regard to the visual NCC, and of what may follow if the hypothesis turns out to be correct.

One could give a similar analysis of much or most work on the visual NCC. When Crick and Koch (1998) propose that the visual NCC lies outside V1, for example, much of the experimental evidence they appeal to involves cases where some content is represented in consciousness but not in V1, or vice versa. For example, Gur and Snodderly (1997) show that for some quickly alternating isoluminant color stimuli, color cells in V1 flicker back and forth even though a single fused color is consciously perceived. And results by He et al. (1996) suggest that orientation of a grating can fade from consciousness even though orientation cells in V1 carry the information. The results are not entirely conclusive, but they suggest a mismatch between the representational content in V1 and the content of consciousness.

One can apply this sort of analysis equally to NCCs in other sensory modalities. An NCC of auditory consciousness, for example, might be defined as a neural representational system whose contents correlate directly with the contents of auditory consciousness: loudness, direction, pitch, tone, and the like. The idea can arguably apply to defining the neural correlates of bodily sensations, of conscious mental imagery, and perhaps of conscious emotion and of the stream of conscious thought. All these aspects of consciousness can be naturally analyzed (at least in part) in terms of their content. In looking for their respective NCCs, we may ultimately be looking for neural systems whose content correlates with the contents of these aspects of consciousness.

Arbitrary Phenomenal Properties

(This section is more technical than those above, and may be skipped by those not interested in philosophical details.)

One might try to give a general definition of an NCC of various states of consciousness, of which each of the above would be a special case. To do this, one would need a general way of thinking about arbitrary states of consciousness. Perhaps the best way is to think in terms of arbitrary *phenomenal properties*. For any distinctive kind of conscious experience, there will be a corresponding phenomenal property: in essence, the property of having a conscious experience of that kind. For example, being in a hypnotic state of consciousness is a phenomenal property; having a visual experience of a horizontal line is a phenomenal property; feeling intense happiness is a phenomenal property; feeling a throbbing pain is a phenomenal property; being conscious is a phenomenal property. Phenomenal properties can be as coarse-grained or as fine-grained as you like, so long as they are wholly determined by the current conscious state of the subject.

With this notion in hand, one might try to define the neural correlate of an arbitrary phenomenal property P:

A state N1 of system N is a neural correlate of phenomenal property P if N's being in N1 directly correlates with the subject having P.

Note that we here talk of a *state* being an NCC. Given a *specific* phenomenal property—experiencing a horizontal line, for example—it is no longer clear that it makes sense to speak of a given system being the NCC of that property. Rather, it will be a particular state of that system. Neural firing in certain horizontal cells in IT (say) might be a neural correlate of seeing a horizontal line, for example; and having one's neurochemical system in a certain region of state-space might be a neural correlate of waking consciousness, on Hobson's hypothesis. These are specific states of the neural systems in question.

Most of the time, we are not concerned with neural correlates of single phenomenal properties, but of *families* of phenomenal properties. Hobson is concerned not just with the neural correlate of waking consciousness, for example, but with the neural correlate of the whole family of background states of consciousness. Work on the visual NCC is not concerned with just the neural correlate of horizontal experience, but with the neural correlates of the whole system of visual experiential contents.

We might say a *phenomenal family* is a set of mutually exclusive phenomenal properties that jointly partition the space of conscious experiences, or at least some subset of that space. That is, any subject having an experience (of a certain relevant kind) will have a phenomenal property in the family, and will not have more than one such property. Specific contents of visual consciousness make a phenomenal family, for example: Any visually conscious subject will have some specific visual content, and it will not have two contents at once (given that we are talking about *overall* visual content). The same goes for contents at a particular location in the visual field: Anyone with an experience of a certain location will have some specific content associated with that location (a red horizontal line, say), and not more than one. (Ambiguous experiences are not counterexamples here, as long as we include ambiguous contents as members of the family in question.) The same goes for color experience at any given location: There will be a phenomenal family (one property for each color quality) for any such location. And the same is true for background states of consciousness. All these sets of phenomenal properties make phenomenal families. We can then say:

A neural correlate of a phenomenal family S is a neural system N such that the state of N directly correlates with the subject's phenomenal property in S.

For any phenomenal family S, a subject will have at most one property in S (one background state, or one overall state of visual consciousness, or one color quality at a location). Neural system N will be an NCC of S when there are a corresponding number of states of N, one for every property in P, such that N's being in a given state directly correlates with the subject's having the corresponding phenomenal property. This template can be seen to apply to most of the definitions given above.

For the neural correlate of creature consciousness, we have a simple phenomenal family with two properties: being conscious and not being conscious. An NCC here will be a system with two states that correlate with these two properties.

For the neural correlate of a background state of consciousness, we have a phenomenal family with a few more properties: dreaming, being in an ordinary waking state, being under hypnosis, and so on. An NCC here will be a neural system with a few states that correlate directly with these properties. Hobson's neurochemical system would be an example.

For the neural correlate of contents of consciousness, one will have a much more complex phenomenal family (overall states of visual consciousness, or states of color consciousness at a location, or particular conscious occurrent thoughts), and a neural representational system to match. The state of the NCC will correlate directly with the specific phenomenal property.

Notice that in the content case, there is an extra strong requirement on the NCC. In the other cases, we have accepted an arbitrary match of neural states to phenomenal states—any state can serve as the neural correlate of a dreaming state of background consciousness, for example. But where content is concerned, not any neural state will do. We require that the *content* of the neural state in question match the content of consciousness. This is a much stronger requirement.

It is arguable that this requirement delivers much greater explanatory and predictive power in the case of neural correlates of conscious content. The systematicity in the correlation means that it can be extended to predict the presence or absence of phenomenal features that may not have been present in the initial empirical data set, for example. And it also will dovetail more nicely with finding a mechanism and a functional role for the NCC that match the role we associate with a given conscious state.

It is this systematicity in the correlation that makes the current work on the neural correlate of visual consciousness particularly interesting. Without it, things would be much more untidy. Imagine that we find arbitrary neural states which correlate directly with the experience of horizontal lines (for example) such that there is no corresponding representational content in the neural state. Instead, we match seemingly arbitrary states N1 with horizontal, N2 with vertical, and so on. Will we count this as a neural correlate of the contents of visual consciousness? If we do, it will be in a much weaker sense, and in a way that will lead to much less explanatory and predictive power.

One might then hope to extend this sort of systematicity to other, noncontent-involving phenomenal families. For example, one might find among background states of consciousness some pattern or some dimension along which they vary systematically (some sort of intensity dimension, for example, or a measure of alertness). If we could then find a neural system whose states do not arbitrarily correlate with the phenomenal states in question, but vary along a corresponding systematic dimension, then the NCC in question will have much greater potential explanatory and predictive power. So this sort of systematicity in phenomenal families is something we should look for, and something we should look to match in potential neural correlates.

Perhaps one could define a "systematic NCC" as a neural correlate of a phenomenal family such that states correlate with each other in some such systematic way. I will not try to give a general abstract definition here, since things are getting complex enough, but I think one can see a glimmer of how it might go. I will, however, keep using the neural correlate of the contents of consciousness (especially visual consciousness) as the paradigmatic example of an NCC, precisely because its definition builds in such a notion of systematicity, with the corresponding explanatory and predictive power.

Direct Correlation

The other thing that we need to clarify is the notion of "direct correlation." We have said that an NCC is a system whose state correlates directly with a state of consciousness, but what does direct correlation involve, exactly? Is it required that the neural system be necessary and sufficient for consciousness, for example, or merely sufficient? And over what range of cases must the correlation obtain for the system to count as an NCC? Any possible case? A relevantly constrained set of cases? And so on.

The paradigmatic case will involve a neural system N with states that correlate with states of consciousness. So we can say that

state of N---state of consciousness

and, specifically,

N is in state N1---subject has conscious state C.

In the case of the contents of consciousness, we have a system N such that representing a content in N directly correlates with representation in consciousness. So we can say

representing C in N---representing C in consciousness.

The question in all these cases concerns the nature of the required relation (represented here as "---"). How strong a relation is required here for N to be an NCC?

Necessity, Sufficiency?

The first question is whether the NCC state is required to be necessary and sufficient for the conscious state, merely sufficient, or something else in the vicinity.

Necessity and sufficiency   The first possibility is that the state of N is necessary and sufficient for the corresponding state of consciousness. This is an attractive requirement for an NCC, but it is arguably too strong. It might turn out that there is more than one neural correlate of a given conscious state. For example, it may be there there are two systems, M and N, such that a certain state of M suffices for being in pain and a certain state of N also suffices for being in pain, where these two states are not themselves always correlated. In this case, it seems that we would likely say that both M and N (or their corresponding states) are neural correlates of pain. But it is not the case that activity in M is necessary and sufficient for pain (since it is not necessary), and the same goes for N. If both M and N are to count as NCCs here, we cannot require an NCC to be necessary *and* sufficient.

Sufficiency   From the above, it seems plausible that we require only that an NCC state be *sufficient* for the corresponding state of consciousness. But is any sufficient state an NCC? If it is, then it seems that the whole brain will count as an NCC of any state of consciousness. The whole brain will count as an NCC of pain, for example, since being in a certain total state of the whole brain will suffice for being in pain. Perhaps there is some very weak sense in which this makes sense, but it does not seem to capture what researchers in the field are after when looking for an NCC. So something more than mere sufficiency is required.

Minimal sufficiency   The trouble with requiring mere sufficiency, intuitively, is that it allows irrelevant processes into an NCC. If N is an NCC, then the system obtained by conjoining N with a neighboring system M will also qualify as an NCC by the previous definition, since the state of N+M will suffice for the relevant states of consciousness.

The obvious remedy is to require that an NCC has to be a *minimal sufficient system*: that is, a *minimal* system whose state is sufficient for the corresponding conscious state. By this definition, N will be an NCC when (1) the states of N suffice for the corresponding states of consciousness, and (2) no proper part M of N is such that the states of M suffice for the corresponding states of consciousness. In this way, we pare down any potential NCC to its core: Any irrelevant material will be whittled away, and an NCC will be required to contain only the core processes that suffice for the conscious state in question.

Note that on this definition, there may be more than one NCC for a given conscious state. It may be that there is more than one minimal sufficient system for a given state, and all of these will count as a neural correlate of that state. The same goes for systems of phenomenal states. This seems to be the right result: We cannot know a priori that there will be only one NCC for a given state or system of states. Whether there will actually be one or more than one for any given state, however, is something that can be determined only empirically.

There is a technical problem for the minimality requirement. It may turn out that there is significant redundancy in a neural correlate of consciousness, such that, for example, a given conscious visual content is represented redundantly in many cells in a given area. If this is so, then that visual area as a whole might not qualify as a minimal sufficient system, since various smaller components of it might themselves correlate with the conscious state. In this case the definition above would imply that various such small components would each be an NCC. One could deal with this sort of case by noting that the problem arises only when the states of the various smaller systems are themselves wholly correlated with each other. (If their mutual correlation can be broken, so can their correlation with consciousness, so that the overall system or

some key subsystem will again emerge as the true NCC). Given this, one could stipulate that where states of minimal sufficient systems are wholly correlated with each other, it is the union of the system that should be regarded as an NCC, rather than the individual systems. So an NCC would be a minimal system whose state is sufficient for a given conscious state and is not wholly correlated with the state of any other system. I will pass over this complication in what follows.

What Range of Cases?

An NCC will be a minimal neural system N such that the state of N is sufficient for a corresponding conscious state C. This is to say: If the system is in state N1, the subject will have conscious state C. But the question now arises: Over what range of cases must the correlation in question hold?

There is sometimes a temptation to say that this question does not need to be answered: All that is required is to say that *in this very case*, neural state N1 suffices for or correlates with conscious state C. But this does not really make sense. There is no such thing as a single-case correlation. Correlation is always defined with respect to a range of cases. The same goes for sufficiency. To say that neural state N1 suffices for conscious state C is to say that in a range of cases, neural state N1 will always be accompanied by conscious state C. But what is the range of cases?

Any possible case   It is momentarily tempting to suggest that the correlation should range across any possible case: If N is an NCC, it should be impossible to be in a relevant state of N without being in the corresponding state of consciousness. But a moment's reflection suggests that this is incompatible with the common usage in the field. NCCs are often supposed to be relatively limited systems, such as the inferior temporal cortex or the intralaminar nucleus. But nobody (or almost nobody) holds that if one excises the entire inferior temporal cortex or intralaminar nucleus and puts it in a jar, and puts the system into a relevant state, it will be accompanied by the corresponding state of consciousness.

That is to say, for a given NCC, it certainly seems *possible* that one can have the NCC state without the corresponding conscious state—for example, by performing sufficiently radical lesions. So we cannot require that the correlation range over all possible cases.

Of course, one could always insist that a *true* NCC must be such that it is impossible to have the NCC state without the corresponding conscious state. The consequence of this would be that an NCC would almost certainly be far larger than it is on any current hypothesis, since we would have to build in a large amount of the brain to make sure that all the background conditions are in place. Perhaps it would be some sort of wide-ranging although skeletal brain state, involving aspects of processes from a number of regions of the brain. This might be a valid usage, but it is clear that this is not what researchers in the field are getting at when they are talking about an NCC.

We might call the notion just defined a *total* NCC, since it builds in the totality of physical processes that are absolutely required for a given conscious state. The notion that is current in the field is more akin to that of a *core* NCC. (I adapt this terminology from Shoemaker's [1981] notion of a "total realization" and a "core realization" of a functional mental state.) A total NCC builds in everything and thus automatically suffices for the corresponding conscious states. A core NCC, on the other hand, contains only the "core" processes that correlate with consciousness. The rest of the total NCC will be relegated to some sort of background conditions required for the correct functioning of the core.

(Philosophical note: The sort of possibility being considered here is natural or nomological possibility, or possibility compatible with the laws of nature. If we required correlation across all *logically* possible cases, there might be no total NCC at all, since it is arguably logically possible, or coherently conceivable, to instantiate any physical process at all without consciousness. But it is probably not naturally possible. It is almost certainly naturally necessary that a being with my brain state will have the same sort as conscious state as I, for example. So natural possibility is the relevant sort for defining the correlation here.)

The question is, then, how to distinguish the core from the background. It seems that what is required for an NCC (in the "core" sense) is not that it correlate with consciousness across any possible conditions, but rather that it correlate across some constrained range of cases in which some aspects of normal brain functioning are held constant. The question then becomes What is to be held constant? Across just what constrained range of cases do we require that an NCC correlate with consciousness?

Ordinary functioning brain in ordinary environments One might take the moral of the above to be that one cannot require an NCC to correlate with consciousness in "unnatural" cases. What matters is that the NCC correlates with consciousness in "natural" cases, those which actually occur in the functioning of a normal brain. The most conservative strategy would be to require correlation only across cases involving a normally functioning brain in a normal environment, receiving "ecologically valid" inputs of the sort received in a normal life.

The trouble with this criterion is that it seems too weak to narrow down the NCC. It may turn out that this way, we find NCCs at all stages of the visual system, for example. In the normal visual environment, we can expect that the contents of visual systems from V1 through IT will all correlate with the contents of visual consciousness, and that even the contents of the retina will do so to some extent. The reason is that in normal cases all these will be linked in a straightforward causal chain, and the systems in question will not be dissociated. But it seems wrong to say that merely because of this, all the systems (perhaps even the retina) should count as an NCC.

The moral of this is that we need a finer-grained criterion to dissociate these systems and to distinguish the core NCC from processes that are merely causally linked to it. To do this, we are have to require correlation across a range of *unusual cases* as well as across normal cases, since it is these cases that yield interesting dissociations.

Normal brain, unusual inputs The next most conservative suggestion is that we still require a normal brain for our range of cases, but that we allow any possible inputs, including "ecologically invalid" inputs. This would cover the Logothetis experiments, for example. The inputs that evoke binocular rivalry are certainly unusual, and are not encountered in a normal environment. But it is precisely these that allow the experiments to make finer-grained distinctions than we normally can. The experiments suggest that IT is more likely than V1 to be an NCC, precisely because it correlates with consciousness across the wider range of cases. If states of V1 truly do not match up with states of consciousness in this situation, then it seems that V1 cannot be an NCC. If that reasoning is correct, then it seems that we require an NCC to correlate with consciousness across all unusual inputs, and not just across normal environments.

The extension of the correlation requirement from normal environments to unusual inputs is a relatively "safe" extension and seems a reasonable requirement, though those who place a high premium on ecological validity might contest it. But it is arguable that this is still too weak to do the fine-grained work in distinguishing an NCC from systems linked to it. Presumably unusual inputs will go only so far in yielding interesting dissociations, and some systems (particularly those well down the processing pathway) may well remain associated with each other

on any unusual inputs. So it is arguable that we will need finer-grained tools to distinguish the NCC.

Normal brain, varying brain stimulation The next possibility is to allow cases involving not just unusual inputs, but also direct stimulation of the brain. Such direct stimulation might include both electrode stimulation and transcranial magnetic stimulation. On this view, we will require that an NCC correlate with consciousness across all cases of brain stimulation, as well as normal functioning. So if we have a potential NCC state that does not correlate with consciousness in a brain stimulation condition, that state will not be a true NCC.

This requirement seems to fit some methods used in the field. Penfield (e.g., Penfield and Rasmussen 1950) pioneered the use of brain stimulation to draw conclusions about the neural bases of consciousness. Libet (1982) has also used brain stimulation to good effect, and more recently Newsome and colleagues (e.g., Salzman et al. 1990) have used brain stimulation to draw some conclusions about neural correlates of motion perception in monkeys. (See also Marge 1991 for a review of transcranial magnetic stimulation in vision.)

Clearly, brain stimulation can be used to produce dissociations that are finer-grained than can be produced with unusual inputs. One might be able to dissociate activity in any system from that in a preceding system by stimulating that system directly, for example, as long as there are not too many backward connections. Given a candidate NCC—inferior temporal cortex, say —one can test the hypothesis by stimulating an area immediately following the candidate in the processing pathway. If that yields a relevant conscious state without relevant activity in IT (say), that indicates that IT is probably not a true NCC after all. Rather, the NCC may lie in a system farther down the processing chain. (I leave aside the possibility that there might be two NCCs at different stages of the chain.)

This reasoning seems sound, suggesting that we may tacitly require an NCC to correlate with consciousness across brain stimulation conditions. There is no immediately obvious problem with the requirement, at least when the stimulation in question is relatively small and localized. If one allows arbitrarily large stimulation, there may be problems. For example, one presumably could use brain stimulation, at least in principle, to disable large areas of the brain (by over-stimulating them, for example) while leaving NCC activity intact. In this case, it is not implausible to expect that one will have the relevant NCC activity without the usual conscious state (just as in the case where one lesions the whole NCC and puts it in a jar), so the correlation will fail in this case. But intuitively, this does not seem to disprove the claim that the NCC in question is a true NCC, at least before the stimulation. If that is so, then we cannot allow unlimited brain stimulation in the range of cases relevant to the correlation; and, more generally, some of the problems with lesions (discussed below) may apply to reasoning that involves brain stimulation. Nevertheless, one might well require that an NCC correlate with consciousness at least across cases of limited stimulation, in the absence of strong reason to believe otherwise.

Abnormal functioning due to lesions In almost all of the cases above, we have retained a normally functioning brain; we have just stimulated it in unusual ways. The next logical step is to allow cases where the brain is not functioning normally, due to lesions in brain systems. Such lesions might be either natural (e.g., due to some sort of brain damage) or artificial (e.g., induced by surgery). On the latest view, we will require that an NCC correlate with states of consciousness not just over cases of normal functioning but over cases of abnormal functioning as well.

This certainly squares with common practice in the field. Lesion studies are often used to draw conclusions about the neural correlates of consciousness. In Milner and Goodale's (1995) work,

for example, the fact that consciousness remains much the same following lesions to the dorsal stream but not to the ventral stream is used to support the conclusion that the NCC lies within the ventral stream. More generally, it is often assumed that if some aspect of consciousness survives relatively intact when a given brain area is damaged, then that brain area is unlikely to be or to contain an NCC.

The tacit premise in this research is that an NCC should correlate with consciousness, not just in cases of normal functioning but in cases of abnormal functioning as well. Given this premise, it follows that if we find an abnormal case in which neural system N is damaged but a previously corresponding conscious state C is preserved, then N is not a neural correlate of C. Without this premise, or a version of it, it is not clear that any such conclusion can be drawn from lesion studies.

The premise may sound reasonable, but we already have reason to be suspicious of it. We know that for any candidate NCC, sufficiently radical changes can destroy the correlation. Preserving merely system N, cut off from the rest of the brain, for example, is unlikely to yield a corresponding conscious state; but, intuitively, this does not imply that N was not an NCC in the original case.

Less radically, one can imagine placing lesions immediately downstream from a candidate NCC N, so that N's effects on the rest of the brain are significantly reduced. In such a case, it is probable that N can be active without the usual behavioral effects associated with consciousness, and quite plausibly without consciousness itself. It's not implausible that an NCC supports consciousness largely by virtue of playing the right functional role in the brain; by virtue of mediating global availability, for example (see Baars 1988 and Chalmers 1998). If that is so, then if the system is changed so that the NCC no longer plays that functional role, NCC activity will no longer correlate with consciousness. But the mere fact that correlation can be destroyed by this sort of lesion does not obviously imply that N is not an NCC in a normal brain. If that inference could be made, then almost any candidate NCC could be ruled out by the right sort of lesion.

It may be that even smaller lesions can destroy a correlation in this way. For example, it is not implausible that for any candidate NCC N, there is some other local system in the brain (perhaps a downstream area) whose proper functioning is required for activity in N to yield the usual effects that go with consciousness, and for N to yield consciousness itself. This second system might not itself be an NCC in any intuitive sense; it might merely play an enabling role, in the way that proper functioning of the heart plays an enabling role for functioning of the brain. If that is so, then if one lesions this single area downstream, activity in N will no longer correlate with consciousness. In this way, any potential NCC might be ruled out by a localized lesion elsewhere.

The trouble is that lesions change the architecture of the brain, and it's quite possible that changes to brain architecture can change the location of an NCC, so that a physical state which was an NCC in a normal brain will not be an NCC in the altered brain. Given this possibility, it seems too strong to require that an NCC correlate with consciousness across arbitrary lesions and changes in brain functioning. We should expect an NCC to be architecture-dependent, not architecture-independent.

So an NCC should not be expected to correlate with consciousness across arbitrary lesion cases. There are now two alternatives. Either we can require correlation across some more restricted range of lesion cases, or we can drop the requirement of correlation in abnormal cases altogether.

For the first alternative to work, we would have to find some way to distinguish "good" lesions from "bad" lesions. An NCC would be expected to correlate with consciousness across the good lesions but not the bad lesions. If one found a "good" lesion case where activity in

system N was present without the corresponding conscious state, this would imply that N is not an NCC; but no such conclusion could be drawn from a "bad" lesion case.

The trouble is that it is not at all obvious that such a distinction can be drawn. It might be tempting to come up with an after-the-fact distinction, defined as the range of lesions in which correlation with a given NCC N is preserved, but this will not be helpful, since we are interested in the criterion that makes N qualify as an NCC in the first place. So a distinction will have to be drawn on relatively a priori grounds (it can then be used to determine whether a given correlation pattern qualifies an arbitrary system as an NCC or not). But it is not clear how to draw the distinction. One might suggest that correlation should be preserved across small lesions but not large ones; but we have seen above that even small lesions might destroy a potential NCC. Or one might suggest that lesions in downstream areas are illegitimate, but upstream and parallel lesions are legitimate. But even here, it is not clear that indirect interaction with an upstream or parallel area might be required to support proper functioning of an NCC. Perhaps with some ingenuity one might be able to come up with a criterion, but it is not at all obvious how.

The second alternative is to hold that correlation across cases of normal functioning (perhaps with unusual inputs and brain stimulation) is all that is required to be an NCC. If this is so, one can never infer directly from the fact that N fails to correlate with consciousness in a lesion to the conclusion that N is not an NCC. On this view, the location of an NCC is wholly architecture-dependent, or entirely dependent on the normal functioning of the brain. One cannot expect an NCC to correlate with consciousness in cases of abnormal functioning or different architecture, so no direct conclusion can be drawn from failure of correlation across lesion cases. Of course, one can still appeal to cases with unusual inputs and brain stimulation to make fine-grained distinctions among NCCs.

The main conceptual objection to the second alternative is that one might *need* lesion cases to make the finest-grained distinctions that are required. Consider a hypothetical case in which we have two linked systems N and M that correlate equally well with consciousness across all normal cases, including all unusual inputs and brain stimulation, but in almost all relevant lesion cases, consciousness correlates much better with N than with M. In this case, might we want to say that N rather than M is an NCC? If so, we have to build some allowance for abnormal cases into the definition of an NCC. An advocate of the second alternative might reply that such cases will be very unusual, and that if N and M are dissociable by lesions, there is likely to be some unusual brain stimulation that will bring out the dissociation as well. In the extreme case where no brain stimulation leads to dissociation, one might simply bite the bullet and say that both N and M are equally good NCCs.

Taking everything into consideration, I am inclined to think the second alternative is better than the first. It seems right to say that "core" NCC location depends on brain architecture and normal functioning, and it is unclear that correlation across abnormal cases should be required, especially given all the associated problems. A problem like the one just mentioned might provide some pressure to investigate the first alternative further, and I do not rule out the possibility that some way of distinguishing "good" from "bad" lesions might be found, but all in all it seems best to say that an NCC cannot be expected to correlate with consciousness across abnormal cases.

Of course this has an impact on the methodology of the search for an NCC. As we have seen, lesion studies are often used to draw conclusions about NCC location (as in the Milner and Goodale research, for example, and also in much research on blindsight), and failure of correlation in lesion cases is often taken to imply that a given system is not an NCC. But we have seen that the tacit premise of this sort of research

—that an NCC must correlate across abnormal as well as normal cases—is difficult to support, and leads to significant problems. So it seems that lesion studies are methodologically dangerous here. One should be very cautious in using them to draw conclusions about NCC location.

This is not to say that lesion studies are irrelevant in the search for an NCC. Even if correlation across abnormal cases is not *required* for system N to be an NCC, it may be that correlation across abnormal cases can provide good *evidence* that N is an NCC, and that failure of such correlation in some cases provides good evidence that N is not an NCC. Say we take the second alternative above, and define an NCC as a system that correlates with consciousness across all normal cases (including unusual input and stimulation). It may nevertheless be the case that information about correlations across all these normal cases with unusual stimulation is difficult to come by (due to problems in monitoring brain systems at a fine grain, for example), and that information about correlation across lesion cases is easier to obtain. In this case, one might sometimes take correlation across abnormal cases as *evidence* that a system will correlate across the normal cases in question, and thus as evidence that the system is an NCC. Similarly, one might take failure of correlation across abnormal cases as evidence that a system will fail to correlate across certain normal cases, and thus as evidence that the system is not an NCC.

The question of whether a given lesion study can serve as evidence in this way needs to be taken on a case-by-case basis. It is clear that some lesion studies will not provide this sort of evidence, as witnessed by the cases of severe lesions and downstream lesions discussed earlier. In those cases, failure of correlation across abnormal cases provides no evidence of failure of correlation across normal cases. On the other hand, it does not seem unreasonable that the Milner and Goodale studies should be taken as evidence that even in normal cases, the ventral stream will correlate better with visual consciousness than the dorsal stream. Of course the real "proof" would come from a careful investigation of the relevant processes across a wide range of "normal" cases involving standard environments, unusual inputs, and brain stimulation; but in the absence of such a demonstration, the lesion cases at least provide suggestive evidence.

In any case, the moral is that one has to be very cautious when drawing conclusions about NCC location from lesion studies. At best these studies serve as indirect evidence rather than as direct criteria, and even as such there is a chance that the evidence can be misleading. One needs to consider the possibility that the lesion in question is changing brain architecture in such a fashion that what was once an NCC is no longer an NCC, and one needs to look very closely at what is going on to rule out the possibility. It may be that this can sometimes be done, but it is a nontrivial matter.

Overall Definition

With all this, we have come to a more detailed definition of an NCC. The general case is something like the following:

An NCC is a minimal neural system N such that there is a mapping from states of N to states of consciousness, where a given state of N is sufficient, under conditions C, for the corresponding state of consciousness.

The central case of the neural correlate of the content of consciousness can be put in more specific terms:

An NCC (for content) is a minimal neural representational system N such that representation of a content in N is sufficient, under conditions C, for representation of that content in consciousness.

One might also give a general definition of the NCC for an arbitrary phenomenal property or for a phenomenal family, but I will leave those aside here.

The "conditions C" clause here represents the relevant range of cases, as discussed above. If the reasoning above is on the right track, then conditions C might be seen as conditions involving normal brain functioning, allowing unusual inputs and limited brain stimulation, but not lesions or other changes in architecture. Of course the precise nature of conditions C is still debatable. Perhaps one could make a case for including a limited range of lesion cases in the definition. In the other direction, perhaps one might make a case that the requirement of correlation across brain stimulation or unusual inputs is too strong, due to the abnormality of those scenarios. But I think the conditions C proposed here are at least a reasonable first pass, pending further investigation.

Of course, to some extent, defining what "really" counts as an NCC is a terminological matter. One could quite reasonably say that there are multiple different notions of NCC, depending on just how one understands the relevant conditions C, or the matter of necessity and sufficiency, and so on; and not much really rests on which of these is the "right" definition. Still, we have seen that different definitions give very different results, and that many potential definitions have the consequence that systems which intuitively seem to qualify as an NCC do not qualify after all, and that NCC hypotheses put forward by researchers in the field could be ruled out on trivial a priori grounds. Those consequences seem undesirable. It makes sense to have a definition of NCC that fits the way the notion is generally used in the field, and that can make sense of empirical research in the area. At the same time we want a definition of NCC to be coherent and well-motivated in its own right, such that an NCC is something worth looking for, and such that the definition can itself be used to assess various hypotheses about the identity of an NCC. It seems to me that the definition I have given here is at least a first pass in this direction.

Methodological Consequences

The discussion so far has been somewhat abstract, and the definitions given above may look like mere words; but from these definitions and the reasoning that went into them, one can straightforwardly extract some concrete methodological recommendations for the NCC search. Many of these recommendations are plausible or obvious in their own right, but it is interesting to see them emerge from the analysis.

Lesion Studies Are Methodologically Dangerous

Lesion studies are often used to draw conclusions about neural correlates of consciousness, but we have seen that their use can be problematic. The identity of an NCC is arguably always relative to specific brain architecture and normal brain functioning, and correlation across abnormal cases should not generally be expected. In some cases, lesion studies can change brain architecture so that a system which was previously an NCC is no longer one. So one can never infer directly from failure of correlation between a system and consciousness in a lesion case to the conclusion that the system is an NCC. Sometimes one can infer this indirectly, by using the failure of correlation here as evidence for failure of correlation in normal cases, but one must be cautious.

There May Be Many NCCs

On the definition above, an NCC is a system whose activity is *sufficient* for certain states of consciousness. This allows for the possibility of multiple NCCs in at least two ways. First, different sorts of conscious states may have different corresponding NCCs; there may be different NCCs for visual and auditory consciousness, for example, and perhaps even for different aspects of visual consciousness. Second, even for a particular sort of conscious state (such as pain), we

cannot rule out the possibility that there will be two different systems whose activity is sufficient to produce that state.

Of course it *could* turn out that there is only a small number of NCCs, or perhaps even one. For all that I have said here, it is possible that there is some central system which represents the contents of visual consciousness, auditory consciousness, emotional experience, the stream of conscious thought, the background state of consciousness, and so on. Such a system might be seen as a sort of "consciousness module," or perhaps as a "Cartesian theater" (Dennett 1991) or a "global workspace" (Baars 1988), depending on whether one is a foe or a friend of the idea (see Chalmers 1998 for some discussion). But it is by no means obvious that there will be such a system, and I think the empirical evidence so far is against it. In any case, the matter cannot be decided a priori, so our definition should be compatible with the existence of multiple NCCs.

Minimize Size of an NCC

We have seen that an NCC should be understood as a *minimal* neural system which correlates with consciousness. Given this, we should constrain the search for the NCC by aiming to find a neural correlate that is as small as possible. Given a broad system that appears to correlate with consciousness, we need to isolate the core relevant parts and aspects of that system which underlie the correlation. And given the dual hypotheses that consciousness correlates with a broad system or with a narrower system contained within it, we might first investigate the "narrow" hypothesis, since if it correlates with consciousness, the broad system cannot be a true NCC.

So to some extent it makes sense to "start small" in the search for an NCC. This fits the working methodology proposed by Crick and Koch (1998). They suggest that an NCC may involve a very small number of neurons (perhaps in the thousands) with certain distinctive properties. There is no guarantee that this is correct (and my own money is against it), but it makes a good working hypothesis in the NCC search. Of course one should simultaneously investigate broad systems for correlation with consciousness, so that one can then focus on those areas and try to narrow things down.

Distinguish NCCs for Background State and for Content

We have seen that there may be different NCCs for different sorts of states of consciousness. An important distinction in this class is that between the neural correlate of background state of consciousness (wakefulness, dreaming, etc.) and the neural correlate of specific contents. It may be that these are quite different systems. It is not implausible, on current evidence, that an NCC for background state involves processes in the thalamus, or thalamocortical interactions, while an NCC for specific contents of consciousness involves processes in the cortex. These different sorts of NCC will require quite different methods for their investigation.

NCC Studies Need to Monitor Neural Representational Content

Arguably the most interesting part of the NCC search is the search for neural determinants of specific contents of consciousness, such as the contents of visual consciousness. We have seen that an NCC here will be a neural representational system whose contents are correlated with the contents of consciousness. To determine whether such a system is truly an NCC, then, we need methods that monitor the representational content of the system. This is just what we find in Logothetis's work, for example, where it is crucial to keep track of activity in neurons with known receptive fields.

This gets at a striking aspect of the NCC search in practice, which is that the most informative and useful results usually come from neuron-level studies on monkeys. Large claims are sometimes made for brain imaging in humans, but it is generally difficult to draw solid conclusions from such studies, especially where an NCC is concerned. We can trace the difference to the fact that neuron-level studies can monitor representational content in neural systems, whereas imaging studies cannot (or at least usually do not). The power of single-cell studies in the work of Logothetis, Andersen, Newsome and colleagues (e.g., the works of Logothetis and Newsome already cited, and Bradley et al. 1998) comes precisely from the way that cells can be monitored to keep track of the activity profile of neurons with known representational properties, such as receptive and projective fields. This allows us to track representational content in these neural systems and to correlate it with the apparent contents of consciousness. This is much harder to do in a coarse-grained brain-imaging study, which generally tells one that there is activity in a region while saying nothing about specific contents.

A moral is that it makes sense to concentrate on developing methods which can track neural representational content, especially in humans (where invasive studies are much more problematic, but where evidence for conscious content is much more straightforward). There has been some recent work on the use of imaging methods to get at certain aspects of the content of visual consciousness, such as colors and shapes in the visual field (e.g., Engel et al. 1997), and different sorts of objects that activate different brain areas (e.g., Tong et al. 1998). There is also some current work using invasive methods in neurosurgery patients to monitor the activity of single cells. One can speculate that if a noninvasive method for monitoring single-cell activity in humans is ever developed, the search for an NCC (like most of neuroscience) will be transformed almost beyond recognition.

Correlation Across a Few Situations Is Limited Evidence

According to the definition above, an NCC is a system that correlates with consciousness across arbitrary cases of normal functioning, in any environment, with any unusual input or limited brain stimulation. In practice, though, evidence is far weaker than this. Typically one has a few cases, involving either a few subjects with different lesions, or a study in which subjects are given different stimuli and one notes an apparent correlation. This is to be expected, given the current technological and ethical constraints on experimental methods. But it does mean that the evidence which current methods give is quite weak. To truly demonstrate that a given system is an NCC, one would need to show correlation across a far wider range of cases than is currently feasible. Of course current methods may give good *negative* evidence about systems that fail to correlate and thus are not NCCs, but strong positive evidence is harder to find. Positive hypotheses based on current sorts of evidence should probably be considered suggestive but highly speculative.

We Need Good Criteria for the Ascription of Consciousness

To find an NCC, we need to find a neural system that correlates with certain conscious states. To do this, we first need a way to know when a system is in a given conscious state. This is famously problematic, given the privacy of consciousness and the philosophical problem of other minds. In general, we rely on indirect criteria for the ascription of consciousness. The most straightforward of these criteria is verbal report in humans, but other criteria are often required. Where nonhuman subjects are involved, one must rely on quite indirect behavioral signs (voluntary bar-pressing in Logothetis's monkeys, for example).

A deep problem for the field is that our ultimate criteria here are not experimentally testable, since the results of any experiment will require such criteria for their interpretation. (First-person experimentation on oneself may be an exception, but even this has limitations.) So any experimental work implicitly relies on pre-empirical principles (even "philosophical" principles) for its interpretation. Given this, it is vital to refine and justify these preempirical principles as well as we can. In the case of verbal report, we may be on relatively safe ground (though even here there may be some grounds for doubt, as witnessed in the debates over "subjective threshold" criteria in unconscious perception research; see, e.g., Merikle and Reingold 1992). In other cases, especially nonhuman cases, careful attention to the assumptions involved are required. I don't think this problem is insurmountable, but it deserves careful attention. Our conclusions about NCC location will be no better than the preexperimental assumptions that go into the search. (I consider this problem, and its consequences for the NCC search, in much more detail in Chalmers 1998.)

Methodological Summary

We can use all this to sketch a general methodology for the NCC search. First, we need methods for determining the contents of conscious experience in a subject, presumably by indirect behavioral criteria or by first-person phenomenology. Second, we need methods to monitor neural states in a subject, and in particular to monitor neural representational contents. Then we need to perform experiments in a variety of situations to determine which neural systems correlate with conscious states and which do not. Experiments involving normal brain functioning with unusual inputs and limited brain stimulation are particularly crucial here. Direct conclusions cannot be drawn from systems with lesions, but such systems can sometimes serve as indirect evidence. We need to consider multiple hypotheses in order to narrow down a set of minimal neural systems that correlate with consciousness across all relevant scenarios. We may well find many different NCCs in different modalities, and different NCCs for background state and conscious contents, although it is not out of the question that there will be only a small number. If all goes well, we might expect eventually to isolate systems that correlate strongly with consciousness across any normally functioning brain.

Should We Expect an NCC?

One might well ask: Given the notion of an NCC as I have defined it, is it guaranteed that there will *be* a neural correlate of consciousness?

In answering, I will assume that states of consciousness depend systematically in some way on overall states of the brain. If this assumption is false, as is held by some Cartesian dualists (e.g., Eccles 1994) and some phenomenal externalists (e.g., Dretske 1995), then there may be no NCC as defined here, since any given neural state might be instantiated without consciousness. (Even on these positions, an NCC *could* be possible, if it were held that brain states at least correlate with conscious states in ordinary cases). But if the assumption is true, then there will at least be some minimal correlation of neural states with consciousness.

Does it follow that there will be an NCC as defined here? This depends on whether we are talking about neural correlates of arbitrary conscious states or about the more constrained case of neural correlates of conscious contents. In the first case, it is guaranteed that the brain as a whole will be a neural system which has states that suffice for arbitrary conscious states. So the brain will be one system whose state is sufficient for a given conscious state; and given that there is at least one such system for a given state, there must be at least one such *minimal* system for that

state. Such a system will be an NCC for that state. Of course this reasoning does not guarantee that there will be only one NCC for a given state, or that the NCC for one state will be the same as the NCC for another, or that an NCC will be simple, but we know that an NCC will exist.

In the case of neural correlates of the content of consciousness, things are more constrained, since a neural correlate is required not just to map to a corresponding state of consciousness, but to match it in *content*. This rules out the whole brain as even a nonminimal neural correlate, for example, since representing a content in the brain does not suffice to represent that content in consciousness (much of the brain's representational content is unconscious). Of course we may hope that there will be more constrained neural systems whose content systematically matches the contents of some aspect of consciousness. But one might argue that it is not obvious that such a system *must* exist. It might be held, for example, that the contents of consciousness are an emergent product of the contents of various neural systems, which together suffice for the conscious content in question, but none of which precisely mirrors it.

I think one can plausibly argue that there is reason to expect that conscious contents will be mirrored by the contents of a neural representational system at *some* level of abstraction. In creatures with language, for example, conscious contents correspond well with contents that are made directly available for verbal report; and in conscious creatures more generally, one can argue that the contents of consciousness correspond to contents which are made directly available for the global voluntary control of behavior (see, e.g., Chalmers 1998). So there is a correlation between the contents of consciousness and contents revealed or exhibited in certain functional roles within the system.

Given that these contents are revealed in verbal report and are exhibited in the control of behavior, there is reason to believe that they are represented at some point within the cognitive system. Of course this depends to some extent on just what "representation" comes to. On some highly constrained notions of representation—if it is held that the only true representation is symbolic representation, for example—then it is far from clear that the content revealed in behavior must be represented. But on less demanding notions of representation—on which, for example, systems are assigned representational content according to their functional role—then it will be natural to expect that the content revealed in a functional role will be represented in a system which plays that functional role.

This does not guarantee that there will be any single neural system whose content always matches the content of consciousness. It may be that the functional role in question is played by multiple systems, and that a given system may sometimes play the role, and sometimes not. If this is so, we may have to move to a higher level of abstraction. If there is no localizable neural system that qualifies as a correlate of conscious content, we may have to look at a more global system—the "global availability" system, for example, whereby contents are made available for report and global control—and argue that the contents of consciousness correspond to the contents made available in this system. If so, it could turn out that what we are left with is more like a "cognitive correlate of consciousness," since the system may not correspond to any neurobiological system whose nature and boundaries are independently carved out. But it can still function as a correlate in some useful sense.

In this context, it is important to note that an NCC need not be a specific anatomical area in the brain. Some of the existing proposals regarding NCCs involve less localized neurobiological properties. For example, Libet (1993) argues that the neural correlate of consciousness is temporally extended neural firing; Crick and Koch (1998) speculate that the NCC might in-

volve a particular sort of cell throughout the cortex; Edelman (1989) suggests that the NCC might involve reentrant thalamocortical loops; and so on. In these cases, NCCs are individuated by temporal properties, or by physiological rather than anatomical properties, or by functional properties, among other possibilities. If that is the case, the "neural representational system" involved in defining a neural correlate of conscious content might also be individuated more abstractly: The relevant neural representational contents might be those represented by temporally extended firings, or by certain sorts of cells, or by reentrant loops, and so on. So abstractness and failure of localization are not in themselves bars to a system's qualifying as an NCC.

It seems, then, that there is a range of possibilities for the brain-based correlates of conscious states, ranging from specific anatomical areas, through more abstract neural systems, to purely "cognitive" correlates such as Baars's (1988) global workspace. Just how specific an NCC may turn out to be is an empirical question. One might reasonably expect that there will be some biological specificity. Within a given organism or species, one often finds a close match between specific functions and specific physiological systems, and it does not seem unlikely that particular neural systems and properties in the brain should be directly implicated in the mechanisms of availability for global control. If that is the case, then we may expect specific neural correlates even of conscious contents. If not, we may have to settle for more abstract correlates, individuated at least partly at the cognitive level, though even here one will expect that some neural systems will be much more heavily involved than others. In any case it seems reasonable to expect that we will find informative brain-based correlates of consciousness at some level of abstraction in cognitive neurobiology.

Some have argued that we should not expect neural correlates of consciousness. For example, in their discussion of neural "filling-in" in visual perception, Pessoa et al. (1998) argue against the necessity of what Teller and Pugh (1983) call a "bridge locus" for perception, which closely resembles the notion of a neural correlate of consciousness. Much of their argument is based on the requirement that such a locus must involve a spatiotemporal isomorphism between neural states and conscious states (so a conscious representation of a checkerboard would require a neural state in a checkerboard layout, for example). These arguments do not affect neural correlates of conscious contents as I have defined them, since a match between neural and conscious content does not require such a spatiotemporal correspondence (a neural representation of a shape need not itself have that shape). Pessoa et al. also argue more generally against a "uniformity of content" thesis, holding that one should not expect a match between the "personal" contents of consciousness and the "subpersonal" contents of neural systems. It is true that the existence of such a match is not automatic, but as before, the fact that conscious contents are mirrored in specific functional roles gives reason to believe that they will be subpersonally represented at least at some level of abstraction.

It has also been argued (e.g., by Güzeldere 1999) that there is probably no neural correlate of consciousness, since there is probably no area of the brain that is specifically dedicated to consciousness as opposed to vision, memory, learning, and so on. One may well agree that there is no such area, but it does not follow that there is no neural correlate of consciousness as defined here. An NCC (as defined here) requires only that a system be correlated with consciousness, not that it be dedicated solely or mainly to consciousness. Güzeldere's alternative conception of an NCC is much more demanding than the conception at issue in most empirical work on the subject, where it is often accepted that an NCC may be closely bound up with visual processing (e.g., Logothetis; Milner and Goodale), memory (e.g., Edelman), and other processes.

This becomes particularly clear once one gives up on the requirement that there be a single NCC, and accepts that there may be multiple NCCs in multiple modalities.

Conclusion

The discussion in the previous section helps bring out what an NCC is not, or at least what it might turn out not to be. An NCC is defined to be a *correlate* of consciousness. From this, it does not automatically follow that an NCC will be a system solely or mainly dedicated to consciousness, or even that an NCC will be the brain system most responsible for the generation of consciousness. It certainly does not follow that an NCC will yield an explanation of consciousness, and it is not even guaranteed that identifying an NCC will be the key to understanding the processes underlying consciousness. If one were to define an NCC in these stronger terms, it would be far from obvious that there must be an NCC, and it would also be much less clear how to search for an NCC.

Defining an NCC solely in terms of correlation seems to capture standard usage best, and it also makes the search more clearly defined and the methodology clearer. Correlations are easy for science to study. It also means that the search for an NCC can be to a large extent theoretically neutral rather than theoretically loaded. Once we have found an NCC, one might hope that it will turn out to be a system dedicated to consciousness, or that it will turn out to yield an explanation of consciousness, but these are further questions. In the meantime the search for an NCC as defined poses a tractable empirical question with relatively clear parameters, one that researchers of widely different theoretical persuasions can engage in.

There are certain rewards of the search for an NCC that one might reasonably expect. For example, these systems might be used to monitor and predict the contents of consciousness in a range of novel situations. For example, we may be able to use them to help reach conclusions about conscious experience in patients under anesthesia, and in subjects with "locked-in syndrome" or in a coma. In cases where brain architecture differs significantly from the original cases (perhaps some coma cases, infants, and animals), the evidence will be quite imperfect, but it will at least be suggestive.

These systems might also serve as a crucial step toward a full science of consciousness. Once we know which systems are NCCs, we can investigate the mechanisms by which they work, and how they produce various characteristic functional effects. Just as isolating the DNA basis of the gene helped explain many of the functional phenomena of life, so isolating NCC systems may help explain many functional phenomena associated with consciousness. We might also systematize the relationship between NCCs and conscious states, and abstract general principles governing the relationship between them. In this way we might be led to a much greater theoretical understanding.

In the meantime, the search for a neural correlate of consciousness provides a project that is relatively tractable, clearly defined, and theoretically neutral, one whose goal seems to be visible somewhere in the middle distance. Because of this, the search makes an appropriate centerpiece for a developing science of consciousness, and is an important springboard in the quest for a general theory of the relationship between physical processes and conscious experience.

References

Anderson, R. A. 1997. Neural mechanisms in visual motion perception in primates. *Neuron* 18: 865–872.

Baars, B. J. 1988. *A Cognitive Theory of Consciousness.* Cambridge: Cambridge University Press.

Bogen, J. E. 1995. On the neurophysiology of consciousness, part I: An overview. *Consciousness and Cognition* 4: 52–62.

Bradley, D. C., Chang, G. C., and Andersen, R. A. 1998. Encoding of three-dimensional structure-from-motion by primate area MT neurons. *Nature* 392: 714–717.

Chalmers, D. J. 1996. *The Conscious Mind: In Search of a Fundamental Theory.* New York: Oxford University Press.

Chalmers, D. J. 1995. Facing up to the problem of consciousness. *Journal of Consciousness Studies* 2: 200–219. Also in S. Hameroff, A. Kaszniak, and A. Scott, eds., 1996, *Toward a Science of Consciousness* (Cambridge, Mass.: MIT Press); and in J. Shear, ed., 1997, *Explaining Consciousness: The Hard Problem* (Cambridge, Mass.: MIT Press).

Chalmers, D. J. 1998. On the search for the neural correlate of consciousness. In S. Hameroff, A. Kaszniak, and A. Scott, eds., *Toward a Science of Consciousness.* Cambridge, Mass.: MIT Press.

Crick, F., and Koch, C. 1990. Towards a neurobiological theory of consciousness. *Seminars in the Neurosciences* 2: 263–275.

Crick, F., and Koch, C. 1995. Are we aware of neural activity in primary visual cortex? *Nature* 375: 121–123.

Crick, F. and Koch, C. 1998. Consciousness and neuroscience. *Cerebral Cortex* 375: 121–123.

Dennett, D. C. 1991. *Consciousness Explained.* Boston: Little Brown.

Dretske, F. 1995. *Naturalizing the Mind.* Cambridge, Mass.: MIT Press.

Eccles, J. C. 1994. *How the Self Controls Its Brain.* New York: Springer-Verlag.

Edelman, G. M. 1989. *The Remembered Present: A Biological Theory of Consciousness.* New York: Basic Books.

Engel, S., Zhang, X., and Wandell, B. 1997. Colour tuning in human visual cortex measured with functional magnetic resonance imaging. *Nature* 388: 68–81.

Flohr, H. 1995. Sensations and brain processes. *Behavioral Brain Research* 71: 157–161.

Gur, M., and Snodderly, D. M. 1997. A dissociation between brain activity and perception: Chromatically active cortical neurons signal chromatic activity that is not perceived. Vision Research 37: 377–382.

Güzeldere, G. 1999. There is no neural correlate of consciousness. Paper presented at Toward a Science of Consciousness: Fundamental Approaches. Tokyo, May 25–28.

He, S., Cavanagh, P., and Intriligator, J. 1996. Attentional resolution and the locus of visual awareness. *Nature* 384: 334–337.

Hobson, J. A. 1997. Consciousness as a state-dependent phenomenon. In J. Cohen and J. Schooler, eds., *Scientific Approaches to Consciousness*. Hillsdale, NJ: Lawrence Erlbaum.

Leopold, D. A., and Logothetis, N. K. 1996. Activity changes in early visual cortex reflect monkeys' percepts during binocular rivalry. *Nature* 379: 549–553.

Libet, B. 1982. Brain stimulation in the study of neuronal functions for conscious sensory experiences. *Human Neurobiology* 1: 235–242.

Libet, B. (1993). The neural time factor in conscious and unconscious events. In *Experimental and Theoretical Studies of Consciousness* (Ciba Foundation Symposium 174). Wiley.

Llinas, R. R., Ribary, U., Joliot, M., and Wang, X.-J. 1994. Content and context in temporal thalamocortical binding. In G. Buzsaki, R. R. Llinas, and W. Singer, eds., *Temporal Coding in the Brain*. Berlin: Springer-Verlag.

Logothetis, N., and Schall, J. 1989. Neuronal correlates of subjective visual perception. *Science* 245: 761–763.

Marge, E. 1991. Magnetostimulation of vision: Direct noninvasive stimulation of the retina and the visual brain. *Optometry and Vision Science* 68: 427–440.

Merikle, P. M., and Reingold, E. M. 1992. Measuring unconscious processes. In R. Bornstein and T. Pittman, eds., *Perception Without Awareness*. New York: Guilford.

Milner, A. D. 1995. Cerebral correlates of visual awareness. *Neuropsychologia* 33: 1117–1130.

Milner, A. D., and Goodale, M. A. 1995. *The Visual Brain in Action*. Oxford: Oxford University Press.

Newman, J. B. 1997. Putting the puzzle together: Toward a general theory of the neural correlates of consciousness. *Journal of Consciousness Studies* 4: 47–66, 100–121.

Newman, J. and Baars, B. J. (1993). A neural attentional model of access to consciousness: A global workspace perspective. *Concepts in Neuroscience*, 4: 255–290.

Penfield, W. 1937. The cerebral cortex and consciousness. In *The Harvey Lectures*. Reprinted in R. H. Wilkins, ed., *Neurosurgical Classics*. New York: Johnson Reprint Corp., 1965.

Penfield, W., and Rasmussen, T. 1950. *The Cerebral Cortex of Man: A Clinical Study of Localization of Function*. New York: Macmillan.

Pessoa, L., Thompson, E., and Noe, A. 1998. Finding out about filling in: A guide to perceptual completion for visual science and the philosophy of perception. *Behavioral and Brain Sciences* 21: 723–748.

Salzman, C. D., Britten, K. H., and Newsome, W. T. 1990. Cortical microstimulation influences perceptual judgments of motion direction. *Nature* 346: 174–187.

Sheinberg, D. L., and Logothetis, N. K. 1997. The role of temporal cortical areas in perceptual organization. *Proceedings of the National Academy of Sciences* 94: 3408–3413.

Shoemaker, S. 1981. Some varieties of functionalism. *Philosophical Topics* 12: 93–119. Reprinted in *Identity, Cause, and Mind*. Cambridge: Cambridge University Press, 1984.

Teller, D. Y., and Pugh, E. N. 1983. Linking propositions in color vision. In J. D. Mollon and L. T. Sharpe, eds., *Color Vision: Physiology and Psychophysics*. London: Academic Press.

Tong, F., Nakayama, K., Vaughan, J. T., and Kanwisher, N. 1998. Binocular rivalry and visual awareness in human extrastriate cortex. *Neuron* 21: 753–759.

3 The Perennial Problem of the Reductive Explainability of Phenomenal Consciousness: C. D. Broad on the Explanatory Gap

Ansgar Beckermann

Broad's Distinction between Emergent and Mechanically Explainable Properties

At the start of the twentieth century the question of whether life could be explained in purely mechanical terms was as hotly debated as the mind–body problem is today. Two factions opposed each other. *Biological mechanists* claimed that the properties characteristic of living organisms (metabolism, perception, goal-directed behavior, procreation, morphogenesis) could be explained mechanistically, in the way the behavior of a clock can be explained by the properties and the arrangement of its cogs, springs, and weights. *Substantial vitalists*, on the other hand, maintained that the explanation envisaged by the mechanists was impossible and that one had to postulate a special nonphysical substance in order to explain life—an entelechy or élan vital. When C. D. Broad developed his theory of emergence in the early 1920s, his aim was to create room for a third position mediating between these two extremes—a position he called *emergent vitalism.*

Broad's first step was to point out that the problem of vitalism is only a special case of a much more general problem—the problem of how the *behavior* of a complex system is related to the *properties and the arrangement of its physical parts*. (According to Broad, living beings differ from nonliving things only in their specific behavior. That is to say, he believed that the property of being alive could be characterized in purely behavioral terms. He strictly distinguished properties of this kind from properties that he called "pure qualities." I will return to this distinction below.)

Regarding this question, there are in principle only two basic types of answers. One can hold the view that the behavior of a complex system cannot be explained by referring exclusively to its physical parts and their arrangement, but only by the assumption that S contains a further, nonphysical component, which is present in all beings that behave in the way characteristic of S and is absent in all other beings. According to Broad, anyone who endorses a theory of this kind is a proponent of a *component theory*. However, one can also hold the opposed view that the behavior of S can, at least in principle, be explained by its physical parts and their arrangement. In this case, however, one has, according to Broad, to distinguish two further possibilities. For even if S's behavior can be explained this way, it may be either *mechanistically explainable* or *emergent*. (Broad strictly distinguishes between mechanism and pure mechanism. According to the latter, the term "mechanistically explainable" means something like "explainable just by reference to the laws of classical mechanics"; according to the former, it means "explainable by reference to all general chemical, physical and dynamical laws" (1925: 46). In the following, "mechanistically explainable" is always meant to have this second, broader meaning.) Mechanistic and Emergent Theories thus concur in denying

that there need be any peculiar *component* which is present in all things that behave in a certain way, and is absent from all things which do not behave in this way. [Both say] that the components may be exactly alike in both cases, and [they] try to explain the difference of behavior wholly in terms of difference of structure. (Broad 1925: 58f.)

However, mechanistic and emergent theories differ fundamentally in their view of the laws that relate the behavior of the components of complex systems to the characteristic behavior of the systems themselves.

On [the theory of emergence] the characteristic behavior of the whole *could* not, even in theory, be deduced from the most complete knowledge of the behavior of its components, taken separately or in other combinations, and of their proportions and arrangements in this whole. (Broad 1925: 59)

Which types of macroscopic behavior are to be regarded as emergent in this sense was controversial even in Broad's day. Broad believed that the behavior of nearly all chemical compounds is emergent in the sense explicated. It was his view, for example,

that so far as we know at present, the characteristic behavior of Common Salt cannot be deduced from the most complete knowledge of the properties of Sodium in isolation; or of Chlorine in isolation; or of other compounds of Sodium, such as Sodium Sulphate, and of other compounds of Chlorine, such as Silver Chloride (Broad 1925: 59).

Naturally, mechanists would disagree. Broad characterizes their theory thus:

On [the mechanistic theory] the characteristic behaviour of the whole is not only completely *determined by* the nature and arrangement of its components; in addition to this it is held that the behaviour of the whole could, in theory at least, be *deduced* from a sufficient knowledge of how the components behave in isolation or in other wholes of a simpler kind. (Broad 1925: 59)

Artificial machines are the best examples of complex objects whose behavior can be completely explained in mechanical terms. For instance, we surely do not have any reason to assume that the behavior of a clock is based on a specific nonphysical component which is present in clocks and only in clocks. Hence, component theories are quite inappropriate for the explanation of the behavior of these machines. However, we do not have any reason to assume that the behavior of clocks is emergent, either. For, obviously, we can completely deduce its behavior from the specific arrangement of the springs, cogs, weights, and so forth.

Put in a nutshell, the difference between emergent and mechanistic theories can be explained as follows:

Put in abstract terms the emergent theory asserts that there are certain wholes, composed (say) of constituents A, B, and C in a relation R to each other; that all wholes composed of constituents of the same kind as A, B, and C in relations of the same kind as R have certain characteristic properties; that A, B, and C are capable of occurring in other kinds of complex where the relation is not of the same kind as R; and that the characteristic properties of the whole $R(A, B, C)$ cannot, even in theory, be deduced from the most complete knowledge of the properties of A, B, and C in isolation or in other wholes which are not of the form $R(A, B, C)$. The mechanistic theory rejects the last clause of this assertion. (Broad 1925: 61)

Broad here stresses two points. First, regardless of whether the characteristic behavior B of a class of systems is mechanistically explainable or emergent, B nomologically depends on the corresponding microstructures. That is to say, if a system S consists of the parts $C_1, \ldots, C_n$ arranged in manner R—for short, if S has microstructure $[C_1, \ldots, C_n; R]$, then the sentence "All systems with microstructure $[C_1, \ldots, C_n; R]$ behave in manner B" is a true law of nature—regardless of whether B is emergent or mechanistically explainable. Obviously, this is the reason for Broad's view that emergent as well as mechanistically explainable properties can be explained by reference to the microstructure of the respective system. However, Broad here employs a comparatively weak notion of explanation.

Second, mechanistically explainable behavior differs from emergent behavior in that the former can, at least in principle, be deduced "from the most complete knowledge of the properties of [the components $C_1, \ldots, C_n$] in isolation or in other wholes," whereas this cannot be done for the latter.

Broad's concepts of mechanistic explainability and emergence can thus be summarized as follows:

(ME) The characteristic behavior B of a complex system S with the microstructure $[C_1, \ldots, C_n; R]$ is *mechanistically explainable* if and only if B can (at least in principle) be deduced from the most complete knowledge of all properties that the components $C_1, \ldots, C_n$ have either in isolation or within other arrangements.

(E) The characteristic behavior B of a complex system S with the microstructure $[C_1, \ldots, C_n; R]$ is *emergent* if and only if the following is true:

(a) The statement "All systems with microstructure $[C_1, \ldots, C_n; R]$ behave in manner B" is a true law of nature, but

(b) B cannot (even in principle) be deduced from the most complete knowledge of all properties that the components $C_1, \ldots, C_n$ have either in isolation or within other arrangements.

The general upshot of these definitions seems to be clear enough. But why does Broad use the complicated clause "from the most complete knowledge of the properties of [the components $C_1, \ldots, C_n$] in isolation or in other wholes"?

To begin with, Broad evidently saw that the notion of an emergent property would, for quite trivial reasons, be empty if one were permitted to use all the properties of the components in the "deduction" of behavior B. Some twenty years after the first publication of *The Mind and Its Place in Nature*, Hempel and Oppenheim, referring to a remark by Grelling, phrased this problem thus:

If a characteristic of a whole is counted as emergent simply if its occurrence cannot be inferred from a knowledge of all the properties of its parts, then, as Grelling has pointed out, no whole can have any emergent characteristics. Thus ... the properties of hydrogen include that of forming, if suitably combined with oxygen, a compound which is liquid, transparent, etc. Hence the liquidity, transparency, etc. of water *can* be inferred from certain properties of its chemical constituents. (Hempel and Oppenheim 1948: 260)

In order to avoid rendering the concept of emergence vacuous, inferences of this kind must be blocked. Broad's formula serves precisely this purpose, since it is obviously designed to guarantee that we cannot have recourse to properties like those mentioned by Hempel and Oppenheim when we attempt to deduce the characteristic behavior B of a complex system from the properties of its parts and its structure. However, the question remains whether this purpose could have been accomplished with a simpler and more lucid formulation. This much seems clear: It is crucial that in our attempts to deduce some behavior B of a complex object from the properties of its parts and their spatial relations, we are not allowed to use ad hoc properties such as the property that certain components, if arranged in a specific way, form a complex object which behaves in manner B. The question, therefore, is how we can guarantee this result without at the same time excluding properties that we may legitimately invoke in such an attempt.

An answer to this question can be found if we consider which laws we may use in deductions of this type. For here we encounter a related possibility of trivializing the concept of emergence. If we were allowed to employ the law mentioned above, the law "All systems with microstructure $[C_1, \ldots, C_n; R]$ behave in manner B," there would be no emergent behavior. Hence, Hempel and Oppenheim could have formulated their point just as well in this way: It is a true law of nature that, if suitably combined with oxygen, hydrogen forms a compound which is liquid, transparent, and so on. Hence the liquidity, transparency, and such of water *can* be derived by means of the laws of nature. Clearly, Broad was aware of both possible ways of trivializing the concept of an emergent property (see, e.g., Broad 1925: 65ff.).

Broad, therefore, must also rule out recourse to laws of this type. That this is something he actually sought to do can be seen from the following passage discussing the properties of clocks:

We know perfectly well that the behavior of a clock can be deduced from the particular arrangement of springs, wheels, pendulum, etc., in it, and from *general laws of mechanics and physics which apply just as much to material systems which are not clocks.* (Broad 1925: 60; italics added)

Obviously, Broad held that if we attempt to deduce some behavior B of a complex object from the properties and arrangement of its parts, we may use only *general laws* that are valid for the parts of a complex system independently of the specific configurations of these parts. However, this constraint provides a way to rule out recourse to ad hoc properties as well. Hence, the most straightforward answer to the question "Which properties of a system's parts may we refer to in such a deduction?" is apparently this: "to those properties which are mentioned in these general laws of nature." I should therefore like to suggest that we replace Broad's clause with the formula "if B can be deduced, by means of the *general* laws of nature that are true of the components $C_1, \ldots, C_n$, from the properties of the components mentioned in these laws." Taken to its logical conclusion, this improved version of Broad's formula renders superfluous any reference to admissible properties; if we specify which laws can figure in the derivations in question, we have implicitly determined which properties may play a role in these derivations.

Even after this point has been clarified, however, the question remains why, according to Broad, we need to know not only how the components of a system behave "in isolation" but also how they behave "in other wholes." As we have already seen, Broad thought that mechanistically explainable behavior differs from emergent behavior in that the former can be deduced, by means of the general laws of nature which are true of the components $C_1, \ldots, C_n$, from the properties of the components mentioned in these laws, whereas the latter cannot. But this provokes the further question of how we can determine which laws are general in the sense required. Broad's own answer to this question has two parts: First, we have to observe how the parts behave in isolation, and second, we have to investigate how they behave in "other" systems.

Why do we have to do both? Broad was quite obviously thinking of the dynamic behavior of systems that are subject to a number of different forces (see Broad 1925: 62, 63f). If we want to find out whether the law that is crucial here, the second Newtonian law $F = m \cdot a$, applies in this case, we have to begin by investigating the behavior of objects that are subject to only *one* force. But if we wish to know how an object behaves generally—that is, how it behaves if more than one force acts on it simultaneously—the knowledge of this law is not enough. We also have to know the law that governs the interaction of the various forces: the law of the vector addition of forces. According to Broad, we always need these two types of laws: (a) laws that state how individual factors separately influence the behavior of an object and (b) laws that state what behavior results if different factors simultaneously act on an object. Laws of the second type Broad terms "laws of composition." Moreover, he emphatically stresses their indispensability:

It is clear that in *no* case could the behavior of a whole composed of certain constituents be predicted *merely* from a knowledge of the properties of these constituents, taken separately, and of their proportions and arrangements in the particular complex under consideration. Whenever this *seems* to be possible it is because we are using a suppressed premise which is so familiar that it has escaped our notice. The suppressed premise is the fact that we have examined other complexes in the past and have noted their behavior; that we have found a general law connecting the behavior of these wholes with that which their constituents would show in isolation; and that we are assuming that this law of composition will hold also of the particular complex whole at present under consideration. (Broad 1925: 63)

However, it is not completely clear what kind of law Broad is alluding to here. The way Broad speaks in the passage just quoted, it seems as if laws of composition are meant to relate the behavior of a *system* to the behavior of its *parts*. (Only the phrase "in isolation" is puzzling in this interpretation.) In this case, laws of composition would have the status of bridge principles relating the level of the parts to the level of the whole. Yet directly after this passage Broad returns to the example of the explanation of the dynamical behavior of objects that are subject to a number of forces:

For purely dynamical transactions this assumption is pretty well justified, because we have found a simple law of composition and have verified it very fully for wholes of very different composition, complexity, and internal structure. It is therefore not particularly rash to expect to predict the dynamical behavior of any material complex under the action of any set of forces, however much it may differ in the details of its structure and parts from those complexes for which the assumed law of composition has actually been verified. (Broad 1925: 63f.)

Obviously, the law of composition he refers to in this passage is the law of the vector addition of forces already mentioned (see Broad 1925: 62).

This law, however, does not state how the behavior of a whole arises from the behavior of its parts, but how the parts of a whole behave if they are subject to a number of forces. Thus it might be more apt to call laws of this type "laws of interaction."

Fortunately, we do not have to decide on one reading, for Broad seems to be right in either case. On the one hand, we of course need laws of interaction since we cannot deduce the behavior of a system from the properties of its parts and their arrangement if we do not know how the parts themselves move if they are arranged in this particular way. On the other hand, we also need laws of composition or bridge principles since we cannot deduce the behavior of a system from the behavior of its parts if we do not know how the behavior of the parts is related to the behavior of the whole. Thus, in order to deduce the behavior of a system from the properties of its parts and their arrangement, we actually need three types of laws:

1. Simple laws, which state how each part of the system S behaves if only a single factor acts on it

2. Laws of interaction, which state how the parts of S behave if a number of factors simultaneously act on them

3. Laws of composition or bridge principles, which state how S behaves as a whole if its parts behave in a specific way.

The fact that any attempt to explain the behavior of a system S by reference to the properties of its parts and their arrangement requires three types of laws is also pointed out by Hüttemann and Terzidis (in press). The indispensability of laws of composition is stressed in McLaughlin (1992).

It should again be noted that all these laws must be general laws or must follow from general laws to be usable in what Broad calls the deduction of the characteristic behavior of a system from the properties and the arrangement of its parts. Put precisely, what Broad's definitions come to, therefore, is the following:

(ME$'$) The characteristic behavior B of a complex system S with the microstructure $[C_1, \ldots, C_n; R]$ is *mechanistically explainable* if and only if the following is true:

(a) The way the components $C_1, \ldots, C_n$ behave when arranged in manner R can be accounted for by the general simple laws and by the general laws of interaction holding for objects of the kind $C_1, \ldots, C_n$; and

(b) there is a general law of composition to the effect that S exhibits behavior B if the components $C_1, \ldots, C_n$ behave in the way they do.

(E$'$) The characteristic behavior B of a complex system S with the microstructure $[C_1, \ldots, C_n; R]$ is *emergent* if and only if the following is true:

(a) The statement "All systems with microstructure $[C_1, \ldots, C_n; R]$ behave in manner B" is a true law of nature, but

(b$_1$) the way the components $C_1, \ldots, C_n$ behave when arranged in manner R cannot be accounted for by the general simple laws and by the general laws of interaction holding for objects of the kind $C_1, \ldots, C_n$; or

(b_2) there is no general law of composition to the effect that S exhibits behavior B if the components $C_1, \ldots, C_n$ behave in the way they do.

Two points should be highlighted here. The first concerns the question of why Broad did not provide a positive example for a law of composition that would render the behavior of a given system mechanistically explainable. My guess is that the laws Broad had in mind are so mundane that he felt no need to mention them. For instance, the following seems to be trivially true of spatial movement:

(P1) If we know how all the components of a complex system move, we also know how the system itself moves.

Think, for example, of a disk whose components all revolve with the same angular velocity and in the same direction around the disk's center. Then it seems quite clear that the disk as a whole spins around its center. Indeed, given the movements of its components, it seems inconceivable that the disk itself moves in any other fashion. (A quite similar point could be made with regard to clocks.)

In much the same way the volume of a system seems to be determined by the places its components occupy, and the shape of a system seems to be determined by the relative positions of its components. The bridge principles Broad must have had in mind thus do not just have the character of very general laws of nature; rather, since we cannot conceive that they could be false, they seem to have the status of a priori truths.

This brings us to the second point. Broad himself emphasizes that the status of the law "All systems with microstructure $[C_1, \ldots, C_n; R]$ behave in manner B" varies remarkably, depending upon whether the behavior in question can be explained in a mechanical way or only in an emergent way. With respect to emergent behavior, this law has the status of a unique and ultimate law. It is (a) not a special case that

can be arrived at by substituting determinate values for determinable variables in general laws. It is (b) not a law that can be generated by combining two or more general laws. And, perhaps most important, (c) the law in question is a law that can be discovered *only* by studying samples of systems with the microstructure $[C_1, \ldots, C_n; R]$ and can be extended inductively *only* to other systems with the same microstructure. Regarding silver chloride Broad writes:

... the law connecting the properties of silver-chloride with those of silver and of chlorine and with the structure of the compound is, so far as we know, an *unique* and *ultimate* law. By this I mean (a) that it is not a special case which arises through substituting certain determinate values for determinable variables in a general law which connects the properties of *any* chemical compound with those of its separate elements and with its structure. And (b) that it is not a special case which arises by combining two more general laws, one of which connects the properties of *any* silver-compound with those of elementary silver, whilst the other connects the properties of *any* chlorine-compound with those of elementary chlorine. So far as we know there are no such laws. It is (c) a law which could have been discovered *only* by studying samples of silver-chloride itself, and which can be extended inductively *only* to other samples of the same substance. (Broad 1925: 64f.)

If, on the other hand, we are concerned with mechanistically explainable behavior, things are very different:

In order to predict the behavior of a clock a man need never have seen a clock in his life. Provided he is told how it is constructed, and that he has learnt from the study of *other* material systems the general rules about motion and about the mechanical properties of springs and of rigid bodies, he can foretell exactly how a system constructed like a clock must behave. (Broad 1925: 65)

If the behavior B of a system S can be explained mechanistically, we are in a position to know that S—like all systems with the microstructure $[C_1, \ldots, C_n; R]$—behaves in manner B without having investigated a single system with this particular microstructure. For in this case the behavior of the system follows directly from the general laws of nature that apply to the components $C_1, \ldots, C_n$. (These general laws of nature comprise the simple laws as well as the laws of interaction and the laws of composition.) This implies that in the case of mechanistically explainable behavior, it is in a certain sense *inconceivable* that a system has the microstructure $[C_1, \ldots, C_n; R]$ but does not exhibit behavior B. For if it follows from the general laws of nature that all systems with that microstructure behave in manner B, then it is impossible—at least *relative to these laws of nature*—that a system possesses the microstructure $[C_1, \ldots, C_n; R]$ but does not behave in manner B. Thus it is a conclusive *test* for the behavior of a system S being mechanistically explainable that it can be predicted before it first occurrs or, in other words, that—relative to the laws of nature—it is inconceivable that it does not occur, given the microstructure of S.

Chemical and Secondary Qualities as Candidates for Emergent Properties

I shall now turn to the following questions: Which properties did Broad take to be emergent and what were his reasons for doing so? We already know what his reasons were with respect to the characteristic behavior of chemical compounds. According to Broad, there are no appropriate laws of composition:

The example of chemical compounds shows us that we have no right to expect that the same simple law of composition will hold for chemical as for dynamical transactions.... It would of course (on any view) be useless merely to study silver in isolation and chlorine in isolation; for that would tell us nothing about the law of their conjoint action. This would be equally true even if a mechanistic explanation of the chemical behavior of compounds were possible. The essential point is that it would also be useless to study chemical com-

pounds in general and to compare their properties with those of their elements in the hope of discovering a *general* law of composition by which the properties of *any* chemical compound could be foretold when the properties of its separate elements were known. So far as we know, there is no general law of this kind.... No doubt the properties of silver-chloride are completely *determined* by those of silver and of chlorine; in the sense that whenever you have a whole composed of these two elements in certain proportions and relations you have something with the characteristic properties of silver-chloride, and that nothing has these properties except a whole composed in this way. But the law connecting the properties of silver-chloride with those of silver and of chlorine and with the structure of the compound is, so far as we know, an *unique* and *ultimate* law. (Broad 1925: 64f.)

Much the same holds, Broad thought, for the characteristic features of living beings:

... it is obviously possible that, just as the characteristic behavior of a [chemical] compound could not be predicted from any amount of knowledge of the properties of its elements in isolation or of the properties of other [chemical] compounds, so the properties of a [compound that is made up of chemical compounds, i.e., a living body] could not be predicted from any amount of knowledge about the properties of its [chemical] constituents taken separately or in other surroundings...; so the only way to find out the characteristic behavior of living bodies may be to study living bodies as such. (Broad 1925: 67)

Nowadays, Broad's treatment of both examples seems outdated. We now know that the electrical conductivity of metals is due to the fact that only a few electrons are located in their outer shell, and these electrons are capable of relatively free movement. We also know that the metal sodium combines with chlorine because chlorine atoms can complete their outer electron shell with the electrons given off by the sodium atoms. In this process sodium and chlorine ions are created; they exert strong electrical forces on each other and, therefore, form a lattice structure. We know, moreover, that sodium chloride is water-soluble because water molecules can—

due to their dipole structure—pull the sodium ions and the chlorine ions from their places within the lattice. And we now also know much about the chemical processes on which the breathing, digestion, and reproduction of living beings are based.

However, it should be noted that Broad did not rule out any of these developments. For example, he writes with regard to the process of breathing:

... since [the process of breathing] is a movement and since the characteristic movements of some complex wholes (*e.g.*, clocks) *can* be predicted from a knowledge of their structure and of other complex wholes which are not clocks, it cannot be positively *proved* that breathing is an "ultimate characteristic" or that its causation is emergent and not mechanistic. Within the physical realm it always remains logically possible that the appearance of emergent laws is due to our imperfect knowledge of microscopic structure and to our mathematical incompetence. (Broad 1925: 81)

Yet Broad immediately adds: "But this method of avoiding emergent laws is not logically possible for trans-physical processes ... (Broad 1925: 81). But what does Broad mean by "trans-physical processes"? And why does he believe that such processes could never be explained mechanistically? In order to understand this, we have to grasp Broad's concept of a pure quality. For Broad considers those laws "to be trans-physical" which relate a system's microstructure to its pure qualities—that is to say, all laws of the form "All systems with microstructure $[C_1, \ldots, C_n; R]$ have pure quality F" (see Broad 1925: 52).

Broad's official definition of "pure quality" is this:

By calling [qualities such as red, hot, etc.] "pure qualities" I mean that, when we say "This is red", "This is hot" and so on, it is no part of the meaning of our predicate that "this" stands in such and such relation to something else. It is *logically* possible that this should be red even though "this" were the only thing in the world. ... (Broad 1925: 52)

This definition, however, is rather puzzling, since for Broad pure qualities seem to be exactly those properties of complex objects which traditionally are called secondary qualities—temperature, color, taste, and smell (see Broad 1925: 46ff., 79f.). Yet secondary qualities are usually characterized as nothing but powers to cause certain sensations in us. So how can an object possess pure qualities unless there are creatures perceiving it? But let us return to the question of why Broad believed that pure qualities are necessarily emergent.

As we have already seen, Broad held the view that "so far as we know at present" most of the *behavior* of chemical compounds is emergent. Yet he thought that scientific progress might prove this view wrong. However, chemical compounds are characterized not only by their specific behavior but also by their pure qualities. May it turn out that these pure qualities, too, are not emergent but mechanistically explainable? Broad's answer to this question was an unequivocal no. (For the following, see Broad 1925: 71f.).

Consider ammonia, for instance. Ammonia is a gas whose molecules consist of three hydrogen atoms and one nitrogen atom. It is readily soluble in water and has a pungent smell. Possibly (according to Broad) we shall one day be able to explain the water solubility of ammonia as well as its other characteristic behavior by reference to the properties of its components and their arrangement. However, this is not true of its smell. Broad thought it to be *theoretically* impossible to explain this smell in a mechanical way. Why? Broad's answer was this: Not even a mathematical archangel—that is to say, a creature who knows all general laws of nature and is able to execute the most complex mathematical calculations in split seconds—could predict what the compound of three hydrogen atoms and one nitrogen atom would smell like.

[Even a mathematical archangel] would be totally unable to predict that a substance with [the microscopic structure of ammonia] must smell as ammonia does when it gets into the human nose. The utmost that he could predict on this subject would be that certain changes would take place in the mucous membrane, the olfactory nerves and so on. But he could not possibly know that these changes would be accompanied by the appearance of a smell in general or the peculiar smell of ammonia in particular, unless someone told him so or he had smelled it for himself. If the existence of the so-called "secondary qualities" ... depends on the microscopic movements and arrangements of material particles which do not have these qualities themselves, then the laws of this dependence are certainly of the emergent type. (Broad 1925: 71f.)

Why would even a mathematical archangel be limited in this way? Considering what we have said so far, the reason can only be that it simply does not follow from the general laws applicable to hydrogen atoms and nitrogen atoms that a compound of three hydrogen atoms and one nitrogen atom smells in the way characteristic of ammonia. From these laws (and the laws of neurophysiology) it follows at best that in the cells of the olfactory nerves and in the brain of a person whose mucous membrane is hit by ammonia molecules, certain electrochemical changes take place. What does not follow is that these changes are accompanied by certain olfactory sensations. In other words, the law which states that certain changes in a person's nervous system lead to such olfactory sensations is not deducible from the general laws of nature. It is an emergent law or, as Broad also calls it, a "transordinal law"—a law that relates a system's microstructure to its nondeducible properties.

Broad's argument for the thesis that pure qualities are necessarily emergent can thus be summarized as follows: Pure qualities are secondary qualities, and it is a characteristic feature of secondary qualities that they cause certain sensations in us. But it does not follow from the general laws of nature that a system S, which has a certain microstructure, will cause a certain sensation in us. At most it follows from these laws that certain changes will be caused in our

nervous system by light reflected from S or by molecules emitted into the air by S. The pivotal point of this argument is Broad's thesis that the laws of composition which relate certain processes in our CNS to our sensations are unique and ultimate laws that cannot be derived from the general laws of nature. Broad's main reason for asserting the emergent character of pure qualities is thus his assumption that sensations cannot be deduced from occurrences in a person's CNS. We must therefore examine the arguments Broad devises to sustain this crucial assumption.

A central reason for his assumption is certainly that Broad believed that sensations—like all other mental states—cannot be analyzed in behavioristic terms. (For the following, see especially Broad 1925: 612–624. Stephan's (1993) analysis of Broad's arguments is similar to my own.)

In Broad's view, this is the main difference between the mind–body problem and the problem of vitalism.

The one and only kind of evidence that we ever have for believing that a thing is alive is that it behaves in certain characteristic ways. *E.g.*, it moves spontaneously, eats, drinks, digests, grows, reproduces, and so on. Now all these are just actions of one body on other bodies. There seems to be no reason whatever to suppose that "being alive" means any more than exhibiting these various forms of bodily behaviour.... But the position about consciousness, certainly seems to be very different. It is perfectly true that an essential part of our evidence for believing that anything but ourselves has a mind and is having such and such experiences is that it performs certain characteristic bodily movements in certain situations.... But it is plain that our observation of the behavior of external bodies is not our only or our primary ground for asserting the existence of minds and mental processes. And it seems to me equally plain that by "having a mind" we do not mean simply "behaving in such and such ways." (Broad 1925: 612f)

For Broad the falsity of behaviorism follows mainly from two considerations: (1) My self-

ascriptions of mental states are not based on observable behavior. Even if my body behaved in
one characteristic way when I see a chair and in
another when I hear a bell

> it is perfectly certain that this is not my ground for
> saying that I see a chair or hear a bell. I often know
> without the least doubt that I am having the experience
> called "seeing a chair" when I am altogether uncertain
> whether my body is acting in any characteristic way.
> And again I distinguish with perfect ease between the
> experience called "seeing a chair" and the experience
> called "hearing a bell" when I am quite doubtful
> whether my bodily behavior, if any, on the two occa-
> sions has been alike or different. (Broad 1925, 614)

(2) Every good actor can behave exactly like
someone who feels pain or great joy. Hence one
cannot conclude from the fact that someone
behaves in a certain way that he really has certain sensations or perceptions. More generally,
this means that even if some creature A always
acts exactly like someone who has real sensations, we can always ask: Does A really have
sensations or does he only behave as if he
had them? With respect to intelligent behavior,
Broad formulates this point as follows:

> However completely the behavior of an external body
> answers to the behavioristic tests for intelligence, it al-
> ways remains a perfectly sensible question to ask: "Has
> it really got a mind, or is it merely an automaton?" It is
> quite true ... that, the more nearly a body answers to
> the behavioristic tests for intelligence, the harder it is
> for us in practice to contemplate the possibility of its
> having no mind. Still, the question: "Has it a mind?" is
> never silly in the sense that it is meaningless. ... it is not
> like asking whether a rich man may have no wealth.
> (Broad 1925: 614)

So Broad was apparently an early proponent
of the argument from absent qualia and believed
in the possibility of philosophical zombies. It
should be noted, however, that even if Broad's
criticism of behaviorism succeeds, this does not
by itself show that every law of the form "If the
neurological process N takes place in person A's
CNS, then A has the sensation E" has to be an
emergent law. Why should not at least some laws
that relate the microstructure of a system to one
of its properties that is *not* behaviorally analyz-
able fail to be emergent?

A part of the answer to this question resides, I
think, in the fact that Broad seems to have
believed laws such as

(1) "Whenever C-fibers fire in a person's CNS,
this person feels pain"

differ in their status from general bridge principles like:

(P1) If one knows how all components of a
complex system S move, one also knows how S
itself moves;

(P2) if one knows the places of all the components of S, one knows what volume is occupied
by S;

(P3) if one knows the relative positions of all the
components of S, one knows the shape of S.

For, in a sense, we simply cannot conceive
that these principles could be false while, by
contrast, we can very well imagine law (1) to be
false. Hence (1) does not have the status that
would be required for it to play the role of a
general bridge principle.

Broad gives another argument, which shows
that he anticipated not only the explanatory gap
but also the knowledge argument:

> We have no difficulty in conceiving and adequately
> describing determinate possible motions which we have
> never witnessed and which we never shall witness....
> But we could not possibly have formed the concept of
> such a colour as blue or such a shade as sky-blue unless
> we had perceived instances of it, no matter how much
> we had reflected on the concept of Colour in general or
> on the instances of other colours and shades which we
> *had* seen. It follows that, even when we know that a
> certain *kind* of secondary quality ... pervades ... a re-
> gion when and only when such and such a *kind* of mi-
> croscopic event ... is going on within the region, we
> still could not possibly predict that such and such a
> determinate event of the kind ... would be connected

with such and such a determinate shade of colour.... The trans-physical laws are then *necessarily* of the emergent type. (Broad 1925: 80)

According to Broad, it is thus crucial that we can form the concept of a certain sensation only after we ourselves have experienced this sensation for the first time. (Although Broad here speaks about secondary qualities, we have seen earlier that the concern really lies with the sensations which are caused by secondary qualities.) However, if it is the case that we can form the concept of a sensation only after experiencing it, then the occurrence of an experience cannot be predicted before it has been experienced at least once. From this alone it follows that sensations are emergent, since for reducible properties—by contrast—it is characteristic that they can be predicted before their first occurrence.

There is one point I should like to add here. Broad obviously thought that sensations are emergent because the laws of composition which connect neural events in the CNS of a person to the person's sensations are unique and ultimate, and therefore lack the status of general bridge laws. At first sight, he seems to have held very much the same view with regard to the emergence of the behavior of chemical compounds. Broad wrote, "The example of chemical compounds shows us that we have no right to expect that the same simple law of composition will hold for chemical as for dynamical transactions" (Broad 1925: 64).

The comparison with the law of dynamical transactions in mechanics, however, makes it quite clear that what is at issue in chemistry is not laws of composition but laws of interaction. According to Broad, the emergent character of the behavior of chemical compounds results from the fact that there are no general laws which tell us how *atoms* behave in all possible arrangements. With regard to definition (E′) the emergent character of the behavior of chemical compounds is thus due to condition (b_1). In the case of sensations, things seem to be different,

even though Broad is not very clear on this point.[1] But he seems to have held that even if there were general laws of interaction which told us everything we wanted to know about the neural events going on in the CNS, we could not predict the sensations connected with these events, because of the lack of suitable laws of composition or bridge principles. Thus, the emergent character of sensations is due to condition (b_2) rather than (b_1).

Broad's Account of the Explanatory Gap

It should have become clear from this account of Broad's position on the emergent character of sensations that his thoughts contain all the essential ingredients of the explanatory gap argument. A direct comparison with Levine's and Chalmers's arguments would make this even clearer. Since I cannot do both, I restrict myself to the work of Levine. Let me briefly rehearse his main line of argument. Consider the two statements (1) Pain in humans is identical to C-fiber firing and (2) Temperature in ideal gases is identical to the mean kinetic energy of their molecules.

According to Levine, there is a fundamental difference between these two statements—the second is "fully explanatory," whereas the first is not. That is to say, on the one hand it is *inconceivable* in a certain epistemological sense that in a gas the mean kinetic energy of the molecules has a certain numerical value (say, $6.21 \cdot 10^{-21}$ Joule), but that the gas does not have the corresponding temperature of 300K. On the other hand, it seems perfectly *conceivable* that I do not feel any pain although my C-fibers are firing. What is the reason for this difference?

Levine's answer is this. If we were asked what we mean by the term "temperature," we would answer: (2′) Temperature is the property of bodies that causes certain sensations of warmth and coldness in us, and that causes the mercury column of thermometers that come into contact with these bodies to rise or fall, and that causes certain chemical reactions, and so forth.

In other words, we would characterize temperature by its causal role alone. However, this would not be a sufficient answer to the question if there were not a second point:

... our knowledge of chemistry and physics makes intelligible how it is that something like the motion of molecules could play the causal role we associate with heat. Furthermore, antecedent to our discovery of the essential nature of heat, its causal role, captured in statements like (2'), exhausts our notion of it. Once we understand how this causal role is carried out there is nothing more we need to understand. (Levine 1983: 357)

Thus the explanatory character of statement (2) is due to two facts: (1) Our concept of temperature is exhausted by the causal role of temperature; (2) Physics can make it intelligible that the mean kinetic energy of the molecules of a gas plays exactly this causal role.

Now it is plain that we also associate a causal role with the term "pain." Pain is caused by injury to tissue, it causes us to scream or whimper, and it causes us to wish to be rid of it as soon as possible. Levine neither disputes this nor denies that the identification of pain with the firing of C-fibers explains the mechanism that underpins this causal role. Nevertheless, there is a crucial difference between the two cases:

However, there is more to our concept of pain than its causal role, there is its qualitative character, how it feels; and what is left unexplained by the discovery of C-fiber firing is *why pain should feel the way it does*! For there seems to be nothing about C-fiber firing which makes it naturally "fit" the phenomenal properties of pain, any more than it would fit some other set of phenomenal properties. Unlike its functional role, the identification of the qualitative side of pain with C-fiber firing ... leaves the connection between it and what we identify it with completely mysterious. One might say, it makes the way pain feels into merely a brute fact. (Levine 1983: 357)

Thus, Levine's first reason for his thesis that (1) is not fully explanatory is the following: Pain is only partly characterized by its causal role. For it is also a characteristic feature of pain that it has a certain qualitative character, namely, that it is painful.

However, this argument on its own does not suffice to demonstrate that (1) is not fully explanatory. For it at least could be the case that it follows from the laws of neurobiology that C-fiber firings also possess this characteristic feature. This is precisely what Levine has to deny. Hence, Levine's second thesis is: It does not follow from the laws of neurobiology that C-fiber firings possess the qualitative character of pain, that is, that C-fiber firings feel painful.

With regard to the latter claim one could ask, however, whether this might not be due to the fact that, at the moment, neurobiological research is not sufficiently advanced. Is it really completely impossible that neurobiology will one day tell us that C-fiber firings in a certain sense must, after all, be connected to the qualitative character of pain?

When answering this question in his article "On Leaving Out What It's Like," Levine begins by stressing that every reduction has to lead to an *explanation* of the phenomenon reduced, and that if this explanation is successful, it is indeed impossible—in an epistemic sense—to conceive of the occurrence of the explanans without the explanandum.

The basic idea is that a reduction should explain what is reduced, and the way we tell whether this has been accomplished is to see whether the phenomenon to be reduced is epistemologically necessitated by the reducing phenomenon, i.e., whether we can see why, given the facts cited in the reduction, things must be the way they seem on the surface (Levine 1993: 129).

Let us try to unpack what Levine has in mind here by means of the example of the macro-property of being liquid. In general, liquids differ from gases in that their volume is (almost) incompressible. They differ from solids in that their shape is changeable and molds itself to the receptacle holding them. This provides us with an—albeit incomplete—list of the features that characterize the property of being liquid. Can we now derive the fact that water is liquid at a temperature of 20° C from the properties of its molecules? Does it follow from the general laws of nature which apply to H_2O molecules that at a temperature of 20° C (and normal pressure) water has all the features which are characteristic of the property of being liquid?

From the laws of nature it follows, first,[2] that the mean distance of H_2O molecules from each other can be reduced further only through great pressure because of the repulsive forces between the molecules. Second, it follows from the laws of nature that the attractive forces between the molecules are not strong enough to fix the molecules in their relative positions. Therefore, the molecules can freely roll over each other. If all molecules are subject to the same force, each molecule will move to the place from which it cannot move any further.

However, this alone does not show that *water* at a temperature of 20° C has all the features which are characteristic of the property of being liquid. For up to now we know only how *the individual H_2O molecules* behave at this temperature. That is to say, in addition we need *bridge principles* (see Levine 1993: 131) which state how the behavior of the liquid as a whole is related to the behavior of the individual molecules. These principles are obviously the following:

(P4) If the mean distance between the molecules of some substance can be reduced only by great pressure, then the volume of that substance can be reduced only by great pressure.

(P5) If the molecules of some substance can freely roll over one another, then the shape of this substance is flexible and molds itself to the shape of the receptacle in which the substance is placed.

This leads us to the following answer to the question why—once this explanation has been given—we cannot conceive that water is *not* liquid at a temperature of 20° C. The first reason is simply that it follows from the general laws of nature that the mean distance between H_2O molecules at a temperature of 20° C can by reduced further only by great pressure and that the attractive forces between the molecules are not strong enough to fix them in their relative positions. The second reason, which is bound up with the special status of the bridge principles (P4) and (P5), is just as important. For obviously this status is responsible for the fact that we *cannot* imagine that the mean distance between the molecules of some substance can be reduced only by great pressure, but that the volume of this substance already decreases under little pressure, or that the molecules of some substance may freely roll over one another but the shape of this substance is inflexible, and therefore does not mold itself to the shape of the receptacle in which it is placed.

According to Levine, things are very different if we consider the relation between pain and C-fiber firings. Even if we know to the smallest detail what neurophysiological processes occur in a person's brain, it is still conceivable (according to Levine) that the person in whose brain these processes occur does not feel any pain. What is the reason for this difference?

If we consider a detailed analysis of the explanation of why it is inconceivable that water is not liquid at a temperature of 20° C, three points stand out:

1. *All* of the characteristic features of the property's being liquid consist in the fact that under certain conditions liquid substances *behave* in a specific way.

2. It follows from the general laws of nature that at a temperature of 20° C certain attractive and repulsive forces obtain between H_2O molecules.

3. There are general bridge principles which state that a substance between whose molecules these forces obtain displays exactly such behavior as is characteristic of the property of being liquid.

Now what about the alleged explanation of pain through the firing of C-fibers? Obviously, when we think about the first point, we immediately encounter a clear difference:

1. Our concept of pain is not exhausted by its causal role, and pain is not characterized by only a certain kind of behavior. Rather, our concept of pain includes a qualitative aspect—what it feels like to be in pain.

However, this point is not the heart of the matter. For pain could still be explained by the firing of C-fibers *if only* there were bridge principles to the effect that the firing of C-fibers feels the way that is characteristic of pain. Therefore the following two points are really crucial here:

2. From the laws of neurobiology it follows *only* under what conditions which neurons fire with what frequency.

3. There are no general bridge principles that connect the firing of neurons with certain qualitative experiences.

Hence Levine's explanatory gap argument, as well as Broad's argument for the emergent character of secondary qualities and sensations, are based on the central thesis:

(T1) Laws like (1), which connect neural processes with sensations, do not have the status of general bridge laws.

For Levine as well as for Broad, the emergent character of sensations thus results from condition (b_2) rather than from condition (b_1) of definition (E'). That is, the problem is not that there are no general laws of *interaction* which tell us how neurons fire if they are connected in the way

they are connected in our CNS. The real problem is that the laws which tell us what goes on in our mind if certain neuron firings take place in our brain, do not have the status they would have to have in order to play the role of suitable bridge principles.

Acknowledgments

I would like to thank Antonia Barke for translating this paper into English and Beth Wilson for copyediting it. I am also indebted to Andreas Hüttemann, who goaded me into reading Broad's *The Mind and Its Place in Nature* even more thoroughly, and to Christian Nimtz, for his useful comments on an earlier draft of this paper.

Notes

1. The reason seems to be that Broad did not clearly distinguish laws of interaction from laws of composition.

2. At least this is generally assumed.

References

Beckermann, A. (1992). Supervenience, emergence, and reduction. In A. Beckermann, J. Kim, and H. Flohr, eds., *Emergence or Reduction?*, 94–118. Berlin and New York: Walter de Gruyter.

Beckermann, A. (1997). Property physicalism, reduction and realization. In M. Carrier and P. Machamer, eds., *Mindscapes: Philosophy, Science, and the Mind*, 303–321. Konstanz: Universitätsverlag; Pittsburgh: Pittsburgh University Press.

Beckermann, A., Kim, J., and Flohr, H., eds. (1992). *Emergence or Reduction?—Essays on the Prospects of Nonreductive Physicalism*. Berlin and New York: Walter de Gruyter.

Broad, C. D. (1925). *The Mind and Its Place in Nature*. London: Routledge and Kegan Paul.

Hempel, C. G., and Oppenheim, P. (1948). Studies in the Logic of Explanation. *Philosophy of Science* 15: 135–175. Reprinted in C. G. Hempel, *Aspects of*

Scientific Explanation and Other Essays in the Philosophy of Science, 245–290. New York: Free Press, 1965.

Hüttemann, A., and Terzidis O. (in press). Emergence in physics. *International Studies in the Philosophy of Science.*

Levine, J. (1983). Materialism and qualia: The explanatory gap. *Pacific Philosophical Quarterly* 64: 354–361.

Levine, J. (1993). On leaving out what it's like. In M. Davies and G. W. Humphreys, eds., *Consciousness: Psychological and Philosophical Essays*, 121–136. Oxford: Basil Blackwell.

McLaughlin, B. (1992). The rise and fall of British emergentism. In Beckermann, Kim and Flohr, eds., *Emergence or Reduction?*, 49–93.

Stephan, A. (1993). C. D. Broads a priori-Argument für die Emergenz phänomenaler Qualitäten. In H. Lenk and H. Poser (eds.), *Neue Realitäten—Herausforderungen der Philosophie. Sektionsbeiträge I zum XVI. Deutschen Kongreß für Philosophie*, 176–183. Berlin: Allgemeine Gesellschaft für Philosophie in Deutschland.

Antti Revonsuo

The field of consciousness studies is full of talk about the *science* of consciousness. For example, the landmark conferences in Tucson strive "Toward a Science of Consciousness"; the professional organization in the field is the Association for the Scientific Study of Consciousness; and the journal *Consciousness and Cognition* offers a "natural-science approach" to consciousness. However, there is little discussion on what it actually requires for a field to constitute a true *science* of consciousness. Indeed, despite all the talk, there is still no such coherent, established branch of science.

In this paper my intention is to explicate what it is we are aiming at when we attempt to establish a science of consciousness. I will argue that the most fruitful approach to actually achieving that goal is currently developing within the cognitive neurosciences. But even there, there are several fundamental obstacles on the way toward a scientific research program on consciousness, since the ontology and methodology of mainstream cognitive neuroscience is not entirely compatible with that required in the science of consciousness.

Scientific Research Programs and the Study of Consciousness

I shall assume that to have a science of consciousness, or indeed of any natural phenomenon, is to have a systematic, scientific *research program* that takes the phenomenon in question seriously as an empirical problem, and attempts to describe and explain it. But what does a systematic research program consist of? Philosophers of science have attempted to explicate what sort of an entity a scientific research program is supposed to be. While there have been considerable disagreements among them about this, there is also substantial agreement on the general characteristics of research programs (or

"research traditions" or "paradigms"). I will mainly follow the ideas of Laudan (1977) on these issues.

A research program is a set of background assumptions that is shared by the community of researchers within the program. The background assumptions involve significant ontological and methodological commitments. These commitments can be thought of as general assumptions concerning the substantive entities and processes in the domain being studied, and the appropriate methods to be used for investigating the phenomena and constructing the theories in that domain (Laudan 1977: 81). The program is not directly empirically testable, but it provides the empirical and conceptual tools for the construction of empirically testable theories. Theories do not exist on their own, but only in the context of a research program that justifies the implicit background assumptions of the theory. The research program outlines the domain of application of the theories belonging to it, indicating which empirical questions are regarded as central, and which belong to foreign domains or are only pseudo problems. There are often several competing specific theories within a research program, presenting more detailed hypotheses of the ontology of the basic entities and their interaction. However, despite the variety of competing theories within a program, there is also significant integrity. The basic assumptions of the research program prevent any scientist working within the program from adopting theories that are incompatible with the metaphysics or methodology of the program. To adopt a view or to advocate a theory that is inconsistent with the metaphysics or methodology of the research program is to put oneself outside the program and reject it.

The sad truth about the current state of consciousness studies appears to be that there is nothing even remotely resembling a scientific research program on consciousness. It is easy to see why this is the case: There are no shared background assumptions on the basic metaphysical and methodological questions of consciousness. Let me mention a prominent example of this metaphysical heterogeneity inherent in consciousness studies. One central figure in the field, Daniel Dennett (1991), basically says that subjective consciousness does not really exist, whereas another, David Chalmers (1996), suggests that consciousness might be everywhere; even very simple physical systems such as electrons, stones, or thermostats have some sort of consciousness. In addition to these rather extreme ideas, a considerable number of other more or less exotic metaphysical views on consciousness can be found in the field.

Most of the hard empirical data on consciousness, however, are coming from the cognitive neurosciences. Might cognitive neuroscience be the research program from which a science of consciousness will emerge? The problem is that neither cognitive neuroscience in general nor specific cognitive or neuroscientific theories provide us with any appropriate ontological account of phenomenal consciousness. The metaphysics of cognitive neuroscience appears to be merely some vague and philosophically outmoded version of functionalism. This is reflected in the words of Michael Gazzaniga as he depicts the goals of the field:

At some point in the future, cognitive neuroscience will be able to describe the algorithms that drive structural neural elements into the physiological activity that results in perception, cognition, and perhaps even consciousness. (Gazzaniga 1995: xiii)

However, as several philosophers have argued, myself included (Revonsuo 1994), functionalistic or computational analyses will not really suffice as genuine explanations of consciousness. Consequently, it is unlikely that "describing the algorithms" (i.e., the formal character of input–output transformations) which are realized simultaneously with conscious phenomena in the brain will be of much help in understanding consciousness. Such algorithms are not descrip-

tions of the actual causal mechanisms and biological processes that constitute phenomenal consciousness in the brain; at best they can capture only the abstract formal features of those processes. If consciousness is a natural biological phenomenon, we primarily need to understand how it is related to and constituted by other natural phenomena in the brain, not how the input–output transformations performed by it could be computationally described.

Although the research program of cognitive neuroscience does not as such offer a viable ontology for consciousness, the volume of empirical research relevant for understanding consciousness within that program is so huge that it is a good place to start charting the prospects for a scientific research program of consciousness. Certainly no science of consciousness can ignore the data emerging from cognitive neuroscience. Perhaps it will eventually be possible to incorporate novel metaphysical assumptions, better suited for explaining consciousness, into cognitive neuroscience.

What we need at present is, then, a formulation of the initial assumptions of a research program on consciousness. The assumptions should be broadly consistent with the main source of empirical data, cognitive neuroscience, and should be sufficiently general and plausible to be acceptable to most empirical cognitive neuroscientists. They should offer clear preliminary answers to such questions as What sort of a phenomenon is consciousness? In what sorts of natural systems is this phenomenon to be found? How does consciousness reveal itself to empirical investigation, and what are the legitimate methods to be used in obtaining data on consciousness?

Toward a Biological Research Program on Consciousness

Instead of adopting the empirically highly implausible views put forward by some philosophers (such as that consciousness doesn't exist, or that it is everywhere, or that it is an algorithm), I believe we should start with a few very simple, clear, and not highly controversial assumptions. Eventually, these assumptions will have to be worked out into a more detailed philosophical theory on consciousness, but for now we can start with something as simple and uncontroversial as possible. My suggestion is the following: Subjective phenomenal consciousness is a real, natural, biological phenomenon that literally resides in the brain.

These assumptions should be taken seriously, as establishing the core of a natural-science, biological research program on consciousness. The program is largely consistent with what empirical cognitive neuroscientists are doing anyway, but when it comes to explaining consciousness, it is not committed to any functionalistic or computational ontology. The task now is to follow the implications that the acceptance of these basic assumptions has.

The first implication is that the "science of consciousness" we are striving at is first and foremost a *biological* science of consciousness; an empirically based, natural-science approach that regards consciousness primarily as a biological phenomenon. The second implication is that such an embryonic research program will have to face several fundamental problems concerning the basic nature of consciousness and its place among other biological phenomena. Let us analyze some of these problems and the challenge they pose for the scientific research program on consciousness.

Problem 1:   How to Establish a Detailed Metaphysical and Ontological Theory of Consciousness That Is Acceptable for the Biological Research Program

What makes this problem especially severe is the fact that many, if not most, philosophers within consciousness studies hold views that are incompatible with the suggested biological research program on consciousness. Consequently, such philosophers have already dismissed this partic-

ular research program and placed themselves outside it. That is a pity, for what would be needed from the philosophers' camp is suggestions as to what sort of metaphysics is consistent with the proposed biological science of consciousness. A general observation of the field reveals that there are still many philosophers who do not take a natural-science approach to consciousness seriously enough. Not surprisingly, many scientists tend to consider philosophers' views as harmless but irrelevant at best, or absurd and potentially harmful at worst. Genuine collaboration between scientists and philosophers in a common effort to develop an empirically based scientific research program on consciousness is still far too infrequent.

Problem 2:   The Ontology of the Research Program in Cognitive Neuroscience, as Such, Is Not Appropriate for a Science of Consciousness

The ontology of the cognitive neurosciences is too narrow and it assumes, at least implicitly, some form of functionalism, computationalism, or representationalism, although such philosophy is infamous for being incapable of explaining consciousness. The current levels of description and explanation in cognitive neuroscience are too limited to account for phenomenal consciousness. This is largely because they focus on describing the currently known computational and neural mechanisms, although those levels of description were never meant to capture phenomenal consciousness. The research program on consciousness needs to introduce novel levels of description and explanation that should capture phenomenal consciousness from the first-person point of view.

Problem 3:   The Paradox of Isomorphism

According to the basic assumptions of our suggested research program, something in the brain literally is consciousness. In other words, consciousness, whatever its ultimate explanation may turn out to be, is a natural phenomenon located in the biological brain. However, the received view seems to be that nothing in the brain exactly (or even remotely) resembles our phenomenal experiences. The problem of isomorphism now becomes apparent: If consciousness resides in the brain, then there must be something in the brain that literally resembles or is similar to consciousness—that is, consciousness itself. Yet we have little idea how this could be the case. Can the research program solve this problem in a satisfactory way?

Problem 4: The Methodological Problems with the Measurement, Observation, and Visualization of Consciousness

If consciousness literally resides in the brain, how should we expect it to reveal itself in the detailed computer-generated images of human brain function constructed from measurements made with PET, fMRI, EEG, and MEG? To put it naively: Why do we not "see" consciousness in functional brain images? Or do we? What is the relation between the neural *correlates* of consciousness and the actual neural *constituents* of consciousness?

I believe that a biological research program on consciousness is what we ought to strive at in order to substantiate all the talk about the "science" of consciousness. In the following I will try to clarify the nature of the task we are facing, and sketch initial strategies to solve some of the problems listed above.

The Problem of Finding an Appropriate Metaphysical Basis for the Biological Research Program on Consciousness

Given the volume of empirical research in the cognitive neurosciences and the relevance of the field for understanding consciousness, why don't we already have a biological research program on consciousness? A research program gains its integrity from the basic metaphysical

assumptions shared by those working within the program. The formulation of such basic metaphysical assumptions would be a suitable job for philosophers involved in the study of consciousness. However, there appears to be a strange gap between the philosophical and the empirical approaches to consciousness: Many current philosophical views that admit the reality of consciousness nevertheless are not consistent with the basic assumptions of a biological research program on consciousness. A number of influential philosophers working within the field of consciousness studies deny that we could ever get an empirical grip on consciousness by studying the brain as a biological system, either because consciousness is not seen as a natural biological phenomenon or because it is not believed to be located in the brain.

For example, Chalmers (1997: 164) thinks that "to explain why and how brains support consciousness, an account of the brain alone is not enough." Dretske (1995: xiv) boldly asserts that "A better understanding of the mind is not to be obtained by knowledge—no matter how detailed and precise—of the biological machinery by which the mind does its job." Tye (1995: 151) informs us that "phenomenology ain't in the head." In the same spirit, Hut and Shepard (1996: 318) tell us that "We should no longer speak of conscious experience as taking place 'in the head' or 'in the brain.'" All of these views deny that consciousness should be thought of as a real biological phenomenon in the brain, or that consciousness could ever be explained by learning more about the brain. Indeed, one is inclined to agree with Mangan's (1998) observation that most philosophy today works *against* viewing consciousness as a biological system.

Why do some philosophers defend such empirically implausible positions, instead of earnestly trying to understand how consciousness *could* be a biological phenomenon in the brain? They usually have strong prior commitments to some fundamental assumptions on the nature of mind such that, having accepted them, one is often forced to resort to antibiological views on consciousness. For example, Dretske and Tye accept representationalism and content externalism. These views lead them to deny that a molecule-by-molecule identical copy of you, if it were suddenly to materialize out of the blue, could have any phenomenal states; or that a brain-in-a-vat physiologically identical with your brain could realize phenomenal states. The premises they have accepted require them to deny that a fully functional biological brain is sufficient for a fully realized subjective phenomenology. Hut and Shepard advocate an instrumentalist interpretation of science, so they basically deny that (or at least are agnostic about whether) the brain really exists. That is why they are reluctant to say that consciousness literally is located in the brain. But one would have a hard time explaining to neuroscientists that the brain doesn't really exist or that a fully functional brain is not sufficient for consciousness. A natural-science approach to consciousness simply has to take some things for granted, including that brains really do exist and that, for all we know, consciousness exists only in virtue of the complex biological processes going on inside the brain.

No wonder empirical scientists may find the philosophy of mind rather worthless, instead of regarding it as a common effort to understand how the brain enables consciousness. This distrust of philosophy is reflected in several comments that empirical consciousness researchers have made on the significance of philosophy for understanding consciousness. Baars and McGovern (1993) wonder whether philosophy helps or hinders scientific work on consciousness, and regard the history of philosophical influence on scientific psychology "worrisome," for philosophers "tend to want to legislate scientists about permissible and impermissible science." Baars and McGovern furthermore regard the results of Dennett's philosophy of consciousness as "strangely unhelpful" to scientific efforts. Zeki (1992) argues that neurobiologists ultimately face the very same problems that have preoccupied philosophers throughout the ages; but fortunately neurobiologists are not philosophers, for if they were, they might find themselves in an endless and ultimately fruitless discussion on the meaning of words such as "unconscious" and "knowledge."

Also, Crick (1994) reminds us of the poor track record that philosophers have shown over the last two thousand years. He furthermore notes that from the point of view of empirical scientists, philosophical functionalism is such a bizarre doctrine that most scientists are surprised to learn that it exists. Crick and Koch (1998) give a piece of practical advice to empirical scientists on how to have tolerance for the views of philosophers: Neuroscientists should listen to the questions philosophers raise, but should not be intimidated by their discussions. Searle (1997) has noticed that Crick is generally hostile to philosophers and philosophy, and comments that the price one has to pay for looking down on philosophy is the inclination to make philosophical mistakes.

The point I want to make is that there is still a deep gap between philosophical and empirical approaches to consciousness.[1] Most empirical scientists would probably accept a biological research program on consciousness; a large proportion of philosophers would not. Many philosophers or theoreticians endorse an antibiological metaphysics of consciousness and place themselves outside a biological research program, while many empirical consciousness researchers openly display a mistrust of philosophers. The net result is that there are very few philosophers deeply involved in empirical cognitive neuroscience as well as in the problem of consciousness, and very few empirical neuroscientists deeply involved both in consciousness research and in the philosophical problems posed by it. Instead, empirical research on consciousness is driven by a pragmatic approach without explicit accounts of the metaphysics of consciousness, and philosophical work on consciousness proceeds on a million different tracks, each inconsistent with the rest, and most of them inconsistent with the empirically based biological reasearch program on consciousness. Consequently, the metaphysical integrity required by a progressive scientific research program on consciousness is still missing. Unless the empirical and the philosophical camps learn to work together in a more fruitful fashion, such an integrity may be difficult to achieve.

Consciousness as a Level of Organization

Admitting the lack of an established philosophical framework for a biological research program on consciousness, how should we proceed with depicting consciousness as a biological phenomenon? The general framework used in understanding complex biological systems conceives of them as composed of several different *levels of organization*. Phenomena at different levels of organization in nature (e.g., molecules, cells, organs) are usually quite different from each other, have distinct causal powers, and require different sorts of approaches to their empirical study. For example, a single cell is quite different from the molecules it is composed of and from the tissues and organs it may be a part of. Levels of organization are seen as really existing in nature. Our biological theories attempt to capture these levels by postulating abstract models and conceptual systems that describe the levels and explain the relations between the different levels. Our theories thus have levels of description and explanation thought to correspond to the levels of organization actually existing in nature.

If this general framework, which is known as the standard hierarchical model of the world, is taken seriously in consciousness research, then the proposed biological research program should *reconceptualize* consciousness as *the phenomenal level of organization in the brain*. The metaphysical and ontological questions concerning consciousness and brain can thus be reconceptualized as regarding the relations between entities, processes, properties, and causal powers at different levels of organization in the brain. Although there are useful conceptual tools developed by philosophers to analyze interlevel micro–macro relations, we should, however, remind ourselves that empirical science has not yet been able to reveal the levels of organization in the brain relevant for understanding the phenomenal level. We should not assume that we will be able to explain consciousness by a purely philosophical analysis of interlevel relations, taking into account only such levels of organization as happen to be known in current cognitive neuroscience. Instead, we should admit from the start that an account of some of the levels of organization unknown to current empirical neuroscience will probably be necessary for the explanation of consciousness. In the absence of knowledge of the actual empirical details, only the general form of the explanatory problem can be figured out.

The characterization of consciousness as the phenomenal level of organization makes it perfectly clear that we are dealing with a real biological phenomenon that definitely resides within the brain; an integral feature of the brain as a biological system. This view leaves no room for arguments that try to separate consciousness from the brain by insisting that we can imagine a complete neurobiological description of the brain that does not tell us anything about consciousness. A complete description of the brain as a biological system *necessarily includes* a description of the phenomenal level of organization in the brain. If we fail to understand subjective phenomenal consciousness, we will have failed to exhaustively understand the brain as a biological system. Once we have accepted the basic assumptions of the biological research program on consciousness, we will realize that it is not possible to have an understanding of all the biological structures, processes, and mechanisms at all the different levels of organization in the brain without having an understanding of consciousness. These basic assumptions of course might be wrong, and the research program may have to be abandoned at some point in the future because of that, but at present such assumptions seem the most reasonable ones on which to start building a scientific research program.

Finding the Appropriate Levels of Description and Explanation for a Scientific Research Program on Consciousness

The first empirical question that we have to face after reconceptualizing consciousness as the phenomenal level of organization is to ask what that level is like. This is the basic question concerning the systematic *description* of the phenomenon we are interested in. Any empirically based scientific discipline must start with systematic description, which is the indispensable foundation of all explanatory research in biology as well (Mayr 1996).

Here we encounter one of the principal problems in current research on consciousness: It seems to operate at two levels of description only—(1) the level of the cognitive or computational information-processing mechanisms and (2) the level of the currently known neural mechanisms or neural correlates of those cognitive mechanisms. Surprisingly, the most important level of description in consciousness research, that of phenomenal organization, has no central role in current theorizing. Without a systematic description of the phenomenal level, however, it does not make much sense to chart the cognitive or neural mechanisms of consciousness, for it remains quite unclear what all those detailed mechanisms are supposed to be mechanisms *of*. The point is that a science of consciousness must first treat the phenomenal level of organization as a proper level of description. The lower levels of explanatory mechanisms can be invoked only after we have a clear conception of the phenomenon that these mechanisms are supposed to explain.

It is not too difficult to see why consciousness research still largely lacks the level of phenomenal description: There is no well-established, empirically based framework of phenomenology

to turn to. In the history of psychology, introspectionism once failed, and many still feel that an empirically based scientific phenomenology is outright impossible. Phenomenology as practiced in philosophical circles seems to be too obscure and conceptually isolated from current cognitive neuroscience to be of any real value for the empirically minded scientist. Furthermore, some philosophers are not too optimistic about the prospects of an "objective phenomenology" (Nagel 1974). Thus, it is no wonder that in consciousness research, conceptual frameworks are primarily taken from the empirically respectable and well-established branches of cognitive science and neuroscience. The problem, however, is that the science of consciousness is not simply a trivial further branch of those fields: Standard mainstream cognitive science and neuroscience largely ignore consciousness; they will not provide us with adequate levels of description for handling phenomenal experience.

I suggest that the science of consciousness needs to develop *a phenomenal level of description* that systematically captures the phenomenal level of organization in the brain. This level of description cannot be imported from any other existing branch of science—it must be contributed by the science of consciousness itself.

Metaphors and Model Systems

How should we go about developing a better understanding of the phenomenal level? I propose that we compare this task with previous attempts to describe and understand other complex biological phenomena. At a stage when there is no well-developed theory of the phenomenon the researchers are interested in, they tend to describe it in terms of a metaphor. A fruitful metaphor typically captures some of the essential features of the phenomenon in an easily comprehensible and visualizable form. Metaphors certainly have been utilized in current consciousness research, but I am afraid that most of them have not been constructed to capture the phenomenal level of organization. The lack of phenomenology is reflected in, for instance, the theater metaphor of consciousness (Baars 1998), which may be a fitting metaphor for the cognitive mechanisms of focal attention, but does not seem to catch the level of phenomenology very well. In the theater metaphor, consciousness resembles a bright spot directed by attention at the theater stage, the rest of the theater being dark but containing unconscious expert systems. This cognitive level of description is worked out in much detail, and then an attempt to map it to brain function is carried out.

Global work space theory (Baars 1988, 1997) attempts to explain a cognitive architecture in neural terms, but neither the cognitive architecture in question nor the theater metaphor used to depict it contains anything like an appropriate description of the phenomenal level, that is, phenomenal consciousness from the first-person point of view. The theory is a paradigm example of theoretical work in cognitive neuroscience, relating the cognitive level of description to the neural levels, but it remains unclear to what extent the theory is a genuine explanatory theory of consciousness as the phenomenal level of organization in the brain.

The main problem with the theater metaphor is that to be conscious does not typically feel like sitting in a dark theater and looking at characters or events appearing on a faraway stage. Rather, my moment-to-moment consciousness feels like being immersed in the center of a multimodal world that is present for me all at once, though I may pay focal attention only to some feature of it. The phenomenal level includes the externalized sensory events, my own body image, and those events which I feel are going on inside my body or my mind (emotions, inner speech). All of these phenomenal contents are highly organized in characteristic ways. Therefore, we need a different kind of metaphor and a different conceptual framework in order to capture the level of phenomenal representation, or consciousness *itself* (but not necessarily its neurocognitive mechanisms).

A *model system* is a system in which the phenomenon of interest manifests itself in a particularly clear form. In the ideal case the phenomenon is clearly isolated from others with which it might otherwise be confused, and is accessible to easy observation or manipulation by the researchers. The model system may not be prominent otherwise; just think of the significance of the lowly fruit fly *Drosophila* for the development of genetics.

I think that the dreaming brain is an excellent source of both a model system and a metaphor of the phenomenal level of organization. We know from empirical dream research that *the phenomenal level of organization is fully realized in the dreaming brain*. The visual appearance of dreams is practically identical with that of the waking world (Rechtschaffen and Buchignani 1992). When we dream, we typically have the experience of being in the center of a spatially extended world of objects and people, with all kinds of events going on around us. We have a body image much like the one we experience when awake, and we apparently can control its actions and sense our own movement through dreamed space. We know that during REM sleep, with which vivid dreaming typically is associated, the brain suppresses the processing of sensory information, but at the same time it activates itself internally. The motor output mechanisms are inhibited and voluntary muscles are virtually paralyzed, although motor commands are actively produced in the brain.

The dreaming brain shows us that sensory input and motor output are not *necessary* for producing a fully realized phenomenal level of organization. The dreaming brain creates the phenomenal level in an isolated form, and in that sense provides us with insights into the processes that are *sufficient* for producing the phenomenal level. At the same time the dreaming brain is an excellent reminder of the subjectivity of conscious states: There is no way we can directly "see" another person's dream world. However, we have a large body of empirical data on the phenomenological contents of dreaming, thanks to the development of quantitative methods in dream content analysis (Domhoff 1996). Quantitative dream content analysis is a rare example of a field in which systematic, empirically based descriptive phenomenology is practiced today.

The dreaming brain is a good model system for consciousness research because it isolates the phenomenal level from other systems that it might be confused with; it underscores the subjectivity of the phenomenon; it invites questions as to the possibilities of directly observing or imaging the phenomenal level in the brain; and it has resulted in empirical research with a systematic methodology and a body of quantitative data based on phenomenological description.

The dreaming brain, furthermore, provides us with a proper metaphor for the phenomenal level itself. When the phenomenal level is fully realized, as it is in the dreaming brain, it is characterized by the *sense of presence in* or *immersion in* a multimodal experiential reality. These terms were originally launched to describe experiences created with the help of a virtual reality (VR) system. However, these terms naturally do not describe the computers or the programs in a VR system, but the subjective *experience* that such systems can at their best create. In developing such vocabulary, I think the VR community has done a valuable service to consciousness research, because they have come up with terms that seem to characterize the realization of the phenomenal level of organization in a very general way.

The Virtual Reality Metaphor of Consciousness

I have proposed (Revonsuo 1995, 1997) that we should take the concept of virtual reality as a metaphor for consciousness. To briefly summarize the ideas behind the VR metaphor, when the brain realizes the phenomenal level, it is actually creating the experience that *I am directly present in a world outside my brain* although the experience itself is brought about by neural systems buried *inside* the brain. The brain is essentially

creating an "out-of-the-brain-experience": the sense of presence in and the immersion in a seemingly real world outside the brain. This is immediately obvious when we consider dreaming: There we are, in the middle of a strange dream world, but it never occurs to us to conceptualize it in any other terms than as a *world* or a *place* we find ourselves in. Almost all dream reports begin by specifying the place in which the subject found himself in the dream. We never come to think about the dream world as showing us how our own brain looks from the inside, although we positively know that's where the whole show is really taking place.

The phenomenal level of organization realizes what I call "virtual presence." Dreaming involves it in two different senses. First, there is the illusion that the experiential events do not take place inside my brain, but somewhere in an externalized perceptual world. Second, dreaming involves the further illusion that I am not present in the environment where my physical body actually is located and sleeping. In this sense, dreaming creates a completely imaginary presence, just as the technological variety of virtual reality does. Waking perception, however, involves only the first kind of illusion, and thus creates a sort of *telepresence* for the brain: the sense of direct presence in the world currently surrounding the body and modulating sensory input. However, the brain and the phenomenal level with it, actually constituting this experience, are deep inside the skull, never actually in direct contact with external objects.

The phenomenal level of organization can thus be seen as the brain's *natural virtual reality system*, a level of organization the purpose of which is to construct a real-time simulation of the organism and its place in the world. This simulation is modulated by sensory information during waking perception, but during dreaming it is realized off-line, by recombining materials from experiences stored in long-term memory. In everyday thinking we rarely realize that what we directly experience is merely a clever *simulation* or *model* of the world, provided by the brain; it is not the world itself. In order for it to be an effective simulation, we are supposed to take it as the real thing, and that is exactly what we do even during dreaming.

Why does the brain bother to create a detailed model of the world for us (or rather for itself)? Obviously in order to guide the organism through paths in the real world that enhance its chances of survival and successful reproduction. An excellent example of the importance of the phenomenal level in the guidance of behavior is a sleep disorder called REM sleep behavior disorder (RBD). Patients with RBD do not become paralyzed during REM sleep as they ought to: the mechanisms of motor inhibition fail. Consequently, the patients act out the behavior they dream about. If they are chased in the dream, they jump out of their beds and start to run for their lives. If they are attacked in the dream, they defend themselves and may kick or throw punches at invisible enemies.

A subject with RBD is phenomenologically immersed in a dream world, but behaviorally interacting with the real physical environment, often with unfortunate consequences. Obviously, one cannot get very far in the real world if one has an entirely erroneous model of the world in consciousness. Thus, these patients often suffer physical injuries during their attempted dream enactments, and may even be seriously injured. For example, a seventy-three-year old man with RBD, while dreaming, attempted to catch a running man. His wife reported that he jumped off the end of the bed and awoke on the floor, badly injured (Dyken et al. 1995). If an epidemic of RBD were suddenly to spread, all of us would behave in bizarre ways every night, guided by whatever the phenomenal level of organization presented to us.

The brain constructs the phenomenal level of organization because it is needed in mediating voluntary behavior. The content of the phenomenal level is ultimately the world as it is *for* the conscious organism: the world that the individual attempts to *interact with* and to which it

attempts to *adapt* through voluntary behavior. This crucial role in mediating voluntary, adaptive behavior, although functioning all the time in waking perception, becomes dramatically revealed when a full-scale hallucinatory world, such as we have during dreaming, guides behavior.

An important implication of the virtual reality metaphor is that it defines a framework for an empirically based phenomenology. The scope of a science of phenomenology could be depicted as the systematic description of the normal structure and the pathological breakdown of the phenomenal level of organization in the brain. We need to develop conceptual frameworks to systematically describe the different ways in which the structure of the phenomenal level can be distorted or break down in consequence of brain injury or in altered states of consciousness. The binding problem can be seen as the question of how the organization at the phenomenal level can become integrated or disintegrated as a result of normal or abnormal functioning of underlying integrative neurocognitive mechanisms. Similarly, the bizarreness of dream images could be conceptualized as specific distortions of the contents at the phenomenal level.

I believe that the critical question for the future of consciousness research is Can we describe consciousness systematically even on its own terms? If not, the prospects for being able to understand its relations to other levels of organization look dim at best. Without a description of the phenomenal level of organization, cognitive neuroscience explanations of consciousness seem rather futile. The virtual reality metaphor is my suggestion as to where we could start looking for such a description.

In sum, the scientific research program on consciousness should seek an initial understanding of consciousness by constructing a metaphor that captures the essential characteristics of the phenomenal level (not the cognitive or neural level) and by identifying model systems in which the phenomenal level is realized in a particularly clear form, isolated from other phenomena.

The Problem of Isomorphism: How to Understand the Claim That Consciousness Is Literally in the Brain

According to the assumptions of the suggested biological research program, some level of organization in the brain is consciousness. Consciousness thus is in the brain, but the received view seems to be that nothing in the brain exactly (or even remotely) *resembles* our phenomenal experiences. If consciousness is in the brain (which is the least incredible hypothesis, for where else should consciousness be?), then we have to choose between the naive view that something in the brain literally resembles phenomenal experience, and the incoherent view which denies that consciousness is similar to phenomenal experience although it is identical with it. The problem of isomorphism is that if consciousness literally resides in the brain, then there must be *something* in the brain that literally resembles or is similar to consciousness—that is to say, consciousness itself. But we have no idea how that could be the case.

The assumptions of the biological research program on consciousness thus entail a certain type of isomorphism between consciousness and brain. But we must clarify the nature of that isomorphism in order to avoid possible misunderstandings. First, it should be noted that our assumptions do not entail any isomorphisms between external stimulus objects and phenomenal states. The phenomenal level need not in any way be isomorphic to external sources of stimulation. Second, do our assumptions entail the doctrine of analytic isomorphism that there is an ultimate neural foundation where an isomorphism obtains between neural activity and the subject's experience? (Pessoa et al. 1998). I think this is a misleading way of formulating the issue, for it implies that the subject's experience and the neural activity are two entirely *different* things that just happen to be isomorphic (at least in some respects).

The biological research program does not have room for such a distinction, for the basic assumptions of the program state that consciousness simply *is* a level of organization in the brain. When it comes to that level of organization, it *is* the neurobiological level that *constitutes* or *is identical with* the phenomenal level. Consequently there *must* be isomorphism between one specific level of organization in the brain and phenomenal consciousness, simply because *these boil down to one and the same thing*. In the biological research program, it makes no sense to separate phenomenal experience from the brain and then ask whether there is anything in the brain isomorphic with experience. Subjective experience is in the brain, and this level of organization of course is isomorphic, indeed identical, with itself.

Formulations of the problem of isomorphism that distinguish between consciousness and neural activity imply a residual dualism which separates subjective experience from the brain. In the suggested biological research program we assume that there is a level of organization in the brain that constitutes consciousness. We may of course ask whether there are *other* levels of organization in the brain that contain features isomorphic with the phenomenal level. Whether or not there are any such levels is an open empirical question. The general lesson that we learn from biological levels of organization is that the constituent parts, residing at a lower level of organization, usually are not isomorphic with the whole that resides at a higher level of organization (e.g., the molecules constituting a continuous cell membrane, taken singly, do not much resemble the membrane that they constitute). The important point in understanding biological levels of organization and their interrelations is not whether one level is isomorphic with another, but whether the units at the lower level of organization can organize themselves in ways that explain how the higher-level phenomenon can emerge from it.

Those who advocate some form of representationalism in the explanation of consciousness often argue that there need be nothing in the brain that resembles the content of experience. This claim is clearly at odds with the biological research program proposed here, and it is important to understand why. The core of the representationalist doctrine can be briefly summarized as follows: The *content* of experience means the *representational* content of experience. Representational content is acquired through the causal-functional role that the representation itself, or in fact the *vehicle* of representation, realizes. The vehicle of representation that plays the causal-functional role correlates or covaries with certain conditions, objects, or whatever else external to the vehicle itself. The representational content resides in those external conditions, and the vehicle of representation need not in any way resemble its content; the vehicle is a sort of empty placeholder that in some way indicates, or whose states correlate or covary with, the presence of whatever it is that the vehicle represents. This idea is clearly expressed by Dretske (1995: 36):

What we find by looking in the brain of a person experiencing blue dogs is neither blue nor doglike. We do not find the content of experience, the properties that make the experience the kind of experience it is.... We find the experience vehicles. What we find, in other words, are the same sort of things we find when we look in books: representational vehicles that in no way resemble what these representations represent.

So, for example, a very simple vehicle can represent an enormously complex content, just as long as it reliably "indicates," or is causally connected and covaries with, the correct external content. Representational vehicles have only an external relation to the content of experience. This leads Dretske (1995: 38) to say that "the mind isn't in the head any more than stories are in books."

Representationalism may be a suitable theory for explaining some aspects of mental phenomena, but it cannot be applied to phenomenal content. Representational content is not at all the same thing as phenomenal content, and the two should not be identified or confused. If I see a blue dog in a dream, then there is something (phenomenally) doglike and something (phenomenally) blue at the phenomenal level of organization in the brain. If there is in my visual awareness a single uncomplicated figure against a uniform background, then the phenomenal content of my visual awareness is relatively simple; but if I see a complex scene of different objects, the phenomenal content is correspondingly complex. Unlike representational content, it makes no difference to phenomenal content how it is connected to the external world or whether it is so connected at all; phenomenal content stands on its own, independent of the contextual relations constituting representational content. The biological research program on consciousness is primarily interested in describing and explaining phenomenal organization as a natural biological phenomenon literally residing in the brain. Denying that the content of experience resides in the brain by identifying phenomenal content with representational content is to deny that consciousness literally resides in the brain and, consequently, to step outside the proposed biological research program on consciousness.

There is at least one level of organization in the brain that is similar to or resembles phenomenal experience, namely, the one that is actually identical with it: the phenomenal level of organization; consciousness itself. But exactly what does it mean to say that something in the brain "resembles" phenomenal experience? I think that the biological research program on consciousness should regard this primarily as an empirical question: How could we test or discover empirically whether or not there are any states in the brain isomorphic with phenomenal experience? If we assume that there are, at which level of organization in the brain should we expect to find such isomorphisms? If consciousness is literally in the brain, and constitutes a level of organization there, then any isomorphisms discovered between phenomenal experience and neural activity serve as indicators that we should be quite close to discovering the phenomenal level of organization in the brain.

It is interesting that, in current cognitive neuroscience, there are empirically based theories which postulate isomorphisms between conscious perception and the corresponding neural states. The theory of synchronizing connections proposed by Wolfgang Singer's group (Roelfsema et al. 1996) suggests specific neural mechanisms that implement the Gestalt principles of perceptual grouping in visual perception in such a manner that the resulting neural states are clearly isomorphic with the contents of visual awareness at the phenomenal level of organization. The local neural elements are hypothesized to link with each other through synchronization, and the global neural assembly is unified through the activity of local synchronizing connections. Even a small local change in the stimulus may result in a large difference in perceptual grouping. The pattern of synchronizing connections postulated by the theory apparently corresponds to the phenomenal content of visual awareness.

We thus have good theoretical reasons to believe that there are levels of organization in the brain showing isomorphisms with the phenomenal content of experience. The really crucial question for the empirically based research program on consciousness is this: Are there any empirical methods that could actually *reveal* such a level of organization in the brain? What does the empirical discovery of levels of biological organization usually require? From the history of biology we learn that discovering novel levels of biological organization is heavily dependent on the available research instruments and methods. For example, without the development of ever more sophisticated microscopes and other related techniques (e.g., staining), our understanding of the inner structure and workings of the living cell could not have made much progress.

Complex levels of biological organization cannot be expected to be visible to the naked eye; on the contrary, they are well hidden in complex, often microscopic, structures and processes. However, those with a representationalist inclination cite it as some sort of empirical evidence for their view that phenomenal content cannot be "seen" with the naked eye by external observers on the exposed surface of the conscious brain (e.g., Dretske 1995: 37). Very few levels of biological organization can be seen by the naked eye on the surface of any given organ, so it is quite odd to regard the fact that consciousness is not directly observable on the surface of the brain as evidence against the view that phenomenal content literally resides in the brain.

This discussion brings us to the last of the four problems mentioned at the outset: How could consciousness—the phenomenal level of organization—be empirically discovered in the brain? Before we go into that topic, let us summarize the main results of our discussion on isomorphism. The proposed biological research program on consciousness entails isomorphism in the sense that it assumes a level of organization in the brain isomorphic with and identical to phenomenal consciousness. However, it is important to understand that this is simply a direct consequence of accepting biological realism with regard to consciousness. Denying this sort of isomorphism amounts to denying that phenomenal consciousness as such really resides in the brain. Representationalists explicitly do deny it, for they mistakenly identify representational content with phenomenal content, and thus set themselves outside the biological research program on consciousness advocated here.

The Problem of the Measurement and the Functional Brain Imaging of Consciousness: Can We Ever "Discover" Consciousness in the Brain?

The phenomenal level of organization is a natural biological phenomenon in the brain. How does that level of organization reveal itself to observation, measurement, and other empirical investigations? The currently fashionable search for the neural correlates of consciousness utilizes such empirical methods as single-cell spike activity recordings and local field potential measurements with invasive microelectrodes in animals. In human subjects, macroelectrodes placed on the scalp are used to reveal the gross electrical activity of the brain (scalp EEG), and superconducting quantum interference devices are used outside the head to detect the tiny magnetic fields evoked by the brain (MEG). Positron emission tomography (PET) and functional magnetic resonance imaging (fMRI) reflect brain activation as revealed by changes in the level of glucose and oxygen metabolism, respectively. A general assumption appears to be that whatever the brain phenomena these methods reflect, there ought to be a detectable difference in them when a conscious process takes place, compared with a control situation when no conscious process takes place (or when the content of consciousness is radically different).

While this assumption may be a fruitful working hypothesis, we should remember that the empirical methods currently available are not likely to directly reflect the levels of organization in the brain that constitute the phenomenal level. Let us assume, just for the sake of argument, that the visual awareness of an object is constituted by complex organized spatial patterns of electrical activity in tens of thousands of neurons that reside somewhere in the visual areas in a distributed manner. These neurons are temporarily linked through activated synchronizing connections firing at high frequencies (see Roelfsema et al. 1996), the organized electrophysiological activity forming higher levels of organization in the brain. In order even to begin to understand consciousness, we ought somehow to discover these levels of organization. However, even if there actually were complex, organized electrophysiological states having fine-grained structure isomorphic with the structure of experience, our current methods of functional brain imaging would be constitutionally incapable of revealing them. We obviously cannot capture those levels of organization in the brain if they are realized at spatial and temporal scales far beyond the powers of resolution of current functional brain imaging.

In fact, the phenomena reflected in our current measurements of brain activation are extremely indirect, far removed from the levels of organization likely to constitute consciousness. PET certainly produces beautiful color-coded images of activated brain areas, but we should remind ourselves what the actual phenomena reflected in those images are. How is a colorful PET image constructed? PET detects gamma rays and thus directly images the sites of origin of those gamma rays in the brain. Those sites are the sites of positron annihilation. The positrons are generated when the radioactive isotope in the blood flow decays. Positron annihilation does not happen in the same location as positron formation does, so a PET image only indirectly depicts changes in local blood flow in the brain. And local blood flow is one step farther removed from any actual neural activity. The PET image is a shadow of changes in local blood flow, which is a rather pale shadow of changes in the level of neural activity. As Stufflebeam and Bechtel (1997) note, multicolored PET images are many steps removed from the phenomena themselves, the activities going on in the human brain. Functional MRI, though based on the detection of completely different phenomena than PET, similarly is far removed from depicting the complex structure of neural activity in real time.

We obviously cannot discover a level of *neural* organization by a method that does not directly reflect it in the first place. If there are higher levels of electrophysiological organization in the brain, and the phenomenal level is closely connected with them, we should have some method that can reflect and preserve the structure and organization of that level. But changes in local blood flow obviously do not reflect such phenomena at all. Why? First, it is obvious that the phenomenal level of organization can be realized or change state many times within a few seconds or minutes, the minimum time required to obtain a PET or an fMRI image. Thus, the time resolution of those methods is too slow. Second, it is quite possible that realizing the phenomenal level of organization does not force the brain to consume more oxygen or glucose than a comparable state without the realization of the phenomenal level. For example, it may be that consciousness is related to synchronous firing. Now if the neurons in the unconscious control condition also fire vigorously, but simply not in synchrony, and in the conscious condition they simply synchronize their activity, it may be that there is little if any difference in the amount of oxygen or glucose needed—in which case PET and fMRI are blind to the realization of the phenomenal level of organization. Even if realizing the phenomenal level does entail increased metabolism, what we at best can see in PET or fMRI images is just that: increased metabolism. We can see neither the phenomenal level itself nor its structure or organization. At best we can observe the smoke (and even that very indirectly) when we would really like to know what the flames and the fire are made of.

EEG and MEG are better, at least in the sense that they reflect the electrophysiological activity of the brain more directly, not via metabolic changes, and they are capable of doing it with high temporal resolution (in the order of one millisecond). However, the sensors detecting traces of brain activity are far removed from the brain: A scalp electrode is separated by at least 1 cm from the cortical surface, and several biological barriers, such as the skull and the membranes between the brain and the skull, lie between it and the cortex. The electrical fields and potentials are much distorted and spatially spread when they finally reach the sensors at the scalp. The "brain maps" of electrophysiological activity directly reflect the *scalp* topography of electrical fields as revealed outside the skull, not the topography of such events directly on the cortical surface. The sensor coils of a SQUID in MEG are even farther from the cortex, for they reside about 1 cm from the scalp, inside a container of liquid helium at a temperature of $-269°$ C.

Both EEG and MEG are sensitive only to synchronous activity in relatively large neural populations near the cortical surface. They are sensitive only to a part of such generators: those which happen to be correctly oriented and near the surface of the cortex (Nunez 1995). EEG and MEG are actually sensitive to differently oriented dipoles, and thus are complementary to one another. Synchronous activity in a neural population creates correlated dipole layers on the cortex. Spatial resolution in detecting such activity is limited to about 1 cm. A cortical area of 1 cm^2 consists of millions of neurons and billions of synapses. The signals are believed to originate as postsynaptic potentials in the apical dendrites of cortical pyramidal cells. Although not all of the synapses need to be synchronously active in order to generate a detectable signal (because the contributions from coherent sources are combined, whereas incoherent sources tend to cancel each other out), it is clear that any signal detectable at the scalp must reflect gross mass action in a huge number of neurons. According to one estimation, the synchronous activation of one synapse in a thousand over an area of 1 cm^2 is enough; this amounts to about 10^7 synapses (Uusitalo 1997). So when we observe even the tiniest electrophysiological event in EEG or MEG, we are actually observing at least 10 million synapses simultaneously activated in a cortical area containing about 10 billion synapses.

In order to reconstruct the anatomical location of the generators in the brain, the sources of the observed evoked fields must be mathematically modeled. Note that the sources are *modeled* (i.e., inferred), not *observed*. Source modeling involves the inverse problem: There is no unique solution to determine the charge distribution inside the brain by observing the pattern on the surface; an infinite number of possible charge distributions can lead to the same pattern. Source modeling requires a large number of background assumptions, which of course need to be correct if the model is to truthfully reflect where the measured electrophysiological activity originated (i.e., where the cell population including those >10 million simultaneously active synapses was located).

Even if the modeling is carried out successfully, and we have correctly inferred the location of activation, we have not succeeded in discovering the fine-grained structure of the levels of organization at which phenomenal experience is likely to be realized. We may have learned that in one particular cortical sulcus, millions of cortical pyramidal neurons must have generated postsynaptic potentials rather synchronously, contributing to the measurable activity outside the skull. However, we have no idea what the *pattern* of activated neurons within that locus was, or what the pattern of activated connections between neurons in that site and several others was. We have only a crude idea of the whereabouts of gross neural activity.

Invasive microelectrode recordings have the drawback that they cannot be used in studies with human subjects, thus largely blocking our access to the contents of the phenomenal level (although ingenious attempts to have animals report the contents of their consciousness have been realized; see, e.g., Sheinberg and Logothetis 1997; Cowey and Stoerig 1995). Although those methods do reveal the activities of single neurons or small groups of neurons, they do not capture the fine-grained complex structure of activated neural networks.

It is not my purpose to dismiss the methods of cognitive neuroscience as useless for the biological research program on consciousness; rather, I want to point out that despite all the technological advances, the available empirical methods are still quite limited and indirect, as far as discovering higher levels of complex organization in the brain is concerned. We should not even expect that these methods will reveal the levels of

phenomenal organization in the brain, since any temporally and structurally fine-grained complex levels of neurobiological organization escape these methods.

It seems that none of the current methods of cognitive neuroscience can be expected to reveal the organization at the phenomenal level in the brain. But can we even imagine any possible future method that could? Can brain imaging ever become "mind imaging"? The answer to this question is one of the key issues in understanding consciousness as a biological phenomenon. I will not attempt to give a full answer here; I will only consider one specific point about biological observation and explanation that I believe is relevant for discovering the phenomenal level in the brain: visualization.

The role of visualization is very important in the description and explanation of all complex biological phenomena. For example, in cytology, data and theoretical models are typically presented in the form of photographs, schematic diagrams, and drawings (e.g., Maienschein 1991). The same is true in neuroscience, where pictures and visualizations undoubtedly have a central role (Sargent 1996). In fact, one branch of neuroscience is called "brain mapping" or even "cartography of the brain." Toga and Mazziotta (1996) note that maps are indispensable in several branches of science, for a map can represent virtually our complete understanding of an object. Cartography has become a way of organizing scientific data, representing it, and communicating results. The visualization of data and phenomena is an essential element in cartography. This view of scientific explanation is remarkably different from the one offered by traditional philosophy of science, which is mostly based on physics and the propositional representation of theories and laws. In biology, visualization and systematized cartography are much more important in the explanation and understanding of phenomena.

Progress in cognitive neuroscience appears to be closely linked to our ability to visualize phenomena with the help of computer technology. In functional brain imaging, the goal seems to be the ever more detailed visualization of data (and phenomena) in a meaningful spatial framework in a 3D volume. The ideal is to construct realistic, visualizable models of the brain and its functions. They should have high temporal and spatial resolution and include several different levels of description at the same time. Currently we can see combinations of anatomical and functional data in a 3D spatial framework, for example, how an electrical field (measured by high-density EEG) develops on the surface of the cortex (as depicted by structural 3D-reconstructed MR image).

In the light of the significance of visualization in the understanding of all complex biological phenomena in general, and the brain in particular, what role might the visualization of phenomena have in the search for the phenomenal level of organization in the brain? I think it is likely that the level of organization we are after in the science of consciousness may require not only more sophisticated instruments of measurement but also more developed technology for the visualization of the data which directly reflect the phenomenon we are attempting to find in the brain. It may be that the conventional methods of visualization are insufficient for this job. Just as our understanding of what the Earth as a physical object truly is like cannot be represented by projecting a flat map of its surface on a two-dimensional surface, so it might be impossible to represent the phenomenal level realistically by means of any currently available method of visualization. A full-scale multimodal virtual reality system may have to be used to "visualize" the phenomenal level of organization, just like a three-dimensional spherical model of the Earth has to be used in order to capture the physical reality of our planet realistically.

If we are on the right track suggesting the above, we end up in an interesting loop: Consciousness is the phenomenal level of organization in the brain; the brain's real-time virtual reality simulation of the world. To depict that level of organization in a way that is true to the phenomenon, we might need to represent it by using a fully immersive virtual reality simulation. Are we just going round in circles? Maybe, maybe not. In any case, that is a different story, not to be elaborated here.

Conclusions

If, instead of just talking about the science of consciousness, the field of consciousness studies truly wants to proceed toward it, then we should realize what is required for a field to constitute a branch science. In this paper I have argued that we need a *biological* research program on consciousness; a systematic, empirically based, natural-science approach which sees consciousness as a real, natural, biological phenomenon in the brain. This program is to include a view of consciousness that can be taken seriously as an empirical hypothesis.

The problems that this research program must face are not insurmountable. I have tried to show how we could start developing a view of consciousness as a biological phenomenon; as the phenomenal level of organization in the brain that first needs to be systematically described on its own terms. In order to start developing a viable metaphysical foundation for the empirically based biological research program, we need close collaboration between philosophy and empirical neuroscience, instead of the two fields finding themselves in opposition to each other. Postulating increasingly bizarre philosophical views of consciousness that could not be taken seriously as empirical scientific hypotheses will not be of much help.

The problem of isomorphism and the problem of observation or measurement of consciousness are essentially questions about *capturing empirically* the relevant levels of organization in the brain. The problem here is not that consciousness or something isomorphic to it hasn't been "found" in the brain (as externalists tend to argue); rather, the problem is that *we do not know how to look for such things empirically*. Current brain imaging methods are not properly sensitive to the relevant levels of organization in the brain.

If we really and truly want to develop a respectable empirically based science of consciousness, the proposed biological research program (or something like it) is what I suggest we should look for. Now we have the opportunity to explore how far that sort of research program could take us in explaining consciousness, and we should not waste it by constantly trying to convince ourselves that we will never understand consciousness anyway because of some deep, dark metaphysical barriers.

Acknowledgment

The writing of this paper was supported by the Academy of Finland (project 36106).

Note

1. But of course I do not deny that great progress has been made during the 1990s in terms of interaction between philosophy and empirical science in the study of consciousness. Furthermore, I do not imply that *all* philosophers should be against a biological approach to consciousness. The most prominent example of a philosopher explicitly advocating a biological view of consciousness, not fundamentally different from the present one, is John Searle (1992, 1997).

References

Baars, B. J. (1988). *A Cognitive Theory of Consciousness*. New York: Cambridge University Press.

Baars, B. J. (1997). *In the Theater of Consciousness: The Workspace of the Mind*. Oxford: Oxford University Press.

Baars, B. J. (1998). Metaphors of consciousness and attention in the brain. *Trends in Neurosciences* 21: 58–62.

Baars, B. J., and McGovern, K. (1993). Does philosophy help or hinder scientific work on consciousness? *Consciousness and Cognition* 2: 18–27.

Chalmers, D. J. (1996). *The Conscious Mind*. Oxford: Oxford University Press.

Chalmers, D. J. (1997). An exchange with David Chalmers. In J. R. Searle, ed., *The Mystery of Consciousness*, 163–176. New York: New York Review.

Cowey, A., and Stoerig, P. (1995). Blindsight in monkeys. *Nature* 373: 247–249.

Crick, F. (1994). *The Astonishing Hypothesis*. London: Simon and Schuster.

Crick, F., and Koch, C. (1998). Consciousness and neuroscience. *Cerebral Cortex* 8: 97–107.

Dennett, D. C. (1991). *Consciousness Explained*. Boston: Little, Brown.

Domhoff, G. W. (1996). *Finding Meaning in Dreams*. New York: Plenum.

Dretske, F. (1995). *Naturalizing the Mind*. Cambridge, MA: MIT Press.

Dyken, M. E., Lin-Dyken, D. C., Seaba, P., and Yamada, T. (1995). Violent sleep-related behavior leading to subdural hemorrhage. *Archives of Neurology* 52: 318–321.

Gazzaniga, M. S. (1995). Preface. In M. S. Gazzaniga, ed., *The Cognitive Neurosciences*. Cambridge, MA: MIT Press.

Hut, P., and Shepard, R. N. (1996). Turning 'the hard problem' upside down and sideways. *Journal of Consciousness Studies* 3: 313–329.

Laudan, L. (1977). *Progress and Its Problems*. London: Routledge and Kegan Paul.

Maienschein, J. (1991). From presentation to representation in E. B. Wilson's *The Cell*. *Biology and Philosophy* 6: 227–254.

Mangan, B. (1998). Consciousness, biological systems, and the fallacy of functional exclusion. In *Consciousness Research Abstracts*, Toward a Science of Consciousness, Tucson III, 52. Thorverton, UK: Imprint Academic.

Mayr, E. (1996). *This Is Biology*. Cambridge, MA: Belknap Press of Harvard University Press.

Nagel, T. (1974). What is it like to be a bat? *Philosophical Review* 83: 435–450.

Nunez, P. L. (1995). *Neocortical Dynamics and Human EEG Rhythms*. New York: Oxford University Press.

Pessoa, L., Thompson, E., and Noë, A. (1998). Finding out about filling in: A guide to perceptual completion for visual science and the philosophy of perception. *Behavioral and Brain Sciences* 21: 723–802.

Rechtschaffen, A., and Buchignani, C. (1992). The visual appearance of dreams. In J. S. Antrobus and M. Bertini, eds., *The Neuropsychology of Sleep and Dreaming*, 143–155. Hillsdale, NJ: Lawrence Erlbaum.

Revonsuo, A. (1994). In search of the science of consciousness. In A. Revonsuo and M. Kamppinen, eds., *Consciousness in Philosophy and Cognitive Neuroscience*, 249–285. Hillsdale, NJ: Lawrence Erlbaum.

Revonsuo, A. (1995). Consciousness, dreams, and virtual realities. *Philosophical Psychology* 8: 35–58.

Revonsuo, A. (1997). How to take consciousness seriously in cognitive neuroscience. *Communication and Cognition* 30: 185–206.

Roelfsema, P. R., Engel, A. K., König, P., and Singer, W. (1996). The role of neural synchronization in response selection: A biologically plausible theory of structured representations in the visual cortex. *Journal of Cognitive Neuroscience* 8: 603–625.

Sargent, P. (1996). On the use of visualizations in the practice of science. *Philosophy of Science* 63 (Proceedings): S230–S238.

Searle, J. R. (1992). *The Rediscovery of the Mind.* Cambridge, MA: MIT Press.

Searle, J. R. (1997). *The Mystery of Consciousness.* New York: New York Review.

Sheinberg, D. L., and Logothetis, N. K. (1997). The role of temporal cortical areas in perceptual organization. *Proceedings of the National Academy of Sciences* 94: 3408–3413.

Stufflebeam, R. S., and Bechtel, W. (1997). PET: Exploring the myth and the method. *Philosophy of Science* 64 (Proceedings): 95–106.

Toga, A. W., and Mazziota, J. C. (1996). *Brain Mapping: The Methods.* San Diego: Academic Press.

Tye, M. (1995). *Ten Problems of Consciousness: A Representational Theory of the Phenomenal Mind.* Cambridge, MA: MIT Press.

Uusitalo, M. A. (1997). *Magnetic Source Imaging of Visual Motion Processing and Neural Activation Traces in the Human Brain.* Doctoral dissertation. Helsinki University of Technology.

Zeki, S. (1992). *A Vision of the Brain.* Oxford: Blackwell.

5 The Evolution and Ontogeny of Consciousness

Gerhard Roth

Introduction

As members of the species *Homo sapiens*, we are the product of biological evolution. More precisely, we are mammals, and within the class Mammalia we are primates (figure 5.1). Among the order Primates, we belong to the Old World primates (Catarrhini). Within this group we are members of the family Hominidae, which comprises the apes (gibbons, orangutans, gorillas, chimpanzees, and man) as opposed to monkeys, the remaining Old World primates (family Cercopithecidae) and all New World primates (suborder Platyrrhini). Among the hominids, we are members of the group great apes, or Homininae, which includes the gorilla (*Gorilla gorilla*), man (*Homo sapiens*), the two chimpanzee species (common chimpanzee, *Pan troglodytes*, and pygmy chimpanzee, *Pan paniscus*) and the orangutan (*Pongo pan*) and excludes the gibbon (*Hylobates*).

Traditionally, gibbons, orangutans, gorillas, and chimpanzees were grouped together into the family Pongidae, while man (with his extinct ancestors) was put into the separate family Hominidae. Such a distinction, though psychologically understandable, is completely unjustified in the light of modern taxonomy and evolutionary biology. Biologically, we *Homo sapiens* are more closely related to the two chimpanzee species than to any other living primate; we share about 99% of our genes with them. Therefore, humans and the chimpanzees should be placed together in a separate taxon, for which no name yet exists. The closest relative of this nameless group is the gorilla, and the closest relative of the African great apes is the orangutan.

The earliest primates originated at least 65 million years (My) ago, the separation between Old and New World primates took place about 40 My ago, and that between Old World monkeys (Cercopithecidae) and apes, including humans, about 30 My (or less) ago. Gibbons branched off at 19–17 My, the orangutan at 16 My, and the gorilla at 9–8 My. Humans and chimpanzees separated 6.7–6.2 My ago (Byrne 1995). Thus, given the evolutionary age of about 65 My of the order Primates, the divergence between *Homo* and *Pan* is relatively recent.

This evolutionary history shows that there can be no doubt that taxonomically and biologically we are (in a nested sense) mammals, primates, apes, and the closest relatives of chimpanzees. Do these evolutionary relationships similarly determine our "higher" cognitive abilities, including consciousness? There are probably the same number of neurobiologists, psychologists, and philosophers who accept as reject the idea that consciousness has evolved in parallel with the biological evolution of *Homo sapiens*, and with the evolution of the human brain in particular. Even if all of us accept the idea that consciousness is strictly bound to brain activity, it still remains undecided whether the brain centers involved in consciousness are shared with at least one other group of animals or are unique to humans. There is, of course, the possibility that some states of consciousness can be found in at least some nonhuman animals, while others are unique to humans.

To prove the presence or absence of states of consciousness directly is impossible, since we are uncertain about consciousness even in our nearest relative. There are, however, indirect ways to determine the presence of consciousness in animals as likely or unlikely. In essence, these are (1) to check in groups of animals for the presence of those cognitive functions which in humans can be exerted only consciously; (2) to examine which parts of the human brain are necessary for (and active during) the various states of consciousness; (3) to examine which of these centers

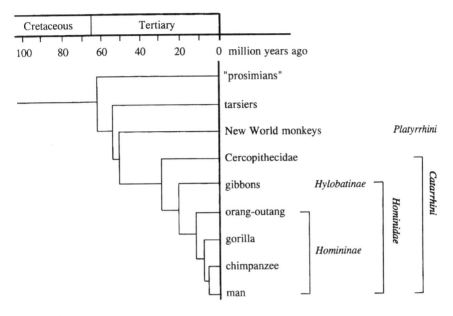

Figure 5.1
Taxonomic relationship (cladogram) of the primates. (Modified from Nieuwenhuys et al. 1998.)

of the human brain are present (and active) in the brains of those animals which—based on behavioral evidence—show certain states of consciousness; (4) to compare the ontogeny of cognitive functions, including states of consciousness in humans, with the ontogeny of the human brain (in the ideal case, the first appearance of certain states of human consciousness should coincide with the maturation of certain centers in the human brain). Taken together, these pieces of evidence should give us a relatively reliable picture of the way different states of consciousness have evolved in parallel to vertebrate, mammalian, primate, and human brain evolution.

Definition of Cognition and Consciousness

In the following, I use the term "cognition" in a wide sense to designate brain functions that ex-clude only primary sensory and motor functions, "autonomic" functions of the brain, reflexes, and reflexlike stereotyped behavior. Cognition, thus, includes such diverse functions as perception, learning, memory, imagination, thinking, expecting, and planning, whether accompanied by consciousness or not. From this it follows that cognition is not necessarily restricted to human beings, nor does it presuppose the existence of consciousness.

In humans, consciousness or awareness varies widely with respect to intensity and content, ranging from deep coma to the highest degree of concentration, from alertness to self-reflection. The most general form of consciousness is wakefulness or vigilance. It is characterized by a general responsiveness to sensory stimuli.

Vigilance is usually combined with subjective awareness or conscious experience of something. This "something" includes external as well as internal bodily stimuli, my own emotions, and my mental activity. From this awareness results the experience of my own presence in the world. Attention is the most characteristic state of increased awareness. A more special type of consciousness is body-identity awareness, the belief that I belong to the body which apparently surrounds me. There is autobiographic consciousness, the conviction that I am the one who existed yesterday. There is reality awareness of what was going on in the past and is happening in the world surrounding me. There is awareness of voluntary control of movements and actions, of being the author of my thoughts and deeds. Finally, there is self-awareness, the ability of self-recognition and self-reflection.

These different aspects of consciousness can dissociate, that is, they can occur independently of each other after damage of different parts of the brain (Kinsbourne 1995; Knight and Grabowecky 1995; Moscovitch 1995). Thus, there are patients who have all normal states of cognition, consciousness, and intelligence except that they deny belonging to their own body, or who do not know who or where they are.

The Neurobiological Basis of the Different States and Appearances of Consciousness

The large human cortex, particularly the so-called associative cortex (see below), has long been called the seat of the soul and of consciousness. It appears indeed that we are aware only of those things which are bound to the activity of the associative cortex. The activity of all subcortical and extratelencephalic centers of the brain, regardless of how important they are for the appearance of consciousness, is never accompanied by consciousness. This is true, above all, for the reticular formation, because its destruction leads to a general loss of consciousness, that is, to coma (Hassler 1978).

The reticular formation consists of three columns of nuclei—a median, a medial, and a lateral column—that extend from the anterior

mesencephalon through the pons to the medulla oblongata and rostral spinal cord (Nieuwenhuys et al. 1988). The medial column receives input from all sensory modalities and the cerebellum, as well as descending cortical input via the pyramidal tract. Its ascending projections form the nonspecific afferent or extralemniscal system, also called the ascending reticular activating system. This system projects directly or indirectly to the intralaminar thalamic nuclei, which, in turn, project in parallel and via different groups of neurons to the striatum and the cortex. The function of the medial reticular formation is the control of the wake-sleep cycle and of general cortical activity.

The median column is formed by the raphe nuclei. These nuclei, predominantly the dorsal raphe nucleus, send serotonergic fibers to all parts of the limbic system that are involved in cognitive functions, such as the hippocampus; amygdala; basal forebrain; limbic thalamic nuclei; cingulate and entorhinal cortex; and frontal, parietal, and occipital cortex. The lateral column contains the noradrenergic locus coeruleus complex, which projects to all parts of the limbic-cognitive system (figure 5.2). The locus coeruleus is supposed to have a role in controlling attention and continuously monitoring the external and internal environments for important events. Its projection to the prefrontal cortex in particular may mediate information about the relevance of complex sensory events and situations (Robbins 1997). The raphe nuclei are supposed to play a modulatory role in the context of behaviorally relevant events, apparently by counteracting and dampening the arousing effect of the other systems.

The next most important brain centers for the control of consciousness are the limbic (intralaminar and midline thalamic nuclei), because they are the most important relay station for the ascending projections of the reticular formation. These thalamic centers receive input from the entire cortex and project, back to it, predominantly to the prefrontal cortex, and additionally

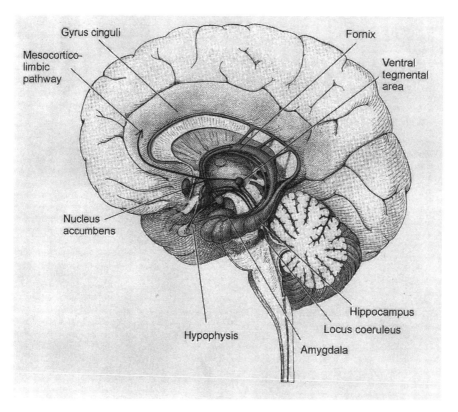

Figure 5.2
Medial view of the human brain showing major limbic centers. (Modified from *Spektrum/Scientific American* 1994.)

to the striatum; they are also connected to the entire limbic system. Damage to these thalamic nuclei leads to impairment of consciousness (Hassler 1978).

The nucleus reticularis thalami surrounds the entire lateral part of the thalamus like a bowl. It receives collaterals from thalamocortical as well as corticothalamic tracts, and has reciprocal connections with the sensory and limbic thalamic nuclei. It does not project to the cortex; rather, it exerts inhibitory control over most thalamic nuclei via GABA-ergic fibers. It is assumed to function as a filter for various kinds of information coming from the sensory periphery and brain

stem, acting under the control of the cortex and the limbic system. It may, therefore, be involved in guidance of attention (Guillery et al. 1998).

The brain centers mentioned so far belong to the limbic system in a wider sense, which in the vertebrate brain is the system that subconsciously controls all aspects of cognitive and emotional states and, accordingly, voluntary behavior. The limbic system evaluates what the organism does, and stores the result of this evaluation in the different kinds of memory. Other parts of the limbic centers discussed in the following contribute in more specific ways to the various states of consciousness (figure 5.2).

The amygdala is a complex of many different nuclei and is reciprocally connected with the associative cortex, particularly with the orbito-frontal prefrontal cortex (either directly or via the mediodorsal thalamic nucleus) and the hippocampal formation (Aggleton 1992). It strongly influences the sensory (visual, auditory, gustatory) cortex. It receives subcortical input from the olfactory system, the limbic thalamic nuclei, and the rest of the limbic system. The amygdala is in control of autonomic responses (via the hypothalamus); regarding cognitive and emotional functions it is an important center (together with the anterior cingulate cortex; see below) for evaluation and perhaps storage of negative experience, such as in the context of fear conditioning and anxiety (Aggleton 1992, 1993). The hippocampal formation (Ammon's horn, subiculum, dentate gyrus) and the surrounding parahippocampal, perirhinal, and entorhinal cortex are important centers for the formation and the consolidation of traces of declarative memory inside the cortex, that is, of those kinds of memory which in principle can be consciously retrieved and reported (Squire 1987; Markowitsch 1992, 1999; Squire and Knowlton 1995).

The dorsal parts of the basal ganglia (the putamen, nucleus caudatus, globus pallidus, nucleus subthalamicus, and substantia nigra) are closely associated with the prefrontal, premotor, and parietal cortex as well as with the entire limbic system. The basal ganglia have to do with subconscious planning and final decisions to take voluntary action under the influence of the limbic system (Passingham 1993).

The basal forebrain-septal nuclei complex is connected reciprocally with the hippocampus and the amygdala, as well as with the centers of the reticular formation already mentioned. Its cholinergic fibers project to all parts of the cortex. The basal forebrain is believed to be involved in the control of attention and of activity of the neocortical neuronal network, primarily in the context of earlier experience (Voitko 1996). The mesolimbic system (nucleus accum-bens, lateral hypothalamus, ventral tegmental area)—like the substantia nigra—is characterized by the neuromodulator dopamine. This system has strong connections with the orbitofrontal cortex and is involved in the formation of positive memories and pleasure, and perhaps in the control of attention in the context of new events (Robbins and Everitt 1995). Its impairment may be involved in cognitive misinterpretation and misevaluation in schizophrenics.

All these parts of the brain outside the cortex contribute substantially to consciousness while their activities remain completely unconscious. Damage to these subcortical centers usually produces either complete loss of consciousness or profound impairment of conscious cognitive and emotional functions. This may include the inability to recognize positive or negative consequences of action, impairment of attention, and/or loss of declarative memory. Importantly, patients usually are unaware of these deficits.

Although activity in the cortex is necessary for consciousness, we are unaware of processes going on in the primary and secondary sensory and motor areas of the cortex, although these processes are necessary for the specific contents of awareness of events inside or outside our body. We are aware only of processes bound to the activity of the cingulate and the associative cortex, and even then of only some of those processes.

The cingulate cortex (areas 23 and 24 in figure 5.3a) is that part of the cortex which surrounds the subcortical parts of the telencephalon and the thalamus. It is tightly connected to the prefrontal and parahippocampal cortex, the basal forebrain-septal region, the amygdala, the limbic thalamic nuclei, and the reticular formation. The anterior part is involved in the sensation of pain (in combination with the somatosensory cortex, the medial thalamic nuclei, and the central tegmental gray) and in memory of painful events. In this sense, it may be the conscious counterpart of the amygdala. It is always active for tasks requiring attention (Posner 1994).

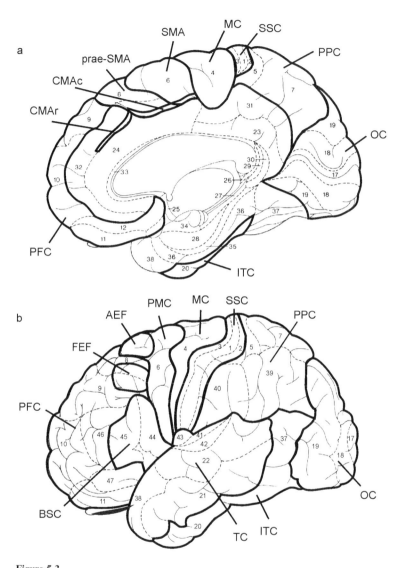

Figure 5.3
(a) Medial view of the human cortex. Numbers refer to cytoarchitectonic cortical fields according to Brodmann. CMAc, caudal cingulate motor area; CMAr, rostral cingulate motor area; ITC, inferotemporal cortex; MC, motor cortex; OC, occipital cortex; prae-SMA, presupplementary motor area; PFC, prefrontal cortex; PPC, posterior parietal cortex; SMA, supplementary motor area; SSC, somatosensory cortex. (b) Lateral view of the human cortex. Numbers refer to cytoarchitectonic cortical fields according to Brodmann. AEF, anterior eye field; BSC, Broca's speech center; FEF, frontal eye field; ITC, inferotemporal cortex; MC, primary motor cortex; OC, occipital cortex; PFC, prefrontal cortex; PMC, dorsolateral premotor cortex; PPC, posterior parietal cortex; SSC, somatosensory cortex; TC, temporal cortex. (Modified from Nieuwenhuys et al. 1988.)

The associative cortex (figure 5.3b) is the portion of the cortex that contains no primary sensory or motor cortical areas, but is involved in "higher" processing of information coming from these areas. It includes the posterior parietal cortex (PPC). The left PPC is involved in symbolic-analytic information processing, mathematics, language, and interpreting drawings and symbols. Lesions impair reading and writing and their respective memory functions. The right PPC deals with real and mental spatial orientation, the control of hand and eye movement, change of perspective, and control of attention. Lesions of inferior right PPC produce neglect (e.g., ignoring the contralateral half of the body or events in the contralateral visual hemifield) or anosognosia (lack of insight or denial of disturbances).

The associative superior and middle temporal cortex houses perception of complex auditory stimuli including (generally left side) Wernicke's semantic speech center, which is crucial for the understanding and the production of meaningful written and spoken language. Perception of music usually involves the right medial temporal cortex. The inferior temporal cortex (ITC) is decisive for complex visual information regarding nonspatial properties of objects and scenes, along with their meaning and correct interpretation. Lesions in ITC produce object agnosia (left ITC); color agnosia (right ITC); prosopagnosia, the inability to recognize faces (right or bilateral ITC); deficits in categorization; changes in personality and emotionality; and deficits in the use of contextual information.

The prefrontal cortex (PFC) includes the largest portion of the cortex (about 30% in man) and has been viewed by many neuroscientists as the highest brain center and the seat of the soul, of consciousness, personality, intelligence, and so on. In contrast to all other parts of the cortex, its anatomical and functional substructures are still a matter of debate (see Roberts et al. 1998). Usually two major parts are distinguished in the primate, including human, brain: a dorsolateral portion and a ventral-orbitofrontal portion. The dorsolateral PFC appears to be involved in (1) attention and selective control of sensory experience; (2) action planning and decision making; (3) temporal coding of events; (4) judgment and insight, particularly with respect to reality; (5) spontaneity of behavior; (6) strategic thinking; (7) associative thinking; and (8) working memory. Thus, the dorsolateral PFC is predominantly, though not exclusively, oriented toward the external world and its demands, including short-term memory. Lesions of the dorsolateral PFC result in perseveration and impairment of making appropriate cognitive or behavioral switches. The orbitofrontal PFC is involved in social and emotional aspects of behavior, ethical considerations, divergent thinking, risk assessment, awareness of consequences of behavior, emotional life, and emotional control of behavior. Accordingly, damage to the orbitofrontal PFC results in loss of interest in important life events, in loss of "ego," in "immoral" behavior, and in disregard of negative consequences of one's own behavior. Thus, the orbitofrontal PFC is predominantly oriented toward the internal emotional and social aspects of life.

The supplementary motor area (SMA) (figure 5.3a) is situated between the medial aspect of the motor cortex and the dorsomedial prefrontal cortex, and represents something like an associative motor cortex. It is active during the preparation and planning of complex movements and during imagined movements (Roland et al. 1980). Together with the prefrontal cortex, it contributes to the awareness of being the author of one's own deeds.

In summary, there is neither consciousness per se nor a highest brain center producing consciousness. Rather, different parts of the associative cortex contribute in different ways to the great diversity and content of consciousness, including awareness of external and internal sensory events; consequences of one's own behavior; autobiographic, body, and ego identity; action planning; and authorship of one's own deeds. The associative cortex does this under the strong influence of the primary and secondary sensory and motor cortices as well as of the subcortical centers mentioned.

Cognition and Consciousness in Animals

After this brief summary of the neural basis of higher cognitive functions and states of consciousness, I turn to the question what kind of cognitive abilities can be found in the different groups of vertebrates and in mammals in particular. Checking recent reviews on the "animal mind" (Stamp Dawkins 1993; Parker et al. 1994; Byrne 1995; Pearce 1997; for criticism see MacPhail 1998), it seems that all vertebrates and probably also invertebrates with large brains (e.g., cephalopods), display sensory or focused attention, extended memory, categorization, and the formation of cognitive maps. Whether this is accompanied by some kind of consciousness is difficult to determine in fishes, amphibians, and reptiles. Many of the so-called higher cognitive functions, such as concept learning, knowledge representation, analogical thinking, the formation of abstract representations, and imitation in the sense of copying behavior are found at least among birds and mammals, and even in humans these higher cognitive functions are not necessarily accompanied by consciousness. There are, however, cognitive functions that in humans require at least some states or levels of consciousness. These functions include the following:

1. Imitation in the sense of task structure or task principle learning and tool learning. This is found in macaque and capuchin monkeys, in apes, and perhaps in some other mammals (e.g., otters).

2. Taking the perspective of the other in deception and counterdeception. This is found in monkeys (e.g., baboons) and great apes.

3. Anticipation of future events (e.g., the preparation of tools in advance). This has been found

in the great apes and may be present in some monkeys.

4. Comprehension of underlying mechanisms, for example, in the use of tools. This has been reported in great apes.

5. Knowledge attribution/theory of mind. This is found in great apes, particularly chimps.

6. Self-recognition in mirror. This is present in great apes and perhaps in dolphins.

7. Teaching. This is found only in chimpanzees.

8. Understanding and use of simple syntactical language (up to three-word sentences). This is found in great apes and dolphins.

9. Use of complex syntactical language. This is found only in humans.

Functions 4, 5, 6, and 8 have been studied extensively in the recent past and are of special interest, because they may draw a line between monkeys and great apes among the primates. Such a line is less emotionally laden than that between humans and nonhuman apes. Primatologists agree almost unanimously that monkeys (e.g., capuchins) exhibit the use of tools (as many other animals do), but without an understanding of the underlying mechanism. They do not seem to "know" why one tool is effective and another is not (Visalberghi and Limongelli 1994). A similar lack of insight has been reported by Kummer (personal communication) among baboons (using a stick to reach apples).

Even more telling are the experiments concerning mirror self-recognition (see Parker et al. 1994). Monkeys are capable of using mirrors, for example, in order to look behind objects that otherwise are inaccessible (Byrne 1995). Kummer reports that baboons recognize a group member on a slide and identify themselves as mother or child on slides without difficulty. Yet primatologists agree that monkeys show no sign of mirror self-recognition. Among apes, chimpanzees and orangutans definitely show mirror self-recognition, while among gorillas only Koko does (it is assumed that gorillas often are too shy). Chimpanzees show great interest in their mirror image and pass the marking test (removing marks of paint from face or body, using the mirror image) well. Interestingly, at least some dolphins are reported to show mirror self-recognition, too, but their behavior appears to be very different from that of apes in front of a mirror. They show no natural interest in their mirror image and dislike the marking test (Marten and Psakaros 1994). The reasons for these differences are unclear, irrespective of the many methodological and conceptual problems.

The attribution of knowledge or theory of mind to others (Baron-Cohen et al., 1985) is difficult to distinguish from the capability of taking the perspective of the other. For most animals with complex behavior, it is important to guess what the other is going to do, for example, in agonistic behavior (see Stamp Dawkins 1993). However, primatologists (e.g., Kummer) state definitely that monkeys (e.g., baboons) do not take into account what the other is "thinking." Important in this context is the performance of very young children. According to Mitchell (1994), in children self-detection starts at 3 months, and mirror self-recognition is shown at 18 months on average. However, little children show embarrassment and coy reactions earlier than that. Self-recognition in photos starts at 24 months, followed by signs of self-evaluative emotions, such as shame and pride. A true theory of mind is said to emerge at four years (Meltzoff and Gopnik 1993). The authors stress that these events occur in the same sequence in apes, though at a much slower rate than in humans.

Much has been written about the presence or absence of "true" (syntactically complex) language in nonhuman primates (and other animals). Monkeys have complex systems for intraspecific vocal communication that can express relatively complicated meaning, including symbolic information (e.g., about objects and events that are not present) or information about relationships between events (e.g., parental relation-

ships). Many of these calls have to be learned by the infant monkey, and—as in songbirds—dialects exist (see Zimmermann et al. 1995). Most authors agree that sentences consisting of up to three words are understood and used by chimpanzees, gorillas, and dolphins. Whether this is a sign of a simple syntax is a matter of debate. Most authors agree that nonhuman primates are unable to infer differences in the meaning of a phrase or sentence from differences in the sequence of words. Chimpanzees do combine "words" to form new words (Gardner et al. 1989), but they do not go beyond the linguistic capabilities of a three-year-old child, even after intense training (Savage-Rumbaugh 1984).

Of great interest in this context is the development of language in human children (Locke 1995). In humans, language learning starts long before speaking: in utero. Vocal learning of the mother's voice begins prenatally; three-day-old neonates show a preference for maternal voice in the way it is transmitted to the fetal auditory system prenatally. Facial learning starts immediately after birth; babies seem to be preadapted to it. At six months after birth, children show a preference for familiar over foreign language. First voweling sounds are produced around 4 to 6 months, when "babbling" starts; first consonant-like sounds occur at 9 to 12 months. Children seem to take great pleasure in producing sounds and speaking. First reproduction of maternal intonation contours takes place around 6 months or even earlier, and first words are produced between 8 and 20 months (average 12 months). Around 18–23 months, children begin to combine words and form two-word utterances. Then they gradually begin to use sentences longer than two words, but typically in a telegraphic style, which—most interestingly—is likewise found in patients with lesions of Broca's speech area (Stromswold 1995). Children use sentences of two or three words without conjugation and declination, and they say little that they have not heard before. In the third year, children start distinguishing singular and plural and asking

"What's that?" From this point on, their language rapidly becomes syntactically more elaborate. Between three and four years, utterances become completely grammatical.

Passive vocabulary is larger than active from the very beginning: at 8 months, infants understand an average of 36 words, but produce fewer than 2; and at 10 months, they understand 67 words on average, but they will not produce that many words until at least 6 months later. At 16 to 18 months, there is a rapid acceleration in the rate at which new words and phrases are comprehended (7–9 words per day until the age of 6 years). Around the end of the second year, the child's vocabulary consists of 150–200 words. At an age of 3–4 years, children have a vocabulary of 1,500 words and understand an additional 3,000–4,000 words. While apes after 4–6 years of intense training may use some hundred words in a meaningful manner, a child of same age has an active vocabulary of 4,500 words. The average adult has an active vocabulary of about 10,000 words, and a passive vocabulary about ten times larger. It has been estimated that during speaking, more than 1000 grammatical rules are applied (Corballis 1991). Thus, it seems that apes have simple linguistic capabilities comparable with those of a human child of two to three years, but from then on, the child rapidly develops a fully syntactical language that is far superior to any communicative system known in animals.

In conclusion, based on the experimental evidence reported above, we may—with some caution—identify several evolutionary steps among tetrapod vertebrates regarding cognitive abilities: (1) among tetrapods from amphibians and reptiles (turtles, snakes, and lizards) to birds and mammals; (2) among mammals from noncetacean and nonprimate mammals to cetaceans (whales and dolphins) and primates; (3) among primates from prosimians and monkeys to apes; (4) among apes from gibbon, orangutan, and gorilla to chimpanzee and man; and (5) from chimpanzee to man. This scenario does not include large land mammals such as elephants, because experiments on cognitive abilities have not been carrried out in these animals.

Animal Brains and the Human Brain

The question now is: Are we able to correlate the differences in higher cognitive functions, including consciousness, among groups of tetrapods and, more specifically, mammals, with properties of their brains? In order to answer this question, we first have to clarify what kinds of differences we need to look for. First of all, differences in cognitive abilities among animals could be simply the result of the presence or absence of major brain structures relevant to cognition (for example, it could be that some animals are less "intelligent," because their brains have no cortex or hippocampus). Second, assuming—as most neurobiologists now do—that all brain functions, including cognition and consciousness, are the result of the anatomy and physiology of networks formed by neurons and their synapses, then structural and physiological differences in these networks should result in different functions.

Thus—given the same overall organization of brains—what should count for cognition, including consciousness, is (1) the number of neurons in the entire brain or in those brain centers necessary for a particular cognitive function or state of consciousness; (2) the number of synapses per neuron in the brain or specific brain centers; (3) short-term plasticity of synapses (i.e., how quickly synapses can change their properties relevant for fast transmission of neuronal activity); (4) plasticity of synapses in the context of memory formation; (5) the ontogenetic dynamics of synapses (i.e., how long synapses retain a high degree of plasticity during their lifetime). If the packing density of neurons and the number of synapses per neuron remained roughly constant, then an increase in brain size would mean a proportional increase in the number of neurons and synapses and, consequently, an increase in the performance of neuronal networks.

Thus, what we have to look for are differences in (1) overall organization of brains, (2) absolute or relative brain size, (3) absolute or relative size of the parts of the brain relevant for higher cognitive abilities, (4) size of the associative cortex and the prefrontal cortex in particular, and (5) differences in physiological properties of the brains under consideration (e.g., neuronal plasticity).

All tetrapod vertebrates (amphibians, reptiles, birds, mammals) have brains that—despite enormous differences in outer appearance, overall size, and relative size of major parts of the brain—are very similar in their general organization and even in many details (Roth and Wullimann 1996). More specifically, all tetrapod brains possess a median, medial, and lateral reticular formation inside the medulla oblongata and the ventral mesencephalon. There is a corpus striatum, a globus pallidus, a nucleus accumbens, a basal forebrain/septum and amygdala within the ventral telencephalon, a lateral pallium homologous to the olfactory cortex of mammals, and a medial pallium homologous to the hippocampal formation (at least Ammon's horn and subiculum). This means that all structures required for attention, declarative memory (or its equivalents in animals), motivation, guidance of voluntary actions, and evaluation of actions are present in the tetrapod brain. These structures essentially have the same connectivity and distribution of transmitters, neuromodulators, and neuropeptides in the various groups of tetrapods.

A more difficult problem is the presence of structures homologous to the mammalian cortex in the telencephalon of nonmammalian tetrapods. Amphibians possess a dorsal pallium, reptiles have a dorsal cortex plus a dorsal ventricular ridge (DVR), and birds have a hyperstriatum and a DVR (here called neostriatum); these structures are believed by many comparative neurobiologists to be homologous to the

cortex of mammals (Karten 1991; Northcutt and Kaas 1995). However, major differences exist between these structures with regard to cytoarchitecture and size. In amphibians, the dorsal pallium is small and unlaminated; in lizards it is relatively larger, and in some groups of reptiles, such as turtles, it shows a three-layered structure. In birds, those parts assumed to be homologous to the mammalian cortex (neostriatum and hyperstriatum) are large but unlaminated. In mammals, excluding insectivores and cetaceans, the dorsal pallium or cortex shows the characteristic six-layered structure. When we compare a bird such as a pigeon or a parrot with a roughly equally intelligent mammal such as a dog, then it becomes apparent that the same or very similar cognitive functions are performed by anatomically very different kinds of pallium/cortex.

Let us now turn to the relevance of absolute and relative brain size, because large brains have often been correlated with "intelligence" or "higher cognitive abilities." Among mammals, very large brains are found in primates (1.4 kg in *Homo sapiens*), in elephants (up to 5.7 kg), and in whales and dolphins (up to 10 kg) (figure 5.4). The reasons for increase in brain size are unclear; body size appears to be the single most important factor influencing brain size (i.e., large animals generally have large brains in absolute terms). However, increase in brain size parallels the increase in body size only to the power of 0.66–0.75 (i.e., 2/3 or 3/4, depending on the statistics used; Jerison 1991)—a phenomenon called "negative brain allometry" (Jerison 1973) (figure 5.5). Consequently, small animals of a given taxon have relatively larger brains and large animals of this group relatively smaller brains. Among mammals, this is reflected by the fact that in very small rodents, brains occupy up to 10% of body mass; in pigs, 0.1%; and in the blue whale, the largest living animal 0.01% (figure 5.6).

In addition, the various groups of vertebrates, while satisfying the principle of negative brain

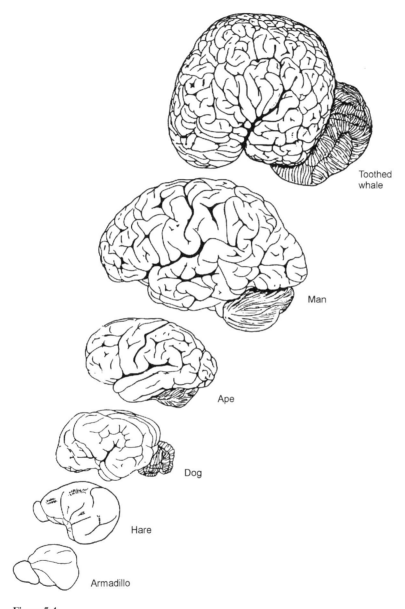

Figure 5.4
Series of mammalian brains, all drawn to the same scale. Man has neither the largest brain nor the most convoluted cortex. Convolution of the cortex as well as of the cerebellum increases monotonically with an increase in brain size.

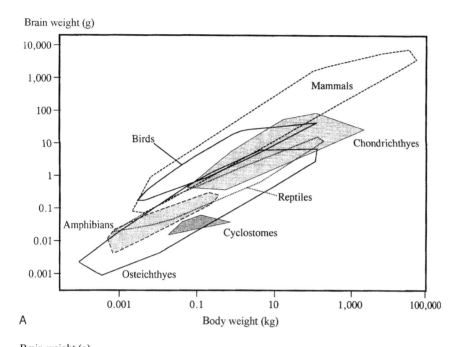

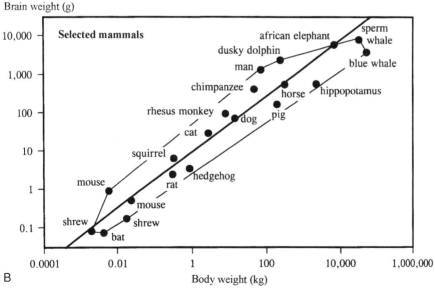

Figure 5.5
Diagrams showing the relationship between body weight and brain weight in a double-logarithmic graph. (A) Convex polygons for brain sizes of the main vertebrate groups. (B) Data from 20 mammalian species. (Modified from Nieuwenhuys et al. 1998.)

Relative brain weight (percentage of body weight)

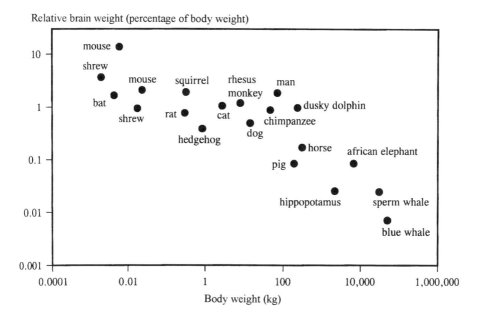

Figure 5.6
Double-logarithmic graph showing brain weight as a percentage of body weight for the same 20 mammalian species as in figure 5.5. (Modified from Nieuwenhuys et al. 1998.)

allometry, exhibit considerable differences in their fundamental brain–body relationship. Among tetrapods, mammals and birds generally have larger brains relative to body volume/weight than amphibians and reptiles, and among mammals, cetaceans and primates have relatively larger brains than the other orders. Thus, during the evolution of birds and mammals, and more specifically of cetaceans and primates, genetic and epigenetic systems controlling brain size have undergone substantial changes in favor of relatively larger brains. These changes resulted in enlargements of brains beyond what would be associated with body size (Jerison 1991).

Thus, man—contrary to a common belief—does not have the largest brain either in absolute or in relative terms. Unless we accept that cetaceans and elephants are more intelligent than

humans and/or have states of consciousness not found in us, the absolute or relative size of the human brain per se cannot account for our factual or alleged superior cognitive abilities. However, among relatively large animals man stands out with a brain that constitutes 2% of body mass. We can quantify this fact by determining the encephalization quotient (EQ), which indicates the ratio between the actual relative brain size of a group of animals and the relative brain size expected on the basis of brain allometry determined by body size alone. Calculating the EQ for man, it turns out that his brain is about seven times larger than that of an average mammal and about three times larger than that of a chimpanzee, if both were the size of a human being (Jerison 1973, 1991). Apparently, during the evolution of *Homo sapiens*, over a period of 3–4 million years, additional genetic and epigenetic processes led to a constant increase in relative (and absolute) brain size. While man stands out in this respect among primates, similar processes must have taken place among cetaceans. Toothed whales, particularly members of the family Delphinidae, exhibit EQs far superior to all primates but *Homo sapiens* (Marino 1998). Man has an EQ of about 7; the dolphins *Sotalia fluviatilis*, *Delphinus delphis*, and *Tursiops truncatus* have EQs of 3.2; and the great apes (except man) have EQs around 2. Thus, man has a much larger brain than expected among primates, but even in this respect his brain is by no means unique, as the example of dolphins shows.

What about the absolute or relative size of the human cortex? There are enormous differences in both absolute and relative brain and pallial/cortical size among tetrapods, and among mammals in particular. For example, man has a brain and a cortex that are roughly 3,000 times larger in volume than those of a mouse. This implies that changes in relative size of cortex are inconspicuous, because in mammals cortical size follows changes in brain size rather strictly; but again there are differences within mammalian groups. Apes (including man) have somewhat larger isocortices than other primates and other mammals, because their forebrains (telencephalon plus diencephalon) are generally somewhat larger, constituting 74 percent of the entire brain as opposed to about 60 percent in other mammals, including mice. At 40 percent of brain mass, the human cortex has the size expected in a great ape (Jerison 1991).

The enormous increase in cortical volume is partly the result of an increase in brain volume and consequently in cortical surface (which is related to an increase in brain volume by the power of 2/3; Jerison 1973), and partly the result of an increase in the thickness of the cortex. The cortex is about 0.8 mm thick in mice and 2.5 mm in man. However, with an increase in cortical thickness and brain size, the number of neurons per unit of cortical volume decreases. While about 100,000 (or more) neurons are

found in one mm^3 of motor cortex in mice, 10,000 neurons are found in the motor cortex of man (Jerison 1991). This decrease in the number of cortical neurons per unit volume is a consequence of a roughly equal increase in the length of axonal and dendritic appendages of neurons, in the number of glial cells, and in the number of small blood vessels. Without such an increase in glial cells and blood vessels, large isocortices would be both architecturally and metabolically impossible.

Thus, the dramatical decrease in nerve cell packing density is at least partially compensated for by an increase in cortical thickness. This could explain why all mammals have a roughly equal number of neurons in a cortical column below a given surface area (e.g., 1 mm^2) (Rockel et al. 1980). Furthermore, as explained above, what should count for the performance of neuronal networks is not so much the number of neurons per se, but the number of synapses their axons and dendrites form or carry (plus the degree of plasticity of synapses). An increase in length of axons and dendrites paralleling a decrease in nerve cell packing density should mean more synapses, and such an increase in the number of synapses could compensate for the strong decrease in nerve cell packing density. It has been estimated that the mouse cortex contains about 10 million (10^7) neurons and 80 billion (8×10^{10}) synapses, and the human cortex about 100 billion (10^{11}) neurons and a quadrillion (10^{15}) synapses, or 10,000 times more (Schüz and Palm 1989; Jerison 1991). These differences certainly have important consequences for differences in the performance of the respective cortices.

What about animals with brains and cortices much larger than those of man, such as elephants or most cetaceans? Shouldn't they be much more intelligent than man or have some superior state of consciousness (a popular assumption for whales and dolphins at least)? As to cetaceans, there is currently a debate on how many neurons their cortices really contain. Their cortex is unusually thin compared with large land mammals and shows a different cytoarchitecture (e.g., no distinct cortical layer IV). Accordingly, experts report a lower number of nerve cells contained in a standard cortical column than in land mammals. However, while Garey and Leuba (1986) report that in dolphins the number of cortical neurons per "standard column" is 2/3 that of land mammals, Güntürkün and von Fersen (1998), after examining the brains of three species of dolphins, reported that this value amounted only to one quarter of that found in land mammals. Accepting this lower value, then—given a cortical surface of about 6,000 cm^2 in dolphins (three times that of man)—the cortex of the bottle-nosed dolphin (*Tursiops truncatus*) should contain three quarters of the corresponding number found in humans (6×10^{10}), which is about equal to the number of cortical neurons estimated for chimpanzees. Calculations of the number of cortical neurons in cetaceans with much larger brains and cortices (e.g., in the sperm whale, with a cortical surface of more than 10,000 cm^2) are difficult, because precise data on cortical nerve cell numbers per "standard" cortical column are lacking. However, even assuming that—due to enormous expansion of the cortex—the respective value is only 1/8 of that found in land mammals, a sperm whale cortex should contain approximately the same number of cortical neurons as that of a dolphin. Based on these calculations, we should expect cetaceans to be roughly as intelligent as nonhuman great apes, which is what cognitive behaviorists have found out about these animals.

The case of elephants remains. They have a similarly enormous brain (around 4 kg) and cortex of about 8,000 cm^2, which is not only thicker than that of cetaceans but also possesses a "normal" six-layered structure. Assuming that the number of cortical neurons is 2/3 the value found in primates, elephants should have at least as many cortical neurons and cortical synapses as humans. Again, we do not know enough about the organization of the cortex of elephants, but

elephants should come close to the cognitive and mental capabilities of man, if only the number of cortical neurons and synapses counted.

Perhaps it might be safer to restrict our consideration to the size of the associative cortex, since—as I mentioned at the outset—different kinds of consciousness are necessarily bound to the activity of specific parts of it. There is a common belief that the associative cortex had increased dramatically in both absolute and relative terms during hominid brain evolution, and that this was the basis for the uniqueness of the human mind. However, such an increase is difficult to assess, since there are no precise criteria for distinguishing primary and secondary sensory cortical areas from true association areas. Kaas (1995) has argued that the number of cortical areas increased dramatically from about 20 such areas in the hypothetical insectivore-like ancestor to more than 60 in primates. However, what increased—according to Kaas—was the number of functionally "intermediate" areas (such as V3 or MT), rather than either the primary or the "highly associative" areas. Furthermore, Kaas is right to warn about the danger of greatly underestimating the number of functionally different cortical areas in small-brained mammals.

Available data suggest that—contrary to common belief—the associative cortex has increased roughly in proportion to an increase in brain and cortical size. This apparently is the case with the prefrontal cortex (PFC) which is regarded by many neuroscientists and neurophilosophers as the true seat of consciousness. Anatomically, the prefrontal cortex is defined as the cortical area with major (though not exclusive) input from the mediodorsal thalamic nucleus (Uylings et al. 1990; Roberts et al. 1998). Using this definition, it turns out that the PFC has increased isometrically with an increase in cortical and overall brain volume within groups of mammals, but here again we find an additional increase in relative PFC size with an increase in absolute brain size across mammalian orders: In rats, PFC constitutes 6.5 percent; in dogs, 8.7 percent; in cows, 9.8 percent; and in man, 10.6 percent of brain mass (Jerison 1997). The human PFC has exactly the size expected according to primate brain allometry. Of course, cetaceans as well as elephants have prefrontal cortices that are much larger in absolute terms than the human PFC, but what they do with this massive "highest" brain center remains a mystery.

We have not yet found anything in brain anatomy that would explain the factual or alleged superiority of humans regarding cognition and consciousness. Given the fact that *Homo sapiens* has an absolutely and relatively large brain and cortex, he appears to be the animal with the highest number of cortical neurons and/or synapses, with the probable exception of elephants. Thus, in this respect he is not extraordinary. What remains is the question of whether there are any anatomical or physiological specializations in the human cortex that could be correlated with the "higher" cognitive abilities and states of consciousness attributed to man. As to the general cytoarchitecture of the human cortex, it is indistinguishable from that of other primates and most other mammals. Likewise, no differences have been discovered so far between humans and nonhuman mammals with respect to short-term or long-term plasticity of cortical neurons, the action of neuromodulators, and so on. Only two things have been discovered that could drastically distinguish the human cortex from that of other primates: (1) differences in growth rate and length of period of growth and (2) the presence of the Broca speech center.

As to (1), maturation of the brain is more or less completed at 2 years after birth in prosimians and 6–8 years in monkeys and and nonhuman apes, but the human brain continues to mature until the age of 20, much longer than in any other primate (Pilbeam and Gould 1974). A critical phase in the development of the human brain seems to occur around the age of 2.5 years. At this time, major anatomical rearrangements

in the associative cortex come to a stop, and the period of "fine-tuning" appears to start, particularly in layer III of the prefrontal cortex (Mrzljak et al. 1990). As mentioned above, at this time human children "take off" cognitively compared with nonhuman primates. Without doubt, the drastically prolonged period of brain development constitutes one important basis for an increased capability of learning and memory formation.

The other exception concerns the presence in the frontal lobe of the Broca speech center (see figure 5.3b), which is responsible for temporal aspects of language including syntax, along with the Wernicke speech center in the temporal lobe, which is responsible for the meaning of words and sentences (although meaning is likewise dependent on syntax and grammar). It is unclear whether these speech centers are true evolutionary novelties. All mammals studied so far have a center for intraspecific communication within the temporal lobe (mostly left) that may be homologous to the Wernicke center. It has been reported that destruction of these areas leads to deficits in intraspecific vocal communication (Heffner and Heffner 1995). In addition, it has long been argued that the posterior part (A 44) of the Broca speech center in humans and the ventral premotor area of nonhuman primates are probably homologous (Preuss 1995). The ventral premotor area controls the movement of forelimbs, face, and mouth, as does the posterior portion of the Broca area.

According to a number of primatologists, nonhuman primates lack a direct connection between the motor cortex and the nucleus ambiguus, where the laryngeal motor neurons are situated. In man, bilateral destruction of the facial motor cortex abolishes the capacity to produce learned vocalization, including speech or humming a melody; a similar destruction in monkeys has no such consequence (Jürgens 1995). According to a number of experts, the evolutionary basis for human language was an emotionally driven stereotyped language typical of nonhuman primates. During hominid evolution, the cortex gained control over this system such that beyond the initiation of hardwired, innate sounds, a "free" production of sounds and their sequences became possible (Deacon 1990; Jürgens 1995). Such an interpretation, however, contrasts with recent evidence of a high degree of sound learning in monkeys (Zimmermann 1995) and the consequences of destruction of left-hemispheric, Wernicke-like temporal areas in all mammals.

Be that as it may, nonhuman primates, including the great apes, are extremely limited, even in nonvocal speech based on the use of sign language or symbols, and these limitations seem to concern mostly syntax. Accordingly, if anything concerning language in the human brain developed relatively recently or underwent substantial modifications, it was probably the Broca center rather than the Wernicke center. Such an assumption is consistent with the fact that the most clear-cut differences between humans and nonhuman primates concern the syntactical complexity of language. Thus, during hominid evolution, the frontal-prefrontal cortex appears to have been reorganized in such a way that the facial and oral motor cortex and the related subcortical speech centers came under the control of a kind of cortex specialized in all aspects of temporal sequence of events, including the sequence of action (Deacon 1990).

Conclusions

Among all features of vertebrate brains, the size of cortex or structures homologous to the mammalian cortex, as well as the number of neurons and synapses contained in these structures, correlate most clearly with the complexity of cognitive functions, including states of consciousness. This would explain the observed differences in cognition between birds and mammals, on the one hand, and the other tetrapod vertebrates, on the other. Furthermore, with the exception of elephants, whose cognition has not been tested sufficiently, apes (at least gorillas and chimpanzees) and cetaceans with large cortices containing 10 to 100 billion (10^{10}–10^{11}) neurons apparently have cognitive abilities superior to those of other mammals. However, this does not explain the superiority (if it truly exists) of chimpanzees over the gorilla, because gorillas have larger brains and cortices than chimpanzees. The superiority of man over all other animals probably results from a very high number of cortical neurons, a drastically prolonged period of ontogenetic plasticity of cortical synapses, and the presence of centers underlying syntactical language.

There are alternative views to what I have presented here. In his book *The Evolution of Consciousness*, published in 1998, the British animal psychologist Euan MacPhail argues that only humans have consciousness, because only they have language. All animals and all young children before developing language are unconscious, regardless of how complex their behaviors and achievements are. After having reviewed the relevant literature supporting the idea of the existence of at least some states of consciousness in at least some animals, he finds it unconvincing at best, and argues that all achievements of animals which indicate consciousness can be explained more parsimoniously by unconscious associative learning. He assumes a big leap in the evolution of man that consists in a fundamental reorganization of the cortico-hippocampal system, leading from merely implicit associative learning and memory ("knowing how") to explicit declarative learning and memory ("knowing that") as the basis of introspection, self-consciousness, and feeling-consciousness. For MacPhail, "true" syntactical language and consciousness are two sides of the same coin; one cannot exist without the other.

While many of MacPhail's critical comments on the relevant literature on animal consciousness are worth considering, I find his own conception inconsistent. There is no neuroanatomical or neurophysiological evidence for a fundamental reorganization of the cortico-hippocampal system from nonhuman primate ancestors to humans; rather, our hippocampus and its connections with the isocortex are very much like those of other primates. Furthermore, if we accept MacPhail's view, we should expect that patients without a hippocampus (like H. M.) should be unconscious and unable to speak; similarly, humans without language should have no consciousness, and autistic children, believed by some psychologists to lack self-consciousness, should have neither language nor consciousness. Both apparently are not the case. Most important, we would be forced to assume that animals are capable of unconsciously mastering cognitive tasks that in humans require highest concentration (e.g., following the track of a tiny spot of light on a screen), while at the same time their brains show the same activation pattern.

Thus, it is fair to assume that all vertebrates with larger cortexlike structures, particularly those with cortices showing cross-modality information transfer, have awareness about what is going on around them. This does not necessarily imply a continuous stream of consciousness, because it may be bound to the existence of an autobiographic memory. Self-recognition (as evidenced by the mirror test) apparently requires a large associative, including prefrontal, cortex. The evolution of a syntactical language may have strongly favored the highest states of consciousness, such as self-reflection, thinking, and action-planning. While thinking is not necessarily bound to language, most people think verbally. Furthermore, many concepts typical of the human mind "exist" only linguistically, because we can talk about them (e.g., future events or abstract entities such as society and freedom). It may well be that the evolution of a special type of prefrontal cortex, that dealing with the analysis of the temporal sequence of events, was at the basis of increased capability for action-planning, syntactical language, imitation, and understanding the behavior of others.

Acknowledgment

I am grateful to Prof. H. J. Jerison, UCLA/Hanse Institute for Advanced Study, for his helpful criticism.

References

Aggleton, J. P. (1992). *The Amygdala: Neurobiological Aspects of Emotion, Memory, and Mental Dysfunction.* New York: Wiley; Chichester, UK: Liss.

Aggleton, J. P. (1993). The contribution of the amygdala to normal and abnormal emotional states. *Trends in Neurosciences* 16: 328–333.

Baron-Cohen, S., Leslie, A. M., and Frith, U. (1985). Does the autistic child have a "theory of mind"? Cognition 21: 37–46.

Byrne, R. (1995). *The Thinking Ape: Evolutionary Origins of Intelligence.* Oxford: Oxford University Press.

Corballis, M. C. (1991). *The Lopsided Ape: Evolution of the Generative Mind.* New York: Oxford University Press.

Deacon, T. W. (1990). Rethinking mammalian brain evolution. *American Zoologist* 30: 629–805.

Gardner, R. A., Gardner, T. B., and van Cantfort, T. E. (1989). *Teaching Sign Language to Chimpanzees.* New York: State University of New York Press.

Garey, L. J., and Leuba, G. (1986). A quantitative study of neuronal and glial numerical density in the visual cortex of the bottlenose dolphin: Evidence for a specialized subarea and changes with age. *Journal of Comparative Neurology* 247: 491–496.

Guillery, R. W., Feig, S. L., and Lozsádi, D. A. (1998). Paying attention to the thalamic reticular nucleis. *Trends in Neuroscience* 21: 28–32.

Güntürkün, O., and Fersen, L. von. (1998). Of whales and myths: Numerics of cetcean cortex. In N. Elsner and R. Wehner, eds., *New Neuroethology on the Move. Proceedings of the 26th Göttingen Neurobiology Conference*, vol. 2, 493. Stuttgart: Thieme.

Hassler, R. (1978). Interaction of reticular activating system for vigilance and the truncothalamic and pallidal systems for directing awareness and attention under striatal control. In P. A. Buser und A. Rougeul-Buser, eds., *Cerebral Correlates of Conscious Experience*, 111–129. Amsterdam: Elsevier/North-Holland.

Heffner, H. E., and Heffner, R. S. (1995). Role of auditory cortex in the perception of vocalization by Japanese macaques. In E. Zimmermann, J. D. Newman, and U. Jürgens, eds., *Current Topics in Primate Vocal Communication*, 207–219. New York: Plenum Press.

Jerison, H. J. (1973). *Evolution of the Brain and Intelligence*. New York: Academic Press.

Jerison, H. J. (1991). *Brain Size and the Evolution of Mind*. New York: American Museum of Natural History.

Jerison, H. J. (1997). Evolution of prefrontal cortex. In N. A. Krasnegor, G. R. Lyon, and P. S. Goldman-Rakic, eds., *Development of the Prefrontal Cortex: Evolution, Neurobiology, and Behavior*, 9–26. Baltimore: Brookes.

Jürgens, U. (1995). Neuronal control of vocal production in non-human and human primates. In E. Zimmermann, J. D. Newman, and U. Jürgens, eds., *Current Topics in Primate Vocal Communication*, 199–206. New York: Plenum Press.

Kaas, J. H. (1995). The evolution of isocortex. *Brain* 46: 187–196.

Karten, H. J. (1991). Homology and evolutionary origins of the "neocortex." Brain, Behavior, and Evolution 38: 264–272.

Kinsbourne, M. (1995). Models of consciousness: Serial or parallel in the brain? In M. S. Gazzaniga et al., eds., *The Cognitive Neurosciences*, 1321–1329. Cambridge, MA: MIT Press.

Knight, R. T., and Grabowecky, M. (1995). Escape from linear time: Prefrontal cortex and conscious experience. In M. S. Gazzaniga et al., eds., *The Cognitive Neurosciences*, 1357–1371. Cambridge, MA: MIT Press.

Locke, J. L. (1995). Linguistic capacity: An ontogenetic theory with evolutionary implications. In E. Zimmermann, J. D. Newman, and U. Jürgens, eds., *Current Topics in Primate Vocal Communication*, 253–272. New York: Plenum Press.

MacPhail, E. (1998). *The Evolution of Consciousness*. Oxford: Oxford University Press.

Marino, L. (1998). A comparison of encephalization between odontocete cetaceans and anthropoid primates. *Brain, Behavior and Evolution* 51: 230–238.

Markowitsch, H. J. (1992). *Neuropsychologie des Gedächtnisses*. Göttingen: Hogrefe.

Markowitsch, H. J. (1999). *Gedächtnisstörungen*. Stuttgart: Kohlhammer.

Marten, K., and Psakaros, S. (1994). Evidence of self-awarenes in the bottlenose dolphin (*Tursiops truncatus*). In T. Parker, R. W. Mitchell, and M. L. Boccia, eds., *Self-Awareness in Animals and Humans: Developmental Perspectives*, 361–379. Cambridge: Cambridge University Press.

Meltzoff, A., and Gopnik, A. (1993). The role of imitation in understanding persons and developing a theory of mind. In S. Baron-Cohen, H. Tager-Flusberg, and D. J. Cohen, eds., *Understanding Other Minds: Perspectives from Autism*, 335–366. Oxford: Oxford University Press.

Mitchell, R. W. (1994). Mental models of mirror-self-recognition: Two theories. *New Ideas in Psychology* 11: 295–325.

Moscovitch, M. (1995). Models of consciousness and memory. In M. S. Gazzaniga et al., eds., *The Cognitive Neurosciences*, 1341–1356. Cambridge, MA: MIT Press.

Mrzljak, L., Uylings, H. B. M., van Eden, C. G., and Judás, M. (1990). Neuronal development in human prefrontal cortex in prenatal and postnatal stages. In H. B. M. Uylings, C. G. van Eden, J. P. C. de Bruin, M. A. Corner, and M. G. P. Feenstra, eds., *The Prefrontal Cortex: Its Structure, Function and Pathology*, 185–222. Amsterdam: Elsevier.

Nieuwenhuys, R., ten Donkelaar, H. J., and Nicholson, C. (1998). *The Central Nervous System of Vertebrates*. Vol. 3. Berlin: Springer-Verlag.

Nieuwenhuys, R., Voogd, J., and van Huijzen, C. (1988). *The Human Central Nervous System*. Berlin: Springer-Verlag. German ed.: *Das Zentralnervensystem des Menschen*. Berlin: Springer-Verlag, 1991.

Northcutt, R. G., and Kaas, J. H. (1995). The emergence and evolution of mammalian isocortex. *Trends in Neurosciences* 18: 373–379.

Passingham, R. (1993). *The Frontal Lobes and Voluntary Action*. Oxford: Oxford University Press.

Pearce, J. M. (1997). *Animal Learning and Cognition*. Exeter: Psychology Press.

Pilbeam, D., and Gould, S. J. (1974). Size and scaling in human evolution. *Science* 186: 892–901.

Posner, M. I. (1994). Seeing the mind. *Science* 262: 673–674.

Preuss, T. M. (1995). Do rats have a prefrontal cortex? The Rose-Woolsey-Akert program reconsidered. *Journal of Cognitive Neuroscience* 7: 1–24.

Robbins, T. W. (1997). Arousal systems and attentional processes. *Biology and Psychology* 45: 57–81.

Robbins, T. W., and Everitt, B. J. (1995). Arousal systems and attention. In M. S. Gazzaniga et al., eds., *The Cognitive Neurosciences*, 243–262. Cambridge, MA: MIT Press.

Roberts, A. C., Robbins, T. W., and Weiskrantz, L. (1998). *The Prefrontal Cortex: Executive and Cognitive Functions*. Oxford: Oxford University Press.

Rockel, A. J., Hiorns, W., and Powell, T. P. S. (1980). The basic uniformity in structure of the neocortex. *Brain* 103: 221–244.

Roland, P. E., Larsen, B., Lassen, N. A., and Skinhut, E. (1980). Supplementary motor area and other cortical areas in organization of voluntary movements in man. *Journal of Neurophysiology* 43: 118–136.

Roth, G., and Wullimann, M. F. (1996). Die Evolution des Nervensystems und der Sinnesorgane. In J. Dudel, R. Menzel, and R. F. Schmidt, eds., *Lehrbuch der Neurowissenschaft*, 1–31. Weinheim: VCH.

Savage-Rumbaugh, S. (1984). Acquisition of functional symbol usage in apes and children. In H. L. Roitblat, T. G. Bever, and H. S Terrace, eds., *Animal Cognition*, 291–310. Hillsdale, NJ: Lawrence Erlbaum.

Schüz, A., and Palm, G. (1989). Density of neurons and synapses in the cerebral cortex of the mouse. *Journal of Comparative Neurology* 286: 442–455.

Squire, L. R. (1987). *Memory and Brain*. New York: Oxford University Press.

Squire, L. R., and Knowlton, B. (1995). Memory, hippocampus, and brain systems. In M. S. Gazzaniga et al., eds., *The Cognitive Neurosciences*, 825–836. Cambridge, MA: MIT Press.

Stamp Dawkins, M. (1993). *Through Our Eyes Only? The Search for Animal Consciousness*. Oxford: W. H. Freeman; Heidelberg, Spektrum. German ed.: *Die Entdeckung des tierischen Bewußtseins*. Heidelberg: Spektrum Akademischer Verlag, 1994.

Stromswold, K. (1995). The cognitive and neural bases of language acquisition. In M. S. Gazzaniga et al., eds., *The Cognitive Neurosciences*, 855–870. Cambridge, MA: MIT Press.

Uylings, H. B. M., and van Eden, C. G. (1990). Qualitative and quantitative comparison of the prefrontal cortex in rat and in primates, including humans. In H. B. M. Uylings et al. (eds.), *The Prefrontal Cortex: Its Structure, Function and Pathology*, 31–62. New York: Oxford University Press.

Visalberghi, E., and Limongelli, L. (1994). Lack of comprehension of cause–effect relationships in tool-using capuchin monkeys (*Cebus apella*). *Journal of Comparative Psychology* 108: 15–22.

Voitko, M. L. (1996). Cognitive functions of the basal forebrain cholinergic system in monkeys: Memory or attention? *Behavioral Brain Research* 75: 13–25.

Zimmermann, E. (1995). Loud calls in nocturnal prosimians: Structure, evolution and ontogeny. In E. Zimmermann, J. D. Newman, and U. Jürgens, eds., *Current Topics in Primate Vocal Communication*, 47–82. New York: Plenum Press.

Zimmermann, E., Newman, J. D., and Jürgens, U., eds. (1995). *Current Topics in Primate Vocal Communication*. New York: Plenum Press.

CANDIDATES FOR THE NCC I: REPRESENTATIONAL DYNAMICS

What the four contributions in this first thematic section have in common is that they investigate certain characteristic features of the representational content activated during the process of conscious experience. Today, one centrally important question is: Are there necessary conditions for any representational state to become a *phenomenal* representational state? What are neurobiological and functional constraints on the space of possible representational architectures for consciousness that could yield the sufficient conditions for the presence of subjective awareness, relative to a certain class of organisms? A classical issue in this debate is constituted by the "homunculus problem": Is there an entity that "interprets" and integrates all currently active representations on the level of consciousness?

Francis Crick and Christof Koch have from the very beginning been at the forefront of the search for a neural correlate of consciousness (NCC). In their contribution to this volume they focus on recent evidence that part of the brain acts in a "zombielike" fashion, producing motor output using visual input that is not available to conscious experience. They start off by reexamining Ray Jackendoff's "intermediate-level theory" of consciousness (1987), and the conceptual distinction between computational and phenomenological mind there introduced. They then attempt to offer a solution to the homunculus problem by postulating an *unconscious homunculus*. This homunculus receives information about the world through the senses, thinks, and plans and executes voluntary actions. However, what generates the contents of our conscious self-experience is only a representation of a subset of the activities of this unconscious homunculus. One of the provocative consequences of this approach is that our thoughts "as such" are never conscious. What we are conscious of is imagery—for instance, a higher-order representation of possible, unexecuted speech acts belonging to the unconscious homunculus. According to the speculative vision proposed by Crick and Koch, what is accessible to consciousness and what is actually given to us in subjective experience are not mental activities like thought, planning, or intentions. What we experience is the phenomenal content of certain sensory representations *associated* with these activities—the cognitive shadow of the zombie within, as it were.

What is the deep representational structure of conscious states? Antonio Damasio in his contribution focuses on a theoretical issue, the importance of which is hard to underestimate: The contents of phenomenal states are never formed by pure perceptual objects or external states of affairs alone. Neither do they solely depict a subject component, an isolated phenomenal self, as it were. In standard situations the representational content of phenomenal experience is a dynamic *relationship*: It portrays the experiencing subject as currently being transformed into a new state by its ongoing interaction with a certain object. (See also chapter 20 in this volume.) It is Damasio's deep sensitivity to the subtlety of the philosophical issues connected with the problem of consciousness that causes him to introduce this second, extended aspect into the empirical debate. In his essay he moves on to another classical motif: consciousness as the result of a higher-order form of mental representation. This is reflected in his concept of a "second-order map." Second-order maps are nonconceptual, neurally realized representations of the causal sequence of events that have led to the organism's being changed by its contact with a given object. These maps then lead to an integrated image of the organism being perturbed, as it were, by objective events in the world, of a unified self *in the act of knowing*. The neural correlates of these second-order mapping processes will clearly constitute a significant portion of the NCC. Based on extensive empirical evidence generated in the context of his research program, Damasio has a number of concrete proposals to make.

One central feature of any successful theory of consciousness will be an explanation for the obvious phenomenological fact that, on numerous levels of analysis, subjective experience consists in the formation of coherent wholes. Conscious representations always are *integrated* representations. (For related perspectives see Metzinger 1995; von der Malsburg 1997.) Wolf Singer offers a series of detailed considerations regarding the structure of neuronal representations underlying phenomenal awareness, focusing on the relevance of synchronicity as a general code for relatedness. He starts off by making the conceptual assumption that consciousness emerges from the transient formation of metarepresentations, then proposes that such metarepresentations are formed by *iterating* precisely the same coding mechanism that is used by the brain to represent features of the external world and bind them into objects. This coding strategy consists in the self-organization of functionally coherent cell assemblies through the transient synchronization of the discharges of all neurons involved. Singer demonstrates that in many cases the conditions necessary for synchronization phenomena to occur and for the activation of a consciously experienced percept are very similar, and that in this respect research programs looking for the neural correlate of consciousness converge with those investigating mechanisms for coherently representing the *external* world.

With regard to strength and temporal precision, there seems to be little difference between neural synchronicity generated by external events and synchronicity caused by internal grouping operations, which in turn might lead to large and widely distributed assemblies of neurons generating the emergence of an *inner* world. However, Singer has an important point to make about self-consciousness: In this case we are confronted with a very special form of phenomenal content, which emerges from social interactions between human beings, and not from internal mechanisms alone (see also chapter 22 in this volume). Therefore, phenomenal self-consciousness carries the status of a cultural construct, which cannot be adequately grasped under a reductionistic neurobiological approach alone.

Conscious experience not only is the result of a highly integrated type of representational dynamics, it is also highly differentiated: Doing phenomenological justice to the target phenomenon means doing justice to the fact that it comes in an inconceivably large number of different forms of contents and sensory nuances. How can we find a theoretical framework that offers the conceptual tools to *simultaneously* capture the holism and the internal complexity of the phenomenon? Gerald Edelman and Giulio Tononi point out that the ability to differentiate among a large repertoire of possibilities—which is one of the most prominent features of conscious experience—clearly constitutes information in the classical sense of a "reduction of uncertainty." Subjective experience in its discriminative structure is not only highly informative; it also renders this information causally relevant by making it available for speech and rationally guided action. Edelman and Tononi conclude that the neural correlate of consciousness must be a distributed neural process which can be described as a *functional cluster*, combining a high internal correlation strength between its elements with the existence of distinct functional borders. They call this the "dynamic core hypothesis." The hypothesis states that any group of neurons can contribute directly to conscious experience only if it is part of a distributed functional cluster which, through reentrant interactions in the thalamocortical system, achieves high integration in a few hundreds of milliseconds. At the same time, it is essential that this functional cluster possess high values of complexity. The authors review recent evidence supporting this new theoretical model. Edelman and Tononi also point out a number of interesting new questions that, under the dynamic core hypothesis, can now be posed and empirically investigated in a precise and promising manner.

Further Reading

Crick, F. (1994). *The Astonishing Hypothesis*. New York: Charles Scribner's Sons.

Crick, F. H. C., and Koch, C. (1990). Towards a neurobiological theory of consciousness. *Seminars in the Neurosciences* 2: 263–275.

Crick, F. H. C., and Koch, C. (1998). Consciousness and neuroscience. *Cerebral Cortex* 8: 97–107.

Damasio, A. (1994). *Descartes' Error*. New York: Putnam/Grosset.

Damasio, A. (1999). *The Feeling of What Happens: Body and Emotion in the Making of Consciousness.* New York: Harcourt Brace.

Damasio, H., Grabowski, T. J., Tranel, D., Hichwa, R., and Damasio, A. R. (1996). A neural basis for lexical retrieval. *Nature* 380: 499–505.

Edelman, G. M. (1987). *Neural Darwinism: The Theory of Neuronal Group Selection.* New York: Basic Books.

Edelman, G. M. (1989). *The Remembered Present: A Biological Theory of Consciousness.* New York: Basic Books.

Edelman, G. M., and Tononi, G. (2000). *Consciousness: How Matter Becomes Imagination.* New York: Basic Books.

Herculano-Houzel, S., Munk, M. H. J., Neuenschwander, S., and Singer, W. (1999). Precisely synchronized oscillatory firing patterns require electroencephalographic activation. *Journal of Neuroscience* 19: 3992–4010.

Jackendoff, R. (1987). *Consciousness and the Computational Mind.* Cambridge, MA: MIT Press.

Koch, C., and Braun, J. (1996). Toward the neuronal correlate of visual awareness. *Current Opinion in Neurobiology* 6: 158–164.

Koch, C., and Davis, J. L., eds. (1994). *Large-Scale Neuronal Theories of the Brain.* Cambridge, MA: MIT Press.

Metzinger, T. (1995). Faster than thought: Holism, homogeneity and temporal coding. In T. Metzinger, ed., *Conscious Experience.* Thorverton, UK: Imprint Academic; Paderborn: Mentis.

Milner, A. D., and Goodale, M. A. (1995). *The Visual Brain in Action.* Oxford: Oxford University Press.

Singer, W. (2000). Response synchronization: A universal coding strategy for the definition of relations. In M. S. Gazzaniga, ed., *The New Cognitive Neurosciences.* 2nd ed. Cambridge, MA: MIT Press.

Singer, W., Engel, A. K., Kreiter, A. K., Munk, M. H. J., Neuenschwander, S., and Roelfsema, P. R. (1997).

Neuronal assemblies: Necessity, signature and detectability. *Trends in Cognitive Sciences* 1: 252–261.

Tononi, G., and Edelman, G. M. (1998a) Consciousness and complexity. *Science* 282: 1846–1851.

Tononi, G., and Edelman, G. M. (1998b). Consciousness and the integration of information in the brain. In H. H. Jasper et al., eds., *Consciousness: At the Frontiers of Neuroscience.* Philadelphia: Lippincott-Raven.

Tononi, G., Sporns, O., and Edelman, G. M. (1994). A measure for brain complexity: Relating functional segregation and integration in the nervous system. *Proceedings of the National Academy of Sciences of the United States of America* 91: 5033–5037.

Tononi, G., Srinivasan, R., Russell, D. P., and Edelman, G. M. (1998). Investigating neural correlates of conscious perception by frequency-tagged neuromagnetic responses. *Proceedings of the National Academy of Sciences of the United States of America* 95: 3198–3203.

von der Malsburg, C. (1997). The coherence definition of consciousness. In M. Ito, Y. Myashita, and E. T. Rolls, eds., *Cognition, Computation, and Consciousness.* Oxford: Oxford University Press.

Zeki, S., and Bartels, A. (1998). The asynchrony of consciousness. *Proceedings of the Royal Society of London* ser. B, 265: 1583–1585.

6 The Unconscious Homunculus

Francis Crick and Christof Koch

It is universally agreed that it is not completely obvious how the activity of the brain produces our sensory experiences and, more generally, how it produces consciousness. This is what Chalmers has dubbed *the hard problem* (Chalmers 1996). Philosophers are divided about the likely nature of the solution to this problem and whether it is, indeed, a problem at all. For a very readable account of the nature of some of their discussions and disagreements, the reader should consult the book edited by Searle (1997), with contributions by Chalmers and Dennett; the anthology edited by Shear (1997); and the collection of essays by Paul and Patricia Churchland (1998).

Our own view is that it is a plausible working assumption that some activity of the brain is all that is necessary to produce consciousness, and that this is the best line to follow unless and until there is clear, decisive evidence to the contrary (as opposed to arguments from ignorance). We suspect that our present ideas about how the brain works are likely to turn out to be inadequate; that radically new ideas may be necessary; and that well-formulated suggestions (even way-out ones) should be carefully considered. However, we also believe that while gedanken-experiments are useful devices for generating new ideas or for suggesting difficulties with existing ideas, they do not lead, in general, to trustworthy conclusions. The problem is one that should be approached scientifically, not logically. That is, any theoretical scheme should be pitted against at least one alternative theory, and *real* experiments should be designed to choose between them. (As an example, see our hypothesis that primates are not directly aware of the neural activity in cortical area V1, the primary visual cortex [Crick and Koch 1995].)

The important first step is to find the neural correlate of consciousness (the NCC) for at least one type of consciousness. We will not repeat here our general approach to the problem, since this has been set out in a recent update of our views (Crick and Koch 1998). In this paper we wish to venture a step further by asking what can be said about the precise nature of qualia from an introspective, first-person perspective. Another way to look at the matter is to emphasize that it is qualia which are at the root of the hard problem, and that one needs to have a clear idea of exactly under what circumstances qualia occur.

The Intermediate-Level Theory of Consciousness

In earlier publications about the visual system of primates (Crick and Koch 1995), we suggested that the biological usefulness of visual consciousness in humans is to produce the best current interpretation of the visual scene in the light of past experience, either of ourselves or of our ancestors (embodied in our genes), and to make this interpretation directly available—for a sufficient amount of time—to the parts of the brain that plan possible voluntary motor outputs of one sort or another, including speech.

Philosophers have invented a creature they call a "zombie," who is supposed to act just as normal people do but to be completely unconscious (Chalmers 1995). While strictly logically possible, this seems to us to be an untenable scientific idea, although there is now suggestive evidence that *part* of the brain does behave like a zombie. That is, in some cases, a person uses current visual input to produce a relevant motor output without being able to say what was seen. Milner and Goodale (1995) point out that a frog has at least two independent systems for action. These may well be unconscious. One is used by the frog to snap at small, preylike objects, and the other is used for jumping away from large, looming objects. Why does our brain not consist simply of a series of such specialized zombie systems? We proposed (Crick and Koch 1995) that such an arrangement is inefficient when very many such systems are required. Better to produce a single but complex representation and make it available for a sufficient time to the parts of the brain that make a choice among many different but possible plans for action. This, in our view, is what seeing is about.

Milner and Goodale (1995) suggest that in primates there are two systems, which we have called the on-line and the seeing systems. The latter is conscious, whereas the former, acting more rapidly, is not. If a bundle of such unconscious, specialized on-line systems could do everything more efficiently than our present arrangement, we would not be conscious of anything.

We decided to reexamine the ideas of Ray Jackendoff (1987) as expressed in his book *Consciousness and the Computational Mind*, in which he put forward the intermediate-level theory of consciousness. Jackendoff's book, which is based on a detailed knowledge of cognitive science, is a closely argued defense of the at-first-sight paradoxical idea that we are not directly conscious of our thoughts, but only of a representation of them in sensory terms. His argument is based on a deep knowledge of modern linguistics and the structure of music, though he also makes some suggestions about the visual system.

Let us first consider Jackendoff's overall view of the mind/brain problem. His analysis postulates three very different domains:

1. The brain

2. The computational mind

3. The phenomenological mind.

The brain domain includes both the neurons (and associated cells) and their activities. The computational mind handles information by doing a series of computations on it. The computational mind is not concerned with exactly how these computations are implemented—this is the standard AI view—but takes for granted that neural instantiation will eventually play an important role in constraining the theory. The phenomenological mind consists of qualia such as blueness, saltiness, painfulness, and so on. Jackendoff confesses he has no idea how blueness and the other experiences arise out of computation (Chalmers's hard problem). What he is concerned with is which types of computations have qualia associated with them. He is less concerned with the main problem that interests us, which is how some activities of the brain correlate with qualia, though he would agree with us that, roughly speaking, it is the transient results of the computations which correlate with qualia; most of the computations leading up to those results are likely to be *un*conscious. But since computations are implemented in neuronal hardware, these two questions can be connected by asking which parts of the brain are responsible for which computations.

Jackendoff remarks that common sense seems to tell us that awareness and thought are inseparable, and that introspection can reveal the contents of the mind. He argues at length that both these beliefs are untrue. They contrast strongly with his conclusion that thinking is largely unconscious. What is conscious about thoughts is akin to having visual images or talking to oneself. He maintains that visual and verbal images are associated with intermediate-level sensory representations, which in turn are generated from thoughts by the fast processing mechanisms in short-term memory. Both the process of thought *and its content* are not directly accessible to awareness.

An example may make this clearer. A bilingual person can express a thought in either language, but the thought itself, which generates the verbal activity or imagery, is not *directly* accessible to him except in these sensory forms.

Another way of stating these ideas is to say that most of what we are directly aware of falls under two broad headings:

1. A representation of the outer world (including our bodies)

2. A representation of the inner world; that is, of our thoughts.

This implies that we are *directly* aware neither of the outer world nor of the inner world, although we have the persistent illusion that we are. Curiously enough, this idea, which seems very appealing to us, has attracted rather little attention from brain scientists.

To appreciate these arguments, the reader should consult Jackendoff (1987) as well as some updates to these ideas (Jackendoff 1996). For the visual system he proposed ideas based on the theories of David Marr. Marr argued in his posthumously published book *Vision* (1982) that it would almost certainly be impossible for the brain to arrive at a visual representation, corresponding to what we consciously see, in only one step. He therefore suggested a hypothetical series of stages. In his analysis he concentrated on the documentation of shape, though he realized that a fuller treatment would include movement, texture, and color.

Marr proposed four possible stages. The first he called "Image" (there might be several such steps). This represents the light intensity value at each point in the visual image. The second he called the "Primal sketch." This makes explicit important information about the two-dimensional image, such as edge segments and terminations. The third stage was the "2-1/2D sketch." This makes explicit the orientation and rough depth of the visible surfaces, as well as discontinuities in orientation and depth, in a *viewer-centered* coordinate frame. The fourth and final step he called the "3D model representation." This describes shapes and their special organization in an *object-centered* frame.

Work on the visual system of the macaque does indeed suggest that it consists of a series of stages (Felleman and Van Essen 1991), and that these follow one another along the broad lines suggested by Marr. The system probably does not display the exact stages he suggested, however, and probably is considerably more compli-

cated. For the sake of convenience, though, we will continue to use his nomenclature.

Jackendoff proposes that we are directly conscious of an extended version of something corresponding roughly to Marr's 2-1/2D sketch but not to his 3D model. For instance, when we look at a person's face, we are directly conscious of the shape, color, movement, and so on, of the front of the face (like the 2-1/2D sketch) but not of the back of the head, though we can imagine what the back of the head might look like, deriving this image from a 3D model of the head of which we are not *directly* conscious.

The experimental evidence shows that the higher levels of the visual system, in the various inferotemporal regions, have neurons that appear to respond mainly to something like an enriched 2-1/2D sketch, and show a certain amount of size, position, and rotation invariance. This has been especially studied for faces and, more recently, for artificial bent-wire 3D shapes (Perrett et al. 1994; Logothetis et al. 1995; Logothetis and Pauls 1995). We will discuss these results more fully later.

Similar Suggestions

We have located three other suggestions along similar lines. There are probably more (for a philosophical perspective, see Metzinger 1995; for a dissenting view, see Siewert 1998), though one should distinguish between suggestions that the *processes* of thought are unconscious, and those which also propose that the contents are unconscious.

The first is due to Sigmund Freud. Consider this quotation from his essay "The Unconscious," published in 1915:

In psycho-analysis there is no choice but for us to assert that mental processes are in themselves unconscious, and to liken the perception of them by means of consciousness to the perception of the external world by means of sense-organs. (Freud 1915: 270).

(The quotation was brought to our attention in a draft paper by Mark Solms.) Freud arrived at this idea from his studies of disturbed patients. He found that without making this assumption, he was unable to explain or even describe a large variety of phenomena he came across.

The second is due to Karl Lashley. In his provocative 1956 book *Cerebral Organization and Behaviour*, he stated:

No activity of mind is ever conscious. This sounds like a paradox, but it is nonetheless true. There are order and arrangement, but there is no experience of the creation of that order. I could give numberless examples, for there is no exception to the rule. A couple of illustrations should suffice. Look at a complicated scene. It consists of a number of objects standing out against an indistinct background: desk, chairs, faces. Each consists of a number of lesser sensations combined in the object, but there is no experience of putting them together. The objects are immediately present. When we think in words, the thoughts come in grammatical form with subject, verb, object, and modifying clauses falling into place without our having the slightest perception of how the sentence structure is produced.... Experience clearly gives no clue as to the means by which it is organized. (Lashley 1956: 4)

In other words, Lashley believed that the processes underlying thoughts, imagery, silent speech, and so on are unconscious; only their content may be accessible to consciousness.

We discovered the third suggestion in a brief report of a meeting on consciousness (*Journal of Consciousness Studies* 4 [1997]: 396), outlining the ideas of Richard Stevens (1997). In brief, from periods of closely observed introspection he concluded that

Conscious awareness is essentially perceptual. It consists entirely of perceptual images. These may be directly stimulated by outside events or internally generated in the more elusive and less well defined form of remembered or imagined percepts.

Among perceptual images Stevens includes unspoken speech. This is in striking agreement with Jackendoff's ideas, which were largely unknown to him. Stevens also makes the point that consciousness is necessary for certain forms of evaluations, because it is only when thoughts and possibilities are conscious, in the form of words and/or images, that we can begin to compare and contrast them.

Though we do not want to endorse all Freud's ideas, nor his unscientific approach to problems, it is remarkable that several authors—Freud, Jackendoff, and Stevens—arrived at broadly the same conclusion from significantly different evidence. The question "How do I know what I think till I hear what I say?" shows that the idea is not unknown to ordinary people.

Let us assume, therefore, that qualia are associated with sensory percepts, and make a few rather obvious points about them. Apart from the fact that they differ from each other (red is quite different from blue, and both from a pain, or a sound), qualia also differ in intensity and duration. Thus the qualia associated with the visual world, in a good light, are more vivid than a recollection of the same visual scene (vivid visual recollections are usually called hallucinations). A quale can be very transient, passing so quickly that we have little or no recollection of it. Neither of these properties is likely to cause any special difficulties when we consider the behavior of neurons, since neurons can easily express intensity and duration.

However, there is a class of conscious percepts that have a rather different character from straightforward sensory percepts. Jackendoff originally used the term "affect" to describe them, though more recently he has used the term "valuation" (Jackendoff 1996). Examples would be a feeling of familiarity or of novelty, or the tip-of-the-tongue feeling, and all the various emotions. It is not clear whether these feelings exist in their own right, or are merely certain mixtures of various bodily sensations. Stevens (1997) discusses "feels" associated with particular percepts, images, or words. We propose to leave these more diffuse percepts on one side for the moment, though eventually they, too, will have to be explained in neural terms.

The Homunculus

The homunculus is usually thought of as a "little man inside the head" who perceives the world through the senses, thinks, and plans and executes voluntary actions. In following up this idea, we came across a "Comment" by Fred Attneave (1961), "In Defense of Homunculi." He lists two kinds of objections to a homunculus. The first is an aversion to dualism, since it might involve "a fluffy kind of nonmatter ... quite beyond the pale of scientific investigation." The second has to do with the supposed regressive nature of the concept; who is looking at the brain states of the homunculus? Attneave notes that "We fall into a regress only if we try to make the homunculus do everything. The moment we specify certain processes that occur outside the homunculus, we are merely classifying or portioning psychoneural functions; the classification may be crude but it is not itself regressive" (Attneave 1961: 778). He puts forward a very speculative overall block diagram of the brain, involving hierarchical sensory processing, an affect system, a motor system, and a part he calls H, the homunculus. It is reciprocally connected to the perceptual machinery at various levels in the hierarchy, not merely the higher ones. It receives input from the affective centers and projects to the motor machinery. (There are other details about reflexes, skills, proprioception, etc.) He emphasizes that his scheme avoids the difficulty of an infinite regress.

Attneave tentatively locates the homunculus in a subcortical area, such as the reticular formation, and he considers it to be conscious. Yet his basic idea is otherwise very similar to the one discussed above. We all have this illusion of a homunculus inside the brain (that's what "I" am), so this illusion needs an explanation. The problem of the infinite regress is avoided in our case because the true homunculus is *un*conscious, and only a representation of it enters consciousness. This puts the problem of consciousness in a somewhat new light. We have therefore named this type of theory as one postulating an *unconscious homunculus*, wherever it may be located in the brain. The unconscious homunculus receives information about the world through the senses, thinks, and plans and executes "voluntary" actions. What becomes conscious, then, is a representation of some of the activities of the unconscious homunculus in the form of imagery and spoken and unspoken speech. Notice that this idea does not, by itself, explain how qualia arise.

The concept of the unconscious homunculus is not a trivial one. It does throw a new light on certain other theoretical approaches. For example, it may make Penrose's worries about consciousness unnecessary. Penrose (1989, 1997) has argued that present-day physics is not capable of explaining how mathematicians think, but if all such thinking is necessarily *un*conscious—and mathematicians have testified (Hadamard 1945) that certainly some of it is—then although something such as quantum gravity may be needed for certain types of thinking, it may not be required to explain consciousness as such. Penrose has given no argument that sensory experiences themselves are difficult to explain in terms of present-day physics.

Possible Experimental Approaches

In approaching a system as complex as the brain, it is important to have some idea, however provisional, of what to look for. Let us therefore follow these authors and adopt the idea of the unconscious homunculus as a tentative working hypothesis, then ask what experiments might be done to support it. For the moment we will concentrate on the visual system.

What we are trying to identify is the activity of the brain that produces visual qualia. We have argued (Crick and Koch 1995, 1998) that whatever other properties are involved, we should expect to find neurons whose firing is in some way correlated with the type of qualia being perceived. So it is not unreasonable to ask which are the neurons whose activity is correlated with Marr's 2-1/2D sketch (roughly speaking, the visual features of which we are directly aware) and which are the neurons whose activity is correlated with Marr's 3D model (of which we are only indirectly aware). For the moment we will assume that this latter activity is represented somewhere in the cortex and leave aside other, less likely possibilities, such as in the reticular formation or the claustrum.

As far as we know, there are only two sets of relevant experimental results. The first is due to Perrett and his coworkers in their study on the neurons in the alert macaque monkey that respond to faces (Perrett et al. 1992). Most of the neurons in the higher levels of the visual system that respond to faces fire only to one aspect of the face, usually a specific view. The firing is somewhat independent of scale, of small translations, and of some degree of rotation (Pauls et al. 1996). These neurons look like members of a distributed representation of a particular view of a face, as suggested by the theoretical work of Poggio (1990; see also Poggio and Edelman 1990; Logothetis et al. 1994) and supported (on a lightly anesthetized macaque) by Young and Yamane (1992).

However, Perrett et al. (1992) reported six neurons (4% of the total) that responded to *all* horizontal views of a head: They are view-invariant. These might be taken to be part of a 3D model representation. However, some of the circuits in the hidden layers of a three-level feed forward neural network, trained by back-projection, often have somewhat unusual properties (Sejnowski and Rosenberg 1987), so one could argue that these apparent 3D model neu-

rons are really only a small, accidental part of a 2-1/2D sketch. Against this interpretation, Perrett et al. (1992) claim that these six neurons have a significantly longer latency (130 msec versus 119 msec), suggesting that they are one step higher in the visual hierarchy. The crucial question is whether these neurons are of a different *type* from the view-specific face neurons (for example, project to a different place). This is not known.

The other example comes from the experiments of Logothetis and Pauls (1995) on the responses of the neurons in an alert macaque, again in the higher levels of the visual hierarchy, to artificial paperclip-like models. Again, a minority of neurons (8 of the 773 cells analyzed) responded in a view-independent manner, but in these experiments the latencies were not measured, nor was it known exactly which type of neuron was being recorded (N. Logothetis, personal communication).

A naive interpretation of our general idea would be that the face representations in prefrontal cortex reported by Scalaidhe et al. (1997), would be implemented solely by view-independent neurons, and without any view-dependent ones. As far as we know, this has not yet been studied. While the activity of view-independent neurons should always be unconscious, it does not follow that the activities of all view-independent ones must always be conscious. Our unconscious thoughts will likely involve neurons of this latter type.

We think this simple guess at the location of these two types of neurons is rather unlikely, though we would not be surprised if the percentage of neurons showing view-invariance turns out to be higher in prefrontal areas than the very small fractions reported in inferotemporal cortex. One might also find a higher percentage in such areas as the parahippocampal gyrus and the perihinal cortex leading to the hippocampus. Whether they will also be found in parts of the thalamus and in the amygdala remains an empirically open question.

Another possibility is that, contrary to Jackendoff's suggestion, there is no true, object-centered (3D) visual representation in an explicit form in the brain. That is, object-centered information is never made explicit at the level of individual neurons, instead being coded in an implicit manner across a distributed set of neurons.

Though there are still unconscious computations that lead up to thoughts, the results of the computations are expressed directly in sensory, viewer-centered terms. If this were true, the search for view-invariant neurons in prefrontal cortex would be unsuccessful.

We have briefly considered the visual system. Though they are outside the scope of this paper, the same analysis should be applied to the other sensory systems, such as audition, somato-sensory, olfaction, and pain. It may not always be completely obvious what the difference is between (unconscious) thoughts and the (conscious) sensory representations of those thoughts in these systems. The crucial test to distinguish between these two is whether any qualia are involved beyond mental imagery and unspoken speech (e.g., the putative *noniconic* thoughts of Siewert 1998). We leave this to future investigators.

Another problem concerns our guess that unconscious thought processes may be located in some places in prefrontal cortex. First, it is not clear exactly where prefrontal cortex ends as one proceeds posteriorly, especially in the general region of the insula. Second, the selection of "prefrontal" cortex (or a subset of thereof) in this way seems rather arbitrary. It would be more satisfactory if there were a more operational definition, such as those cortical areas receiving a projection from the basal ganglia via the thalamus (usually thalamic area MD). It is conceivable that the rather rapid sequential winner-take-all operations performed by the basal ganglia may not be compatible with consciousness, but are frequently used by more rapid, unconscious thought processes.

Conclusion

As Stevens (1997) has stated, the picture that emerges from all of this is quite surprising. We are not directly aware of the outer world of sensory events. Instead, we are conscious of the results of some of the computations performed by the nervous system on the various neural representations of this sensory world. These results are expressed in various cortical areas (excluding primary visual cortex; Crick and Koch 1995). Nor are we directly aware of our inner world of thoughts, intentions, and planning (that is, of our unconscious homunculus), but only of the sensory representations associated with these mental activities. What remains is the sobering realization that our subjective world of qualia—what distinguishes us from zombies and fills our life with color, music, smells, and other vivid sensations—is possibly caused by the activity of a small fraction of all the neurons in the brain, located strategically between the outer and the inner worlds. How these act to produce the subjective world that is so dear to us is still a complete mystery.

Acknowledgments

We thank Dave Chalmers, Patricia Churchland, Ray Jackendoff, Thomas Metzinger, Graeme Mitchinson, Roger Penrose, David Perrett, and Tomaso Poggio. We also thank the J. W. Kieckhefer Foundation, the National Institute of Mental Health, the Office of Naval Research, and the National Science Foundation.

References

Attneave, F. (1961). In defense of homunculi. In W. A. Rosenblith, ed., *Sensory Communication*, 777–782. Cambridge, MA.: MIT Press.

Chalmers, D. (1996). *The Conscious Mind: In Search of a Fundamental Theory*. New York: Oxford University Press.

Churchland, P. M., and Churchland, P. S. (1998). *On the Contrary: Critical Essays, 1987–1997.* Cambridge, MA: MIT Press.

Crick, F., and Koch, C. (1995). Are we aware of neural activity in primary visual cortex? *Nature* 375: 121–123.

Crick, F., and Koch, C. (1998). Consciousness and neuroscience. *Cerebral Cortex* 8: 97–107.

Felleman, D. J., and van Essen, D. (1991). Distributed hierarchical processing in the primate cerebral cortex. *Cerebral Cortex* 1: 1–47.

Freud, S. (1915). Das Unbewusste. *Internationale Zeitschrift für Psychoanalyse.* 3, no. 4: 189–203, and 3, no. 5: 257–269.

Hadamard, J. (1945). *The Mathematician's Mind.* Princeton, NJ: Princeton University Press.

Jackendoff, R. (1987). *Consciousness and the Computational Mind.* Cambridge, MA: MIT Press.

Jackendoff, R. (1996). How language helps us think. *Pragmatics and Cognition* 4: 1–34.

Lashley, K. S. (1956). Cerebral organization and behavior. In *The Brain and Human Behavior, Proceedings of the Association for Nervous and Mental Disease,* pp. 1–18. New York: Hafner.

Logothetis, N. K., and Pauls, J. (1995). Psychophysical and physiological evidence for viewer-centered object representations in the primate. *Cerebral Cortex* 3: 270–288.

Logothetis, N. K., Pauls, J., Bülthoff, H. H., and Poggio, T. (1994). View-dependent object recognition by monkeys. *Current Biology* 4: 401–414.

Logothetis, N. K., Pauls, J., and Poggio, T. (1995). Shape representation in the inferior temporal cortex of monkeys. *Current Biology* 5: 552–563.

Marr, D. (1982). *Vision.* San Francisco: W. H. Freeman.

Metzinger, T. (1995). Introduction: The problem of consciousness. In T. Metzinger, ed., *Conscious Syperience.* Paderborn: Mentis.

Milner, A., and Goodale, M. (1995). *The Visual Brain in Action.* Oxford: Oxford University Press.

Pauls, J., Bricolo, E., and Logothetis, N. (1996). View-invariant representations in monkey temporal cortex: Position, scale, and rotational invariance. In S. K. Nayar and T. Poggio, eds., *Early Visual Learning,* 9–41. New York: Oxford University Press.

Penrose, R. (1989). *The Emperor's New Mind.* Oxford: Oxford University Press.

Penrose, R. (1997). *The Large, the Small and the Human Mind.* Cambridge: Cambridge University Press.

Perrett, D. I., Hietanen, J. K., Oram, M. W., and Benson, P. J. (1992). Organization and functions of cells responsive to faces in the temporal cortex. *Philosophical Transactions of the Royal Society of London* ser B., 335: 23–30.

Perrett, D. I., Oram, M. W., Hietanen, J. K., and Benson, P. J. (1994). Issues of representation in object vision. In ed. M. J. Farah and G. Ratcliff, *The Neuropsychology of High-Level Vision,* 33–61. Hillsdale, NJ: Lawrence Erlbaum.

Poggio, T. (1990). A theory of how the brain might work. *Cold Spring Harbor Symposia on Quantitative, Biology* 55: 899–910.

Poggio, T., and Edelman, S. (1990). A network that learns to recognize three-dimensional objects. *Nature* 343: 263–266.

Scalaidhe, S. P. O., Wilson, F. A. W., and Goldman-Rakic, P. S. (1997). Areal segregation of face-processing neurons in prefrontal cortex. *Science* 278: 1135–1138.

Searle, J. R. (1997). *The Mystery of Consciousness.* New York: New York Review of Books.

Sejnowski, T. J., and Rosenberg, C. R. (1987). Parallel networks that learn to pronounce English text. *Complex Systems* 1: 145–168.

Shear, J. (1997). *Explaining Consciousness: The Hard Problem.* Cambridge, MA: MIT Press.

Siewert, C. P. (1998). *The Significance of Consciousness.* Princeton, NJ: Princeton University Press.

Stevens, R. (1997). Western phenomenological approaches to the study of conscious experience and their implications. In J. Richardson and M. Velmans, eds., *Methodologies for the Study of Consciousness: A New Synthesis,* 100–123. Kalamazoo, MI: Fetzer Institute.

Young, M. P., and Yamane, S. (1992). Sparse population coding of faces in the inferotemporal cortex. *Science* 256: 1327–1331.

7 A Neurobiology for Consciousness

Antonio R. Damasio

In this brief survey of my views on the neurobiology of consciousness, I begin by stating what I see as the consciousness problem. I see the problem of consciousness as a combination of two closely related problems. The first is that of understanding how the brain constructs the mental patterns I designate, for short, as the images of an "object." By "image" I mean a mental pattern in any of the sensory modalities, not just visual but also auditory or tactile; by "object" I mean entities as diverse as a person, a place, a song, or a state of sadness. In the simplest of formulations, this first problem of consciousness is the problem of how we get, so to speak, an integrated "movie-in-the-brain," a movie with as many sensory tracks as our nervous system has sensory portals—sight, sound, taste and olfaction, touch, inner body senses, and so forth.

From the perspective of neuroscience, solving this first problem at its roots requires the discovery of how neural patterns are implemented in nerve cell circuits and, eventually, how those neural patterns become the explicit mental patterns or images that I regard as the highest level of biological phenomena. (I take the process of mind to be made of a continuous flow of mental patterns or images, available only in a first-person perspective. For that reason mental patterns or images are distinguishable from neural patterns, which are available to observations made in a third-person perspective. This distinction does not imply a substance dualism, however, since I regard *both* mental patterns and neural patterns as biological phenomena. The level of complexity of the two kinds of phenomena is different but their substance is the same—a biological substance.)

To arrive at the solution of this first problem of consciousness, it is thus necessary to address the philosophical issue of qualia because the fundamental components of the images in the movie metaphor are made of qualia, the simple sensory qualities to be found in the blueness of the sky or in the sound produced by a violin. I believe the mechanism whereby these qualities arise will come to be explained in neurobiological terms, although their current account is quite incomplete and the explanatory gap remarkable.

In many contemporary treatments, some version of this first problem of consciousness is taken to be the *whole* problem of consciousness. As I indicated, however, I believe there is a second problem. This is the problem of how, along with constructing mental patterns for a given object, the brain also constructs a sense of self in the act of knowing the object. It is the problem of how, in parallel with representing the printed words on this page and displaying the conceptual knowledge required to understand those words, your brain also displays something sufficient to indicate, moment by moment, that *you* are doing the reading and the understanding of the text rather than someone else. Besides the images of what you perceive and recall there is this other presence that signifies you as observer and owner of the things imaged, as potential actor on the things imaged. There is a presence of you in a particular relationship with some object. If there were no such presence, your thoughts would not belong to you.

The solution for this second problem requires the understanding of how the images of an object and of the complex matrix of relations, reactions, and plans related to it are sensed as the mental property of an automatic owner, observer, perceiver, knower, thinker, and potential actor. We can be certain that the solution traditionally proposed for the second problem—a homunculus creature in charge of knowing—is not correct, and not acceptable. The mechanism for achieving a sense of self that I shall propose does not use a homunculus at all.

The neurobiology of consciousness faces two problems, then: the problem of how the movie-in-the-brain is generated, and the problem of how the brain also generates the sense that there is an owner and observer of that movie. The second problem is intimately related to the first, which is nested within it. From my standpoint, the second problem is that of generating the appearance of an owner and observer of the movie and placing that owner *within the movie*. In short, solving the problem of consciousness consists of discovering the biological underpinnings not just of the mental patterns of an object but also of the mental patterns that convey the sense of a self in the act of knowing, *such that an owner-based unified perspective can be created regarding events occurring within the organism and in its surroundings*. The unified inner mental pattern we know as consciousness must include, in a blended form, these two primary ingredients—objects and a sense of self.

Some Important Facts from the Neuropsychological Investigation of Consciousness

The ideas surveyed in this paper were inspired largely by observations of neurological patients with disorders of mind and behavior, and by findings from the experimental neuropsychological investigation of those disorders. The results of such studies, along with evidence from general biology, neuroanatomy, and neurophysiology, were used to construct a theory and to design testable hypotheses regarding the neuroanatomical underpinnings of consciousness. The detailed analysis of the pertinent evidence is presented in my book *The Feeling of What Happens*, which lists the supporting references and outlines an ongoing research program in this area.[1] In the pages that follow, I summarize the theoretical framework, the hypotheses, and the available evidence.

The facts revealed by neurological observations and neuropsychological experiments were the starting point for the work reviewed here. A roundup of those facts is in order at this point.

The first fact is that some aspects of the processes of consciousness can be related to the operation of specific brain regions and systems. In the case of the problem of self, the regions and systems are located in a restricted set of neural territories and, just as with functions such as memory or language, promise to yield a neuroanatomy for consciousness.

The second fact is that consciousness can be separated from wakefulness and low-level attention, as is shown by patients who can be awake and attentive without having normal consciousness. Both wakefulness and attention are often taken as synonymous with consciousness, but there are good grounds to separate them as contributive functions instead.

The third fact is that consciousness and emotion are *not* separable. It is usually the case that consciousness and emotion are impaired together, which suggests, at the very least, a contiguity of the neural systems that support consciousness and emotion, and that may be indicative of an ever closer anatomical and functional connection.

The fourth fact is that consciousness can be separated into simple and complex kinds. The simple kind, which I term *core consciousness*, provides the organism with a sense of self about the here and now. Core consciousness does not pertain to the future or the past—the only past briefly illuminated in core consciousness is what occurred in the immediately preceding instant. On the other hand, the complex kind of consciousness, which I term *extended consciousness*, has many levels and grades. Extended consciousness provides the organism with an identity and a person, an elaborate sense of self, and places that self at a specific point in individual historical time. Extended consciousness offers awareness of the lived past and of the anticipated future, along with the objects in the here and now.

Core consciousness is a simple, biological phenomenon. It has one level of organization, it is stable across the lifetime of the organism, and it is not dependent on conventional memory, working memory, reasoning, or language. I believe it is not exclusively human. On the other hand, extended consciousness is a complex biological phenomenon. It has several levels of organization, and it evolves across the lifetime of the organism. It depends on conventional memory and working memory, and when it reaches its peak, it depends on language as well. I believe that simple levels of extended consciousness are present in some nonhumans, but extended consciousness attains its maximal development only in humans.

Core consciousness is the first step in the process of knowing and does not permit the knowledge of a whole being. Extended consciousness, on the other hand, allows a whole being to be known, and both the past and the anticipated future are sensed along with the here and now.

Neurological observations reveal that when extended consciousness is impaired, core consciousness remains unscathed. By contrast, impairments that begin at the level of core consciousness demolish the entire edifice of consciousness, and extended consciousness collapses as well. Extended consciousness is thus not an independent variety of consciousness: It is built on the foundation of core consciousness.

The two kinds of consciousness are associated with two kinds of self. The sense of self that emerges in core consciousness is the *core self*, a transient and repeatedly re-created entity for each and every object with which the brain interacts. The traditional notion of self, however, the self we link to the idea of identity, is the *autobiographical self*, and corresponds to a nontransient collection of unique facts and ways of being that characterize a person. The autobiographical self depends on systematized memories of situations in which core consciousness was involved in the knowing of the most invariant characteristics of an organism's life, but occurs only in extended consciousness.

A fifth fact concludes the list. Consciousness is often explained in terms of other cognitive functions, such as language, memory, reason, attention, and working memory. Yet the study of neurological patients suggests that those functions are not required for core consciousness, and that such functions appear necessary only for the higher reaches of extended consciousness. Thus, a theory of consciousness should *not* be just a theory of how those functions help construct, from the top down, an interpretation of what goes on in brain and mind. For example, memory, intelligent inferences, and language are critical to the generation of the autobiographical self and the process of extended consciousness. Some interpretation of the events that take place in an organism can surely arise after autobiographical self and extended consciousness are in place. But consciousness is unlikely to have begun at that high level in the hierarchy of cognitive processes. I assume that the earliest forms of consciousness precede inferences and interpretations.

Likewise, a theory of consciousness should *not* be just a theory of how the brain attends to the image of an object. In my view, natural low-level attention precedes consciousness, and focused attention follows the unfolding of consciousness. Attention is as necessary for consciousness to occur as having images is. But attention is not sufficient for consciousness to occur, and is not the same as consciousness.

Finally, although the production of unified mental scenes is an important aspect of consciousness, a theory of consciousness should *not* be just a theory of how the brain creates unified mental scenes, an operation that requires the cooperation of numerous neural/cognitive functions, and in particular, the participation of working memory. Those scenes do not exist in a vacuum. I believe images are integrated and unified for the benefit of the organism within which they occur. The mechanisms that prompt the integration and unification of the scene require an explanation that goes beyond a large-scale application of working memory.

A comprehensive theory of consciousness should address the two problems I outlined, and from my standpoint, it might well begin by focusing on the problem of self. Such a focus might be criticized on the grounds that it addresses *just* the problem of so-called self-consciousness and neglects the remainder of the consciousness problem, the issue of qualia. The following should be noted, however. First, the biological state I describe as the sense of self, and the biological machinery responsible for constructing it, may participate in optimizing the processing of the objects that come to be known in consciousness. In other words, having a sense of self may influence the processing of whatever gets to be known. This is accomplished by promoting the enhancement of the object to be known and the unification of the mental scene. The mysterious biological processes that pose the second problem of consciousness may play a role in the biological processes that pose the first. Second, having a sense of self may be necessary for *knowing*, in the proper sense. The creation of a first-person perspective, of subjectivity, is the puzzle on which consciousness hinges, and as far as I can see, accounting for subjectivity is necessary to deal with the matter of consciousness in a comprehensive way. Finally, addressing the problem of self from my theoretical perspective also addresses the qualia issue relative to the images of the organism having consciousness.

The Organism, the Object, and Their Relationship

My proposal to treat the problem of consciousness calls for seeing it in terms of two key players, the *organism* and the *object*, and in terms of the *relationships* of those players in the course of their natural interactions. In this perspective, consciousness consists of constructing knowledge about two facts: that the organism is involved in relating to some object, and that the object in the relation is causing the organism to change.

The process of knowledge construction requires a brain, a system endowed with the sig-

naling properties with which brains can assemble neural patterns about objects external to it, and the ability to turn neural patterns into images and, eventually, to assemble neural patterns and images *about* its own neural patterns and images. The neural patterns and the images necessary for consciousness are those which constitute proxies for the organism, for the object, and for the relationship between the two. Placed in this framework, understanding the biology of consciousness becomes a matter of discovering how the brain can construct neural patterns that map *both* the two players and their relationships.

Thinking along these lines led me to concentrate on a number of fundamental facts. First, the mapping of the object and of the organism are relatively separable in neuroanatomical terms. Second, the mapping of the object and of the organism is profoundly asymmetric.

Let us consider first the case of an external object. Within the limits of its sensory and motor devices, the brain constructs maps of an object by mapping the sensory and motor interactions that take place between the object and the body, and records such interactions. This allows the object to exist in two varieties: actually present and interacting with the organism now, or present as an activated memory recalled from past occasions on which the object has interacted with the organism. In either variety, the brain can deploy neural patterns for the object. When it does so, it deploys a proxy for the object.

As we consider the neurobiological basis for the two critical players in consciousness, the problem of representing the object is less mysterious than the problem of representing the organism. Neuroscience has been dedicating a considerable effort to understanding the neural basis of the "something-to-be-known." Studies of perception, learning and memory, and language have given us a rough idea of how the brain processes an object, in sensory and motor terms, and an idea of how knowledge about an object can be stored, categorized, and retrieved.

On the side of the organism, however, matters are quite different. The organism in the relationship is the entire unit of our living being—our body, as it were—and yet, as it turns out, a part of the organism called brain already holds a naturally constructed set of maps which stand for that whole organism. On the side of the object there is virtually infinite variation, while on the side of the organism there are highly constrained circumstances, mandated by the invariant structures of the living body and by the narrowly limited natural conditions under which a living body must operate. On the object side, the constructions have many degrees of freedom; on the organism side, there is a largely preset model of the organism-in-the-brain, on which ever-changing states of the organism are mapped within a limited dynamic range of perturbations.

The reasons behind the limited range of body state variation are simple. The body must operate within a narrow range of parameters if it is to survive. In comparison with the environment surrounding it, the body's internal state must be relatively stable. That stability is achieved by an elaborate neural machinery designed to detect minimal variations in parameters of the internal chemical profile and to command actions aimed at correcting the detected variations, directly or indirectly.

I see the organism "model" inside the brain of the organism as a likely biological forerunner for what eventually becomes the elusive sense of self. I believe the deep roots for the sense we subsume under the term "self," including the elaborate self that encompasses identity and personhood, can be found in the ensemble of brain devices which continuously maintain the body state within the narrow range and relative stability required for survival (i.e., the process known as homeostasis), and continually represent, *nonconsciously*, in dynamic body maps, the state of the living body in its many dimensions. The ensemble of such devices is the basis for the *protoself*, the nonconscious foundation for the levels of self that appear in our minds as the conscious

protagonists of consciousness: core self and autobiographical self.

Neither the protoself nor the core and autobiographical selves are all-knowing homunculi ready to produce consciousness. They are important references in the process of constructing consciousness, but they are not the producers of consciousness. The sense of self does not correspond, in neurobiological terms or in terms of cognitive operation, to the usual intuitions of self as knower, or of self as homunculus interpreter. This distinction is critical because, as a consequence of the justified rejection of homuncular explanations for consciousness, the notion of self was unjustifiably eliminated from polite conversation on the topic. The precious baby self was thrown away with the homunculus bathwater. It was wrong, no doubt, to imagine a self creature making consciousness and interpreting the world inside the brain—there is no such creature in biological terms. Yet the self sense is so central to our experience that its mental appearance is the reality that requires explanation. There is nothing satisfactory about attempts to explain consciousness that begin by excluding self on the grounds that the experience of self is illusory. Illusion or no illusion, a satisfactory account of consciousness should explain how the sense of self comes to mind.

The Protoself

Knowledge about the neuroanatomy underlying both the regulation of the life state and the transmission of signals from body to brain led me to propose a list of neural devices to support the protoself. The list begins with nuclei located at the brain stem level, such as the *parabrachial nuclei* and the *periaqueductal gray*. The list also includes neural devices located at higher levels: the *hypothalamus*, the *basal forebrain*, and *somatosensory cortices* such as the *insula* and S_2. All of these structures are involved in regulating the life state, or representing the life state, or both.

The presumed relation between specific brain regions and a proposed function such as protoself should be qualified at this point. The nonconscious protoself is not produced in any of the single regions mentioned above. Such functions as protoself or the core self and autobiographical self, to be introduced later, are not "located" in one particular brain region, or in one set of regions, but are the product of the interaction of neural and chemical signals among a set of regions. Phrenological thinking, which consists of attributing complicated mental functions to simple brain regions on the basis of correlative evidence, is a natural tendency in mind and brain research. But there are no single "centers" responsible for the sort of complex functions that are part of mind processes.

Assembling Consciousness

I propose that there are three steps behind the assembling of consciousness. The first step leads to constructing an account of what happens within the brain when the organism interacts with an object, be it within body boundaries (e.g., pain) or outside of them (e.g., a landscape). The mapped account is a simple narrative without words that allows the sense of self—the feeling of self-knowing—to emerge as the apparent protagonist of the events, as the subject changed by the object in a natural causal relationship. The phenomenon is transient, emerging incessantly for brief periods of time on the order of fractions of a second, for as long as there are objects to provoke the narrative process.

The second step requires the gradual buildup of memories of many instances of a special class of "objects": *the objects of the organism's own past experience, reactivated in recall and illuminated by core consciousness.* This second step requires conventional memory for facts, in this case the "objects" of one's autobiography. Once autobiographical memories are formed, clusters of those memories can be consistently and continuously activated whenever any object is being processed. Each of those autobiographical memories is treated by the brain as an object, and each becomes an inducer of core consciousness along with the particular nonself object that is being processed. This second step is the basis for extended consciousness, which relies on the same fundamental mechanism—the creation of mapped accounts of relationships between an organism and an object—but applies the mechanism to a consistent set of previously memorized objects pertaining to the organism's history rather than to a single nonself object X. An autobiographical self is created in this process.

The third step in the assembly of consciousness consists of simultaneously holding active, for a substantial amount of time, the many images whose collection defines the autobiographical self and the images that define the object. The reiterated components of the autobiographical self and the object are affected by the feeling of self-knowing that arises in core consciousness. As a consequence, this large compass of mind contents becomes *known* in an integrated perspective unified around an "owner." A grand unified mental pattern is created.

When an organism such as ours interacts with a given object—for instance, an object that you can see and touch, and that also can make a sound—the brain uses its sensory systems to make neural maps of the object (maps, for short). The maps construct the form, color, sound, and touch of the object in dynamic neural patterns laid out in neuron circuits. Because the neural patterns are immediately related to the object, I shall call them first-order maps. In addition, the organism also makes first-order maps for the movements it must carry out to apprehend the object, such as eye or hand movements, and, no less important, for the obligate emotional reactions we have to any object. As opposed to the maps of the object, these "reaction" maps are constructed in the regions I identified as supporting the protoself, and they map the organism in the process of being changed as a consequence of interacting with the object.

All the first-order maps I have mentioned—those of the object and those of the organism reacting to the object—are the source of mental images whose flow constitutes the thought process. That is not sufficient to generate consciousness. In fact, if this process were all that a brain could do, the organism would not *know* that it had such images and consciousness would be missing.

Consciousness occurs when an organism can form yet another level of mapping with a particular sort of content and when that content is introduced into mind in imaged form. The higher-level maps describe what goes on in the first-order maps just enumerated, and do so by means of signals received from first-order maps via neuron projections. Because the mapping occurs after the first-order mapping, and relies on signals coming from the first-order maps, I call it second-order mapping.

These second-order maps describe the relationship between the object and the organism—the organism is represented by an integrated pattern of the nonconscious protoself. In that relationship the object *causes* the organism (i.e., the protoself) to change. Put in other words, the second-order maps represent the organism engaged in the process of making first-order sensory maps related to the apprehension of a given object. Second-order maps are also the source of mental images, as is the case with first-order maps, and thus they also contribute those images to the thought process. I propose that a significant part of what we call *consciousness is constituted by the images that these second-order maps contribute to the mind, in the form of a sense of self knowing.* Consciousness consists of newly constructed knowledge about a specific topic—information, if you will, introduced into the natural process of making images.

In short, the presence of an object causes the organism to respond to it and, by so doing, to form first-order sensory maps for the object and for the changes the organism undergoes during object processing (e.g., motor accommodations and emotional reactions). Mental images arise from these first-order sensory maps, and in yet another brain sector—which is interconnected with the first—second-order sensory maps are being formed that "represent" the events which are occurring in the first-order sensory maps. These second-order maps signify without words the organism's relationship with the object, and specifically the fact that an object has caused the organism to change. These second-order maps thus signify to an organism that interacting with a given object or thinking a given thought modifies that organism. The second-order maps achieve this by signaling the modifications that the protoself undergoes and that are caused by the interaction of the organism with the object. And, because both the protoself and the second-order maps are constructed with the vocabulary of body signals, the images that result from such second-order mappings take the form of feelings. *Knowing begins as a feeling because its substrate is built from body signals.*

The feeling of knowing is the answer to an imaginary and never-posed question: To whom do these thoughts belong? The answer is that the thoughts belong to the organism, as deputized by the protoself. The story of the organism–object relationship is the first of all stories ever told, evolutionarily and individually, a primordial narrative without words. Only as the story is told do sense of self and knowing begin.

The Sites for Second-Order Maps

I proposed neural sites in which the first-order maps of object and protoself are formed, and I also proposed sites for these second-order maps in brain regions whose neuroanatomical design allows signals from multiple first-order sources to be received by means of neural connections. Candidate sites include the superior colliculus, the thalamus, the cingulate cortices, some medial parietal association cortices, and the prefrontal cortices. Not all of these sites are equally likely contributors. For example, I regard the *cingulate cortices* and the *thalamus* as far more likely sites than the others. Moreover, it must be clear that these neural sites are richly interconnected, sometimes directly, sometimes via relays in the thalamus, and that the second-order neural pattern I am hypothesizing occurs as a result of the interactions among the several candidate sites rather than happening in any one of them alone.

Closing the Assembly of Consciousness

Although the images arising in second-order mappings constitute a significant part of core consciousness, they do not constitute all of it. The sense of self and knowing is necessary but not sufficient for an entirely normal core consciousness to emerge. What else is needed to complete core consciousness? The processes behind the second-order mapping provide a cue for the integration and enhancement of the neural patterns that describe the causative object. The result is a "unified field of consciousness": a salient mental image of the object placed in its spatial and temporal context *and* in the "self" context. In short, the process through which the mapping of an object causes changes in the mapping of the organism's state, generates *both* a second-order mapping of the object–organism relationship, and a subsequent high-order integration and enhancement of the object mapping. Core consciousness is the outcome of this elaborate arrangement, and thus includes two components: an *image of the self knowing* (the feeling of knowing) and a *salient image of the causative object* in the context that led to it.

As long as the brain is awake and making images, core consciousness occurs continuously and abundantly, because any object, actually present or recalled from memory, can precipitate the process. But in spite of its seeming continuity, I suspect that the process is transient and pulselike. Interaction with an object causes the rise of the core consciousness over a fraction of a second, but before that pulse of core consciousness decays, another object causes another pulse of core consciousness to begin. The apparent continuity of core consciousness comes from the abundant production of such pulses along with the fact that we have no device to detect the breaks. Neither conventional long-term memory nor language is needed for this process.

To conclude, core consciousness emerges from a nonverbal second-order account of what happens to protoself maps when object maps modify them, and from an integration of the salient images of an object in the context that led to them. We become conscious when the imaged narrative becomes part of the mind; the process of consciousness is further advanced by the enhancement of the image of the object that initiated the chain of events.

Concluding Remarks

The theoretical framework and hypotheses surveyed above are the basis for an ongoing research program that has already disclosed some facts and pointed to some provisional conclusions. The most intriguing fact is that consciousness depends most critically on evolutionarily old regions. The structures without which consciousness cannot operate are all largely located in the depth of the brain and near its midline rather than on its surface. Consciousness does not depend primarily on the modern brain achievements of the neocortex, those on which fine perception, language, and high reason most directly depend. All but one of the anatomical structures that I hypothesize as supportive of the protoself and of the second-order mappings of core consciousness are evolutionarily older and anatomically deep, central, and paramidline; the insular and S_2 cortices, the one partial exception, are not part of the external neocortical surface. All of these structures are primarily involved in the representation and regulation of the organism state. In short, notwithstanding the fact that even the simplest form of core consciousness involves varied neocortical regions, depending on the sort of object that is being made conscious, the structures indispensable for the operations of consciousness are not located in neocortex.

The neocortical regions (i.e., the evolutionarily modern early sensory structures) are also involved in the process of making consciousness. Yet for almost every object, the early sensory cortices are involved in processing separate aspects of objects, and the disabling of one of those regions, even if extensive, does not compromise the central resource of consciousness but only a sector of it; on the other hand, the regions that support the protoself and second-order structures constitute a central resource, and their dysfunction causes a disruption of the process of consciousness.

The above facts are especially important when we consider the future directions of research in the neurobiology of consciousness. They are also relevant when we consider consciousness from an evolutionary perspective and wonder about the possible onset of consciousness in evolution.

There is a remarkable and not previously emphasized overlap of biological functions within the neuroanatomical structures that support the protoself and the second-order mappings. Taken individually, most of these structures are involved in most of the following functions: (a) regulating organism homeostasis, signaling body structures, and signaling body states, including those related to pain, pleasure, drives, and motivations; (b) participating in the processes of emotion and feeling; (c) participating in the processes of attention; (d) participating in the processes of wakefulness and sleep; (e) participating in the learning process. The current survey suggests that these areas, beyond the above quintet of functions, also participate in the construction of core consciousness. Again, there are important implications for this fact from a general, biological standpoint.

These conclusions do not deny that some brain stem structures are involved in the processes of wakefulness and attention, and that they modulate the activity of the cerebral cortex via the intralaminar thalamic nuclei, the nonthalamic cortical projections of monomines, and the thalamic projections of acetylcholine nuclei. What the conclusions suggest is that nearby brain stem structures, and perhaps even some of the very same structures, also have other activities, such as managing body states and representing current body states; and those activities are not incidental to the brain stem's activation role. Rather, they may be the reason why such an activation role has prevailed in evolution and why that role is primarily operated from that brain region.

The current formulation for the neurobiology of consciousness is not in conflict with those which concern the brain stem's "ascending reticular activating system" and its extension in the thalamus.[2] The activity of those regions is likely to contribute to creating the selective, integrated, and unified contents of the conscious mind. The current formulation simply suggests that such a contribution is not sufficient to explain the emergence of consciousness, and recommends a more comprehensive neurobiological perspective to undertake the investigation of consciousness.

Notes

1. For theoretical background, hypotheses, and discussion of evidence, see Antonio R. Damasio, *The Feeling of What Happens: Body and Emotion in the Making of Consciousness* (New York: Harcourt Brace, 1999). For other views on the neurobiological basis of consciousness, see Gerald Edelman, *The Remembered Present* (New York: Basic Books, 1989); and Francis Crick, *The Astonishing Hypothesis* (New York: Scribner's, 1994; see also chapters 6 and 9 in this volume). For a review of the philosophical background to this proposal, see T. Metzinger, ed., *Conscious Experience* (Paderborn, Germany: Mentis/Thorverton, UK: Imprint Academic, 1995), and chapter 20 in this volume; Paul Churchland, *The Matter of Conscious-*

ness (Cambridge, MA: MIT Press, 1983); John Searle, *The Rediscovery of the Mind* (Cambridge, MA: MIT Press, 1992).

2. See R. Llinás and D. Paré, "Of Dreaming and Wakefulness," *Neuroscience* 44 (1991): 521–535; M. Steriade, "New Vistas on the Morphology, Chemical Transmitters, and Physiological Actions of the Ascending Brainstem Reticular System," *Archives italiennes de biologie* 126 (1988): 225–238; J. Allan Hobson, *The Chemistry of Conscious States: How the Brain Changes Its Mind* (New York: Basic Books, 1994).

Wolf Singer

The term *consciousness* has a number of different connotations, ranging from awareness of one's perceptions and sensations to self-awareness, the perception of oneself as an agent endowed with intentionality and free will. In this paper I take the position that the first connotation of consciousness, phenomenal awareness, should in principle be tractable within neurobiological description systems because the problem of its relation to neuronal processes can probably be reduced to the question of how neuronal representations are organized. The latter connotation, by contrast, transcends purely neurobiological descriptions, because it has a social, a cultural, and a historical dimension.

The Inner Eye

Brains capable of processing signals at a conscious level appear to have the ability to represent the outcome of their distributed computational operations in a common format. These metarepresentations comprise protocols not only of sensory and motor processes but also of the state of value-assigning systems. Thus, brains that have consciousness possess a representational metalevel at which internal states are explicitly represented; they have what one might call an "inner eye" function. They can compare protocols of their own performance with incoming signals and from the outcomes of these internal deliberations derive decisions for future acts. This allows them to respond more flexibly to changing conditions than brains that lack consciousness and are confined to reacting to stimuli without the option of further reflection and internal deliberation. The intercalation of a further processing step between primary sensory computations and the programming of motor responses has obvious adaptive functions and may have contributed to the evolution of brains capable of being conscious of their own performance.

In order to run protocols of processes occurring within the brain, additional cognitive structures are required that analyze these processes and generate neuronal representations of them. Thus, implementation of monitoring functions requires second-order processing levels that generate metarepresentations of the computational results provided by first-order processes. The most likely substrates for such operations are cortical areas that have been added in the course of evolution and that treat the output of lower-order cortical areas in the same way as the latter treat input from the sensory periphery (Krubitzer 1998). The inner-eye function could thus be realized by a reflexive iteration of self-similar cortical functions. This interpretation is compatible with the neuroanatomical evidence that the phylogenetically more recent cortical areas are remote from primary sensory input and interact mainly, either through the thalamus or directly through cortico-cortical connections, with areas of lower order.

If these more recent monitoring structures in turn have access to the motor system—and available evidence indicates that this is the case —then brains endowed with such monitoring functions would in addition have the possibility to signal the result of the internal monitoring to other organisms. Through facial mimicry, gestures, vocalizations, and (in humans) language, such brains could signal to others what their perceptions, intentions, value assignments, and action plans are. Since such information dramatically increases the predictability of future actions of the respective other, it is likely to have an important function in the stabilization of labor-sharing societies; yet another adaptive function of consciousness that could have favored its evolution.

Two arguments, one based on evolution and the other on ontogeny, suggest that consciousness is a graded phenomenon whereby the gradations are correlated with the phylogenetic and ontogenetic differentiation of the cerebral cortex. The evolutionary argument is derived from the evidence that brains have evolved gradually, the most recent evolutionary changes being confined to an expansion of cerebral cortex and the addition of new cortical areas. This suggests that consciousness evolved as a consequence of cortical expansion and therefore is probably not an all-or-none phenomenon. The ontogenetic argument is based on the observation that the various manifestations of consciousness, from rudimentary awareness of sensations to the fully expressed self-consciousness of the adult, go in parallel with the gradual maturation of cerebral structures, in particular of the phylogenetically more recent cortical areas.

If one accepts that the aspect of consciousness which we address as phenomenal awareness results from an iteration of the same cognitive operations that support primary sensory processing, the explanatory gap reduces itself to the question of how the cerebral cortex processes signals and generates representations. If this question is answered with respect to primary sensory functions, the discovered strategies should be generalizeable to the formation of meta-representations, the representation of the brain's own computational operations that assume the postulated inner-eye function.

Self-Consciousness

However, there are other aspects of consciousness, such as self-awareness and the experience of individuality, that seem to require explanations which transcend purely neurobiological reductionism. It is my perception that the ontological status of these phenomena differs from that of the qualia of phenomenal awareness, and that it is these aspects of consciousness which give rise to the hard problems in the philosophy of mind and provide the incentive for adopting dualistic positions. The most challenging phenomenon in this context is that we perceive

ourselves as agents who are endowed with the freedom to decide, implying that the self is capable of controlling, by will, processes in the brain. We experience these aspects of consciousness as immaterial mental entities that are capable of influencing the neuronal processes required for execution of actions, and hence we perceive them as different from the material processes in the brain.

I propose that these latter connotations of consciousness are perceived as different because they require for their development interactions among brains that are sufficiently differentiated as to have phenomenal awareness and to signal to one another that they are endowed with this capacity. Such brains are able to enter dialogues of the kind "I know that you know how I feel" or "I know that you know what my intentions are," and so on. My proposal is that the experience of the "self" with all its subjective mental attributes emerges from such dialogues among human beings, above all from the early interactions between caregivers and babies. The experience of individuality and responsibility, and as a consequence the intuition that one is endowed with intentionality and free will, would then have to be considered as a product of social interactions. The subjective attributes of consciousness would have the ontological status of social realities, of cultural constructs, and would therefore, transcend pure neurobiological description systems that focus on individual brains.

The mechanisms that enable us to experience ourselves as endowed with mental capacities do, of course, reside in individual brains, but the contents of this experience are derived from social interactions. But why then should the experience of the self be so obviously different from other experiences that we also derive from social interactions? One explanation could be that the dialogue that leads to the experience of the self is initiated during an early developmental stage, before episodic memory matures and begins to keep track of what the brain experiences. If so, there would be no conscious record of the processes that led to the experience of the self and the associated subjective connotations of consciousness. Because of this amnesia these early experiences would lack causation; they would appear to be timeless and detached from any real world context. In consequence, the subjective connotations of consciousness, although acquired by learning, would be perceived as having transcendental qualities that resist reductionistic explanations.

Two Representational Strategies

If the argument is valid that the internal monitoring functions which lead to metarepresentations rest on the same cognitive operations as the sensory processes that deal with signals conveyed by the sense organs, search for the neuronal substrate of phenomenal awareness converges with the search for the structure of neuronal representations in general. In the following paragraphs I shall, therefore, present hypotheses on the putative structure of neuronal representations.

The working hypothesis proposed here is that evolved brains use two complementary strategies in order to represent contents (see also Singer 1995). The first strategy is thought to rely on individual neurons that are tuned to particular constellations of input activity. Through their selective responses these neurons establish explicit representations of particular constellations of features. It is commonly held that the specificity of these neurons is brought about by selective convergence of input connections in hierarchically structured feedforward architectures. This representational strategy allows for rapid processing and is ideally suited for the representation of frequently occurring stereotyped combinations of features; however, it is expensive in terms of the number of required neurons and is not suited to cope with the virtually infinite diversity of possible feature constellations encountered in real-world objects.

The second strategy consists of the temporary association of neurons into functionally coherent assemblies that as a whole represent a particular content whereby each participating neuron is tuned to one of the elementary features of composite perceptual objects. This representational strategy is more economical with respect to neuron numbers because a particular neuron can, at different times, participate in different assemblies, just as a particular feature can be part of many different perceptual objects. Moreover, this representational strategy is more flexible. It allows for the rapid de novo representation of constellations that have never been experienced before because there are virtually no limits to the dynamic association of neurons in ever-changing constellations, provided the participating neurons are interconnected. Thus, for the representation of highly complex and permanently changing contents, this second, implicit strategy appears to be better suited than the first, explicit strategy.

The mechanism that generates the metarepresentations required for phenomenal awareness has to cope with contents that are particularly unpredictable and rich in combinatorial complexity. Such metarepresentations are necessarily polymodal, and need to reconfigurate themselves at the same pace that the contents of phenomenal awareness change. It appears, then, that the second representational strategy, based on the formation of dynamic assemblies, would be more suitable for the implementation of metarepresentations than the explicit strategy. Further support for this view can be derived from the argument that conditions required for the formation of metarepresentations ought to be the same as those required for awareness to occur. Neuronal codes that are readily observable in deep anesthesia, or during slow-wave sleep, or in the absence of attention should not be accepted as correlates of awareness or consciousness. Since the receptive fields of individual neurons tend to differ only little in awake and anesthetized brains, it is unlikely that the explicit representations encoded by individual neurons are the substrate of the metarepresentations that support consciousness. As detailed below, brain states that are compatible with the manifestation of consciousness also favor the emergence of ordered spatiotemporal activity patterns which could serve as substrate for the formation of assemblies.

The following sections will, therefore, focus on the question of whether there is any evidence that contents are represented not only explicitly, by tuned neurons, but also implicitly, by dynamically associated assemblies; and if so, what the electrophysiological manifestations of such assemblies might be. The hypothesis will be put forward that one signature of assemblies is the synchronization of responses of participating neurons, and data will be reviewed that suggest a correlation between the occurrence of response synchronization, on the one hand, and brain states favorable for the occurrence of awareness, on the other.

The Signature of Assemblies

In assembly coding, two important constraints need to be present. First, a selection mechanism is required that permits dynamic yet consistent association of neurons into distinct, functionally coherent assemblies. Second, responses of neurons that have been identified as groupable must be labeled so that they can be recognized by subsequent processing stages as belonging together. This is necessary in order to assure that responses, once they are bound together, are evaluated jointly as constituents of a coherent code and do not get confounded with responses of cells belonging to other, simultaneously formed assemblies which represent different contents. Numerous theoretical studies have addressed the question of how assemblies can self-organize on the basis of cooperative interactions within associative neuronal networks (Braitenberg 1978; Edelman 1987; Palm 1990; Gerstein and Gochin 1992).

Here I shall focus on the second problem of assembly coding: the question of how responses of cells that have been grouped into an assembly can be tagged as related. An unambiguous signature of relatedness is absolutely crucial for assembly codes because, in contrast to explicit single-cell codes, the meaning of responses changes with the context in which they are interpreted. Hence, in assembly coding, false conjunctions are deleterious. Tagging responses as related is equivalent to assuring that they are processed and evaluated together at the subsequent processing stage. This, in turn, can be achieved only by raising their saliency jointly and selectively. There are three options. First, nongrouped responses can be inhibited; second, the amplitude of the selected responses can be enhanced; and third, the selected cells can be made to discharge in precise temporal synchrony. All three mechanisms enhance the relative impact of the grouped responses at the next higher processing level. Selecting responses by modulating discharge rates is common in labeled line coding, where a particular cell always signals the same content.

However, this strategy may not always be suited for distinguishing assemblies because it introduces ambiguities (von der Malsburg 1985) and reduces processing speed (Singer et al. 1997). Ambiguities could arise because discharge rates of feature-selective cells vary over a wide range as a function of the match between stimulus and receptive field properties, and these modulations of response amplitude would not be distinguishable from those signaling the relatedness of responses. Processing speed would be reduced because rate-coded assemblies can be identified only after a sufficient number of spikes have been integrated to distinguish high rates from low rates. Therefore, they need to be maintained for some time in order to be distinguishable. However, rate-coded assemblies cannot overlap in time within the same processing stage, because it would be impossible to distinguish which responses belong to which assembly. Together, these factors severely reduce the rate of succession with which different contents can be represented by a given population of neurons.

Both the ambiguities resulting from stimulus-related rate fluctuations and the temporal constraints can be overcome if the selection and labeling of responses is achieved through synchronization of individual discharges (von der Malsburg 1985; Gray et al. 1989; Singer and Gray 1995). Expressing the relatedness of responses by synchronization resolves the ambiguities resulting from stimulus-dependent rate fluctuations because synchronization can be modulated independently of rates. Response amplitudes could thus be reserved to signal how well particular features match the preferences of neurons, and synchronicity could be used in parallel to signal how these features are related. Defining assemblies by synchronization also accelerates the rate at which different assemblies can follow one another because the selected event is the individual spike or a brief burst of spikes; saliency is enhanced only for those discharges which are synchronized precisely and generate coincident synaptic potentials in target cells at the subsequent processing stage. The rate at which different assemblies can follow one another without being confounded is limited, then, only by the duration of the interval over which synaptic potentials summate effectively (for a detailed discussion, see Singer 1999).

Another advantage of selecting responses by synchronization is that the timing of input events is preserved with high precision in the output activity of cells because synchronized input is transmitted with minimal latency jitter (Abeles 1982; Softky 1994; König et al. 1996). This, in turn, can be exploited to preserve the signature of relatedness across processing stages, thus further reducing the risk of getting false conjunctions. Finally, synchronization enhances processing speed by accelerating synaptic transmission per se because synchronized excitatory postsynaptic potentials (EPSPs) trigger action potentials with minimal delay.

Cellular Prerequisites for Selection by Synchronization

At the level of cellular mechanisms two prerequisites need to be fulfilled in order to exploit synchronization as a coding mechanism. First, neurons must be able to act as coincidence detectors, that is, they must be particularly sensitive to coincident synaptic inputs. Second, mechanisms must exist that permit rapid and context-dependent temporal coordination of distributed discharge patterns.

The question of whether neurons in the central nervous system are capable of performing coincidence detection with the required precision is controversial because both theoretical arguments and simulation studies have led to opposite conclusions (Softky 1994; König et al. 1996; Shadlen and Newsome 1994). However, experimental evidence indicates clearly that neurons can evaluate temporal relations among incoming activity with sometimes surprising precision. In the auditory system, coincidence detection is used to locate sound sources. Neurons in auditory nuclei of the brain stem evaluate the delays among incoming signals from the two ears with a precision in the submillisecond range (for review see Carr 1993). Another example is the oscillatory responses of retinal ganglion cells that can be synchronized over large distances with close to zero phase lag (Neuenschwander and Singer 1996). Because of the high frequency of these oscillations (up to 100 Hz), the neuronal mechanism responsible for synchronization must operate with time constants in the millisecond range. This time-modulated activity is reliably transmitted up to cortical neurons, as indicated by cross-correlation analysis between retinal ganglion cells and cortical neurons (Castelo-Branco et al. 1998).

The implication is that neurons along the transmission chain must have operated with integration time constants no longer than half a cycle of the oscillation, and hence no more than

5 ms. The ability of cortical networks to handle temporally structured activity with high precision can also be inferred from the abundant evidence on the oscillatory patterning and synchronization of neuronal responses in the neocortex (reviewed in Singer and Gray 1995). Such temporally coordinated discharge patterns can emerge and stabilize only if the temporal structure of activity is preserved during synaptic transmission, and does not get dispersed and smeared too much by temporal integration. In the awake, performing brain the oscillatory patterning of cortical responses is typically in the gamma frequency range (30 to 60 Hz), and synchronization peaks often have a width at base in the range of 10 to 15 ms, indicating that temporal integration intervals should be on average no longer than 10 ms.

Rapid Synchronization

If synchronization is to play a role as signature of assemblies, it must be possible to synchronize discharges rapidly because of the constraints set by processing speed.

Early simulation studies that used harmonic oscillators rather than single spiking neurons showed that it may take a few cycles before synchronicity is established through phase locking (König and Schillen 1991). However, later simulations with spiking neurons revealed that networks of appropriately coupled units can undergo sudden state changes whereby the synchronization of discharges and their oscillatory patterning occur promptly and virtually simultaneously (for review, see Singer et al. 1997).

Very rapid synchronization has been observed in the visual cortex of cats. When neurons were activated by the onset of an appropriately oriented grating, their initial responses were better synchronized than expected from mere stimulus locking (Fries et al. 1997b). Comparison of actual response latencies and immediately preceding fluctuations of the local field potential revealed that the response latency shifted as a function of

the polarity of the preceding field potential fluctuation. Because these fluctuations were not independent between the different recording sites, response latencies became synchronized. Thus, coordinated fluctuations of excitability act like a dynamic filter and cause a virtually instantaneous synchronization of the very first discharges of responses (Fries et al. 1997b). Since the spatiotemporal patterns of these fluctuations reflect the architecture of intracortical association connections, grouping by synchronization can be extremely fast and still occur as a function of the prewired associational dispositions of the cortical network.

Evidence suggests that an oscillatory patterning of responses may be instrumental for the internal synchronization of neurons, in particular when interactions comprise substantial conduction delays or occur across polysynaptic pathways (König et al. 1995). In vitro experiments in slices of the visual cortex support this conjecture, showing that subthreshold oscillatory modulation of the membrane potential is ideally suited to establish synchronization (Volgushev et al. 1998). In cells with oscillating membrane potential, responses can become delayed considerably, whereby the maximally possible delay interval depends on oscillation frequency and can amount to nearly the duration of one cycle. With such a mechanism, responses to temporally dispersed EPSPs can become synchronized within less than an oscillation cycle in cells exhibiting coherent fluctuations of their membrane potential.

Functional Correlates of Response Synchronization

Perceptual Grouping

Following the discovery of stimulus-related response synchronization among neurons in the cat visual cortex (Gray and Singer 1987, 1989), numerous experiments have been performed in the search for a correlation between the occurrence of response synchronization and particular stimulus configurations. The prediction to be tested was that synchronization probability should reflect some of the gestalt criteria according to which the visual system groups related features during scene segmentation. Among the grouping criteria examined so far are continuity, vicinity, similarity in the orientation domain, collinearity, and common fate in the motion domain (Gray et al. 1989; Engel et al. 1991b, 1991c; Freiwald et al. 1995 for the cat; Kreiter and Singer 1996 for the monkey). So far, the results of these investigations are compatible with the hypothesis that the probability of response synchronization reflects the gestalt criteria applied to perceptual grouping (figure 8.1). Stimulus-specific response synchronization has been found within and across different areas, and even between hemispheres (for review, see Singer and Gray 1995); most important, none of these synchronization phenomena were detectable by correlating successively recorded responses. This indicates that they were not due to stimulus locking but to internal dynamic coordination of spike timing. Thus, the observed temporal coherence among responses is much greater than expected from mere covariation of event-related rate changes.

Studies involving lesions (Engel et al. 1991a; Nowak et al. 1995) and developmental manipulations (Löwel and Singer 1992; König et al. 1993) indicate that the interactions responsible for these dynamic synchronization phenomena are mediated to a substantial extent by cortico-cortical connections. The criteria for perceptual grouping should then be reflected in the architecture of these connections. This postulate agrees with the evidence that cortico-cortical connections preferentially link neurons with related feature preferences (for review, see Schmidt et al. 1997).

Response Synchronization and Behavioral States

Most of the early experiments in search of synchronization phenomena were performed on lightly anesthetized animals. It was important,

therefore, to investigate whether response synchronization also occurs during states where the EEG is actually desynchronized, as is characteristic of the awake, attentive brain. Evidence from cats and monkeys indicates that high-precision, internally generated synchrony is considerably more pronounced in the awake than in the anesthetized brain. Whenever tested—data are available from the primary visual cortex of cats and monkeys, the motion-sensitive areas MT and MST in monkeys and infero-temporal cortex of monkeys—the synchronization phenomena were readily demonstrable and showed a dependence on stimulus configuration similar to the synchronization measured under anesthesia (for review, see Singer et al. 1997).

Of particular interest in this context is the finding that response synchronization is especially pronounced when the global EEG desynchronizes and when the animals are attentive. Stimulating the mesencephalic reticular formation in anesthetized animals leads to a transient desynchronization of the EEG resembling the transition from slow-wave sleep to REM sleep. Munk et al. (1996) have shown that stimulus-specific synchronization of neuronal responses is drastically facilitated when the EEG is in a desynchronized rather than in a synchronized state.

Direct evidence for an attention-related facilitation of synchronization has been obtained from cats trained to perform a visually triggered motor response (Roelfsema et al. 1997). Simultaneous recordings from visual, association, somatosensory, and motor areas revealed that the cortical areas involved in the execution of the task synchronized their activity, predominantly with zero phase lag, as soon as the animals prepared themselves for the task and focused their attention on the relevant stimulus. Immediately after the appearance of the visual stimulus, synchronization increased further over the visual areas, and these coordinated activation patterns were maintained until the task was completed. However, once the reward was available and the animals engaged in eating behavior, these

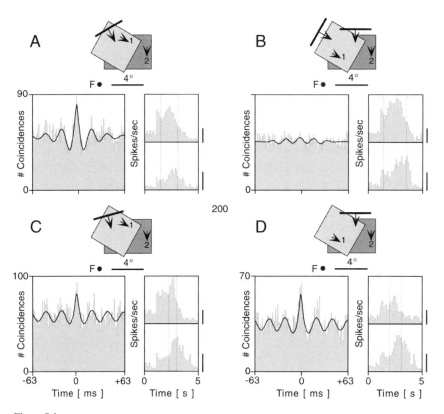

Figure 8.1
Stimulus-dependence of neuronal synchronization in area MT of the visual cortex of a macaque monkey carrying out a fixation task. Neuronal responses were obtained from two cell groups with different directional preferences. The figure shows cross-correlograms and peristimulus-time histograms for four different stimulation conditions. The small insets indicate the receptive field locations (1, 2) with respect to the fixation point (F) and the directional preference of the neurons (small arrows). (A) A single moving stimulus bar, whose direction of motion was intermediate between the neurons' preferences, led to a pronounced synchronization of the two cell groups, as indicated by the central maximum in the cross-correlogram. (B) Presentation of two stimuli moving in the respective preferred directions of cell groups 1 and 2 abolishes synchronization. (C, D) The synchronization observed with a single stimulus does not depend on its particular orientation. (C) Changing orientation and direction of motion by 15° or (D) using one of the bars from the configuration in (B) had little influence on synchronization. Scale bars for the peristimulus-time histograms correspond to 40 spikes/sec. The continuous line superimposed on the correlograms represents a damped cosine function that was fitted to the data to assess the significance of the correlogram modulation. (Modified from Kreiter and Singer 1996.)

coherent patterns collapsed and gave way to low-frequency oscillatory activity that did not exhibit any consistent phase relations.

This close correspondence between the execution of an attention-demanding visuomotor performance and the occurrence of zero phase-lag synchrony suggests a functional role of this temporal patterning. One possibility is that the synchronization observed during the preparatory period reflects an entrainment of activity into a temporal pattern that is common to selected cortical areas in order to facilitate rapid temporal coordination of signals once the stimulus has become available. Attentional mechanisms could impose a coherent subthreshold modulation on neurons in cortical areas that need to participate in the execution of the anticipated task, and thereby permit rapid synchronization of selected responses using the synchronizing mechanisms described above. According to this scenario, the attentional mechanisms would induce what one might call a state of expectancy in the respective cortical areas by imposing on them a specific, task-related, dynamic activation pattern that, once stimulus-driven input becomes available, acts like a dynamic filter which causes rapid synchronization of selected responses, thereby accomplishing the required grouping and binding of responses, and, in addition, ensuring rapid transmissions.

Perception

In a series of visual experiments, attempts have been made to find correlations between perceptual disturbances and abnormalities in neuronal synchronization. Kittens were made strabismic shortly after eye opening, which leads to an inability to group signals generated by the two eyes into a coherent percept.

This inability is reflected by the failure of neurons driven by the two eyes to synchronize their responses even if these are evoked by a single object (König et al. 1993). A likely reason for the disruption of response synchronization is that the tangential intracortical connections between neurons driven by different eyes are lost during early development due to consistent decorrelation of the responses evoked from the two eyes (Löwel and Singer 1992).

A subgroup of the strabismic animals developed in addition a syndrome called strabismic amblyopia. Subjects suffering from strabismic amblyopia, both animals and humans, have reduced visual acuity in the amblyopic eye. Moreover, they have difficulty identifying figures embedded in a contour-rich background (suggesting problems with perceptual grouping). In these amblyopic animals there was a close correlation between perceptual deficits and abnormalities in response synchronization, but there was no evidence for abnormalities of the response properties of individual cells. Quite unexpectedly, neurons in the primary visual cortex responded equally well to visual stimuli irrespective of whether these were shown to the normal or to the amblyopic eye. Thus, neurons driven by the amblyopic eye continued to respond vigorously to gratings that the animals had not been able to resolve with this eye during previous behavioral testing. Responses mediated by the normal and the amblyopic eye showed no difference in their amplitude or feature-specific tuning, irrespective of the spatial frequency of the applied test gratings. The only significant difference was the reduced ability of neurons driven by the amblyopic eye to synchronize their responses; this difference was particularly pronounced when the spatial frequency of the grating stimuli approached the range beyond which the animals had no longer been able to resolve gratings with the amblyopic eye (Roelfsema et al. 1994). In primary visual cortex, there is, thus, a close correlation between a specific perceptual deficit and alterations in synchronization; and this relation could very well be causal.

If synchronization is used to group responses together and to label them for further joint processing, then one expects that disturbances in synchronization should lead to disturbances in perceptual grouping such as occur for interocular binding operations in all strabismic animals and for monocular grouping operations in animals suffering from strabismic amblyopia. Since reduced synchronization is likely to reduce the saliency of responses conveyed by the amblyopic eye, it can also account for the fact that the amblyopic eye consistently loses in interocular competition when both eyes are open. Here, then, is a clear case where the firing of neurons in a cortical area does not correspond to perception, suggesting that the firing of individual neurons is a necessary but not a sufficient condition to support perception. Additional, and in this case indispensable, information appears to be conveyed by the precise temporal relations among the discharges of simultaneously active neurons.

Another close correlation between response synchronization and perception and a remarkable dissociation between individual responses and perception has been found in experiments on binocular rivalry. When the two eyes are presented with patterns that cannot be fused into a single coherent percept, the two patterns are perceived in alternation rather than as a superposition of their components. This implies that there is a central gating mechanism which in alternation selects the signals arriving from the two eyes for further processing. Interocular rivalry is thus a suitable paradigm to investigate the neuronal correlates of dynamic response selection, a process closely related to the formation of assemblies.

This paradigm has been applied to investigate how neuronal responses that are selected and perceived differ from those which are suppressed and excluded from supporting perception. Multiunit and field potential responses were recorded with chronically implanted electrodes from up to 30 sites in cat primary visual cortex while the animals were exposed to rivalrous stimulation conditions (Fries et al. 1997a). Because the animal performs tracking eye movements only for the pattern that is actually perceived, patterns

moving in opposite directions were presented dichoptically in order to determine, from the optokinetic tracking response, which of the two eyes is selected. The outcome of these experiments was surprising; it turned out that the discharge rate of neurons in primary visual cortex failed to reflect the suppression of input from the respective nondominant eye. A close and highly significant correlation existed, however, between changes in the strength of response synchronization and the outcome of rivalry. Cells mediating responses of the eye that won in interocular competition increased the synchronicity of their responses upon introduction of the rivalrous stimulus, whereas the reverse was true for cells driven by the eye that became suppressed. Thus, in this particular case of competition, selection of responses for further processing appears to be achieved by raising their saliency through synchronization rather than enhancing discharge frequency. Likewise, suppression is not achieved by inhibiting responses but by desynchronization (figure 8.2).

As in the amblyopic animals, there is thus a remarkable dissociation, at least in primary visual areas, between perception and the discharge rate of individual neurons. Cells whose responses are not perceived and are excluded from controlling behavior respond as vigorously as cells whose responses are perceived and support behavior. This dissociation is particularly stringent in the case of rivalry, because here responses to physically unchanged stimuli were recorded from the same neurons before and after introducing the rivalrous stimulus. Responses could be followed continuously while they passed from a condition where they were readily perceivable to a condition where they either continued to support perception despite rivalry or became excluded from perception. Another puzzling result of the rivalry study is that responses which win the competition increase their synchronicity upon presentation of the rivalrous stimulus. This suggests the action of a mechanism that enhances the saliency of the selected

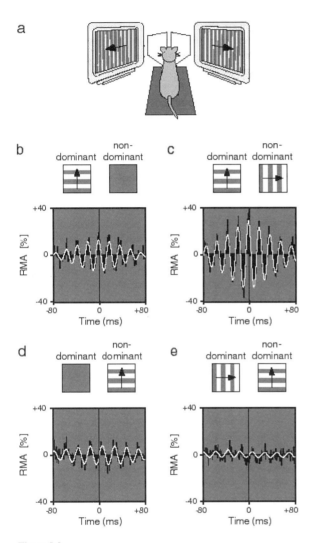

Figure 8.2
Neuronal synchronization under conditions of binocular rivalry. (A) Using two mirrors, different patterns were presented to the two eyes of strabismic cats. Panels (B–E) show normalized cross-correlograms for two pairs of recording sites activated by the eye that won (B, C) and lost (D, E) in interocular competition, respectively. Insets above the correlograms indicate stimulation conditions. Under monocular stimulation (B), cells driven by the winning eye show a significant correlation that is enhanced after introduction of the rivalrous stimulus to the other eye (C). The reverse is the case for cells driven by the losing eye (compare conditions D and E). The white continuous line superimposed on the correlograms represents a damped cosine function fitted to the data. Relative modulation amplitude (RMA) of the center peak in the correlogram, was computed as the ratio of peak amplitude over offset of correlogram modulation. This measure reflects the strength of synchrony. (Modified from Fries et al. 1997a.)

responses by improving their synchronicity in order to protect them against the interference caused by the rivalrous stimulus.

These results provide direct support for the hypothesis that precise temporal relations between the discharges of spatially distributed neurons matter in cortical processing, and that synchronization may be exploited to jointly raise the saliency of the responses selected for further processing. The important point here is that this selection can be achieved without inhibiting the nonselected responses. Thus, in principle, it should be possible to select a second group of responses by synchronizing them independently of the first. The result would be two coexisting, but functionally distinct, assemblies at the same processing level. The example of rivalry also illustrates how synchronization and rate modulation depend on each other. The signals from the suppressed eye failed to induce tracking eye movements, indicating that eventually the vigorous but poorly synchronized responses in primary visual areas failed to drive the neurons responsible for the execution of eye movements. Direct evidence for the failure of neurons at subsequent processing stages to respond to the input from the respective suppressed eye has been obtained in behaving monkeys trained to indicate which eye they were actually using (Logothetis and Schall 1989; Logothetis et al. 1996). This convertibility provides the option to use both coding strategies in parallel in order to encode complementary information (see above).

In conclusion, the data reviewed in this section indicate that evaluation of internally generated correlation patterns between responses of simultaneously recorded neurons permits the extraction of information about stimulus configurations, behavioral states, and perception that cannot be obtained by analyzing the responses of individual neurons sequentially. The relevant variable containing this additional information is the rather precise synchronization of a fraction of the discharges constituting the respective responses. The data indicate, further, that

responses containing synchronized epochs have a higher probability of being processed further and eventually being perceived than responses lacking such synchronized epochs, thereby supporting the hypothesis that synchronization is used as a mechanism for response selection. Since synchronization necessarily involves at least two neurons, it inevitably and simultaneously raises the saliency of more than one response. It is thus well suited to select subsets of responses for further joint processing, thereby defining the group of selected responses as related. Thus, synchronization fulfills the requirements postulated for a binding mechanism that selects a subset from a larger number of simultaneously active neurons, and labels the responses of this subset in a way that favors joint processing at the subsequent processing stage. The evidence that synchronization probability reflects gestalt criteria which guide perceptual grouping supports the hypothesis that synchronization serves as a binding mechanism in the context of assembly formation by jointly raising the saliency of selected subsets of responses.

The Generality of Synchronicity

Studies in nonvisual sensory modalities and in the motor system indicate that synchrony and oscillatory activity may be quite ubiquitous in the nervous system. Synchronization in the gamma frequency range occurs in the olfactory system of various vertebrate and invertebrate species, where it has been related to the processing of odor information (for review, see Laurent 1996). In the auditory cortex, synchronized gamma oscillations have been described both in humans (for review, see Joliot et al. 1994) and in animals (Eggermont 1992; de Charms and Merzenich 1996). In the somatosensory system, synchronized oscillatory activity in the gamma frequency range has been described both in the cat (Steriade et al. 1996) and in the monkey (Murthy and Fetz 1996). Furthermore, synchronized oscillatory firing has been observed in other systems, such as the hippocampus (Buzsáki and Chrobak 1995) and the frontal cortex (Vaadia et al. 1995).

Similar evidence is available for the motor system, where neural synchronization in the gamma frequency range has been discovered in cats (Steriade et al. 1996), monkeys (Murthy and Fetz 1996; Sanes and Donoghue 1993), and humans (Kristeva-Feige et al. 1993).

Synchrony may also play a role in sensorimotor integration. In awake, behaving monkeys, task-dependent synchronization between units distributed across sensory and motor cortical areas and within motor cortex itself has been reported (Murthy and Fetz 1996; Sanes and Donoghue 1993; Hatsopoulos et al. 1997; Ojakangas et al. 1997; Riehle et al. 1997). Thus, synchrony also seems to play a role in visuomotor coordination and in the programming of motor responses. As proposed previously, it may be instrumental in the flexible channeling (binding) of sensory signals to particular motor programs (Roelfsema et al. 1996).

Synchronization also seems to play a role in the linkage between cortical assemblies and subcortical target structures such as the superior colliculus. This possibility is suggested by the existence of precise temporal relationships between the discharges of neurons in areas of the visual cortex and the superior colliculus (Brecht et al. 1998). In these experiments, it could be shown that corticotectal interactions are strongly dependent on the temporal coherence of cortical activity. If cortical neurons engage in synchronous oscillatory activity either with partners within the same cortical area or with cells in other cortical areas, their impact on tectal cells is enhanced, indicating that tectal cells are driven more effectively by synchronous than by asynchronous cortical activity. This finding is consistent with the idea that the temporal organization of activity patterns plays an important role in defining the output of the cortex.

Taken together, available evidence suggests that comparable synchronization phenomena are found in a large number of different functional systems. Thus, it seems justified to generalize the results obtained in the visual cortex and to suggest that temporal coordination of discharges may be of general relevance for neural information processing. Importantly, there is increasing evidence that dynamic synchronization, in particular at frequencies in the gamma band, also occurs in the human brain. EEG studies have provided evidence for precise synchronization of activity in the gamma-frequency range in human visual cortex that is related to perception and reflects the subjective coherence of stimulus arrangements (Tallon-Baudry et al. 1996, 1997, 1998; Rodriguez et al. 1999; Miltner et al. 1999).

Synchronicity as a General Code for Relatedness

If synchronicity serves as the signature of relatedness, then synchronized responses should be interpreted as being related, irrespective of the cause of synchronization. Psychophysical evidence supports this conjecture, indicating that synchronously presented stimuli are bound perceptually and interpreted as elements of the same figure with greater probability than asynchronously appearing texture elements (Leonards et al. 1996; Leonards and Singer 1997, 1998; Alais et al. 1998; Usher and Donnelly 1998; but see Kiper et al. 1996). Hence, the synchronicity of responses imposed by simultaneously appearing texture elements (stimulus-locked synchronization) seems to be exploited for perceptual grouping. With respect to their strength and temporal precision, the externally induced and internally generated synchrony are virtually indistinguishable. Since the psychophysical results indicate that the former is interpreted as a signature of relatedness, it would be puzzling if this were not the case for internally generated synchrony as well. Synchronization could, thus serve as a general tag of relatedness irrespective of whether it results from coincidence of external events or from internal grouping operations.

Conclusion

The hypothesis defended here made the following assumptions: (1) phenomenal awareness necessitates and emerges from the formation of meta-representations; (2) the latter are realized by the addition of cortical areas of higher order that process the output of lower-order areas in the same way as the latter process their respective input; (3) in order to account for the required combinatorial flexibility, these metarepresentations are implemented by the dynamic association of distributed neurons into functionally coherent assemblies rather than by individual specialized cells; (4) the binding mechanism that groups neurons into assemblies and labels their responses as related is the transient synchronization of discharges with a precision in the millisecond range; (5) the formation of such dynamically associated, synchronized cell assemblies requires activated brain states characterized by "desynchronized" EEG and is facilitated by attentional mechanisms. The first assumption differs from the others because it is a conceptual premise that by itself does not provide any experimentally testable predictions; each of the following subordinate assumptions leads to predictions about structural and functional features of brains that are capable of generating meta-representations.

The data reviewed above illustrate that there is supportive experimental evidence for many of these features. However, we lack the proof that the observed features actually serve the functions that our theories assign to them. This is the case not only for the more recently discovered functional properties, such as the transient synchronization of distributed neuronal responses, but also for the rate-modulated discharges of individual neurons. As long as we have no complete theory of the structure of neuronal representations, it cannot be decided whether a sequence of discharges of a particular unit signifies that this unit participates in an assembly that lasts as long as the sequence of discharges, or whether the unit participates in several different, successively organized assemblies, or whether it represents a content on its own. This uncertainty is due to the difficulty of identifying assemblies. Assemblies can be identified only if one succeeds in recording simultaneously from a sufficiently large fraction of neurons actually participating in a particular assembly. For reasons detailed elsewhere (Singer et al. 1997), this is technically very demanding, and therefore attempts to identify assemblies are still at the very beginning. Thus, if it is the case that the generation of the metarepresentations required for consciousness involves the organization of highly distributed assemblies, we are a long way from the direct identification of the neuronal correlates of even the simplest forms of consciousness.

As long as analysis remains confined to the activity of individual neurons, it will be difficult to decide whether a recorded response is only a necessary, or whether it is a sufficient, condition for consciousness. Obviously, neurons need to discharge in order to convey information; if a group of neurons in a particular transmission chain stops responding, the content conveyed by that group of neurons cannot be perceived. Hence, correlations between perceptual awareness and cellular responses indicate only that the discharges of cells at a particular processing stage are necessary for a particular content to reach the level of awareness. In order to find out whether additional prerequisites have to be fulfilled (e.g., the binding of these responses into widely distributed assemblies), variables need to be determined that permit assessment of order parameters beyond the level of single units. This can be achieved only with recording techniques that disclose the spatiotemporal activation profile of large numbers of neurons.

The fact that the most global of these methods, the EEG, differentiates rather reliably between brain states where consciousness is or is not possible favors the hypothesis that the generation of consciousness-supporting metarepresentations requires coordination of activity well beyond the level of single-cell firing. Consciousness manifests itself only during brain states characterized by "desynchronized" EEG. These states, in turn, favor the occurrence of gamma oscillations and long-distance synchronization of neuronal responses with a precision in the millisecond range. It seems not unreasonable, therefore, to pursue the hypothesis that the metarepresentations required for phenomenal awareness to manifest itself consist of large assemblies of distributed neurons whose signature of relatedness is the internally generated synchronicity of discharges.

References

Abeles, M. (1982). Role of the cortical neuron: Integrator or coincidence detector? *Israel Journal of Medical Sciences* 18: 83–92.

Alais, D., Blake, R., and Lee, S.-H. (1998). Visual features that vary together over time group together over space. *Nature Neuroscience* 1(2): 160–164.

Braitenberg, V. (1978). Cell assemblies in the cerebral cortex. In R. Heim and G. Palm, eds., *Architectonics of the Cerebral Cortex. Lecture Notes in Biomathematics 21, Theoretical Approaches in Complex Systems*, 171–188. Berlin-Heidelberg-New York: Springer-Verlag.

Brecht, M., Singer, W., and Engel, A. K. (1998). Correlation analysis of corticotectal interactions in the cat visual system. *Journal of Neurophysiology* 79: 2394–2407.

Buzsáki, G., and Chrobak, J. J. (1995). Temporal structure in spatially organized neuronal ensembles: A role for interneuronal networks. *Current Opinion in Neurobiology* 5: 504–510.

Carr, C. E. (1993). Processing of temporal information in the brain. *Annual Review of Neuroscience* 16: 223–243.

Castelo-Branco, M., Neuenschwander, S., and Singer, W. (1998). Synchronization of visual responses between the cortex, lateral geniculate nucleus, and retina in the anesthetized cat. *Journal of Neuroscience* 18: 6395–6410.

De Charms, R. C., and Merzenich, M. M. (1996). Primary cortical representation of sounds by the coordination of action-potential timing. *Nature* 381: 610–613.

Edelman, G. M. (1987). *Neural Darwinism: The Theory of Neuronal Group Selection*. New York: Basic Books.

Eggermont, J. J. (1992). Neural interaction in cat primary auditory cortex. Dependence on recording depth, electrode separation, and age. *Journal of Neurophysiology* 68: 1216–1228.

Engel, A. K., König, P., Kreiter, A. K., and Singer, W. (1991a). Interhemispheric synchronization of oscillatory neuronal responses in cat visual cortex. *Science* 252: 1177–1179.

Engel, A. K., Kreiter, A. K., König, P., and Singer, W. (1991b). Synchronization of oscillatory neuronal responses between striate and extrastriate visual cortical areas of the cat. *Proceedings of the National Academy of Sciences of the USA* 88: 6048–6052.

Engel, A. K., König, P., and Singer, W. (1991c). Direct physiological evidence for scene segmentation by temporal coding. *Proceedings of the National Academy of Sciences of the USA* 88: 9136–9140.

Freiwald, W. A., Kreiter, A. K., and Singer, W. (1995). Stimulus dependent intercolumnar synchronization of single unit responses in cat area 17. *Neuroreport* 6: 2348–2352.

Fries., P., Roelfsema, P. R., Engel, A. K., König, P., and Singer, W. (1997a). Synchronization of oscillatory responses in visual cortex correlates with perception in interocular rivalry. *Proceedings of the National Academy of Sciences of the USA* 94: 12699–12704.

Fries, P., Roelfsema, P. R., Singer, W., and Engel, A. K. (1997b). Correlated variation of response latencies due to synchronous subthreshold membrane potential fluctuations in cat striate cortex. *Society for Neuroscience Abstracts* 23: 1266.

Gerstein, G. L., and Gochin, P. M. (1992). Neuronal population coding and the elephant. In A. Aertsen and V. Braitenberg, eds., *Information Processing in the Cortex, Experiments and Theory*, 139–173. Berlin-Heidelberg-New York: Springer-Verlag.

Gray, C. M., König, P., Engel, A. K., and Singer, W. (1989). Oscillatory responses in cat visual cortex exhibit inter-columnar synchronization which reflects global stimulus properties. *Nature* 338: 334–337.

Gray, C. M., and Singer, W. (1987). Stimulus-specific neuronal oscillations in the cat visual cortex: A cortical functional unit. *Society for Neuroscience Abstracts* 13: 1449.

Gray, C. M., and Singer, W. (1989). Stimulus-specific neuronal oscillations in orientation columns of cat visual cortex. *Proceedings of the National Academy of Sciences of the USA* 86: 1698–1702.

Grillner, S., Wallen, P., Brodin, L., and Lansner, A. (1991). Neuronal network generating locomotor behavior in lamprey: Circuitry, transmitters, membrane properties, and simulation. *Annual Review of Neuroscience* 14: 169–199.

Hatsopoulos, N. G., Ojakangas, C. L., and Donoghue, J. P. (1997). Planning of sequential arm movements from simultaneously recorded motor cortical neurons. *Society for Neuroscience Abstracts* 23: 1400.

Joliot, M., Ribary, U., and Llinás, R. (1994). Human oscillatory brain activity near 40 Hz coexists with cognitive temporal binding. *Proceedings of National Academy of Sciences of the USA* 91: 11748–11751.

Kiper, D. C., Gegenfurtner, K. R., and Movshon, J. A. (1996). Cortical oscillatory responses do not affect visual segmentation. *Vision Research* 36: 539–544.

König, P., Engel, A. K., Löwel, S., and Singer, W. (1993). Squint affects synchronization of oscillatory responses in cat visual cortex. *European Journal of Neuroscience* 5: 501–508.

König, P., Engel, A. K., and Singer, W. (1995). The relation between oscillatory activity and long-range synchronization in cat visual cortex. *Proceedings of the National Academy of Sciences of the USA* 92: 290–294.

König, P., Engel, A. K., and Singer, W. (1996). Integrator or coincidence detector? The role of the cortical neuron revisited. *Trends in Neurosciences* 19: 130–137.

König, P., and Schillen, T. B. (1991). Stimulus-dependent assembly formation of oscillatory responses: I. Synchronization. *Neural Computation* 3: 155–166.

Kreiter, A. K., and Singer, W. (1996). Stimulus-dependent synchronization of neuronal responses in the visual cortex of awake macaque monkey. *Journal of Neuroscience* 16: 2381–2396.

Kristeva-Feige, R., Feige, B., Makeig, S., Ross, B., and Elbert, T. (1993). Oscillatory brain activity during a motor task. *Neuroreport* 4: 1291–1294.

Krubitzer, L. (1998). Constructing the neocortex: influence on the pattern of organization in mammals. In M. S. Gazzaniga and J. S. Altman, eds., Brain and Mind: Evolutionary Perspectives, 19–34. Strasbourg: HFSP.

Laurent, G. (1996). Dynamical representation of odors by oscillating and evolving neural assemblies. *Trends in Neurosciences* 19: 489–496.

Leonards, U., Singer, W., and Fahle, M. (1996). The influence of temporal phase differences on texture segmentation. *Vision Research* 36: 2689–2697.

Leonards, U., and Singer, W. (1997). Selective temporal interactions between processing streams with differential sensitivity for colour and luminance contrast. *Vision Research* 37: 1129–1140.

Leonards, U. and Singer, W. (1998). Two segmentation mechanisms with differential sensitivity for colour and luminance contrast. *Vision Research* 38: 101–109.

Logothetis, N. K., Leopold, D. A., and Sheinberg, D. L. (1996). What is rivalling during binocular rivalry? *Nature* 380: 621–624.

Logothetis, N. K., and Schall, J. D. (1989). Neuronal correlates of subjective visual perception. *Science* 245: 761–763.

Löwel, S., and Singer, W. (1992). Selection of intrinsic horizontal connections in the visual cortex by correlated neuronal activity. *Science* 255: 209–212.

Miltner, W. H. R., Braun, C., Arnold, M., Witte, H., and Taub, E. (1999). Coherence of gamma-band EEG activity as a basis for associative learning. *Nature* 397: 434–436.

Munk, M. H. J., Roelfsema, P. R., König, P., Engel, A. K., and Singer, W. (1996). Role of reticular activation in the modulation of intracortical synchronization. *Science* 272: 271–274.

Murthy, V. N., and Fetz, E. E. (1996). Synchronization of neurons during local field potential oscillations in sensorimotor cortex of awake monkeys. *Journal of Neurophysiology* 76: 3968–3982.

Neuenschwander, S., and Singer, W. (1996). Long-range synchronization of oscillatory light responses in the cat retina and lateral geniculate nucleus. *Nature* 379: 728–733.

Nowak, L. G., Munk, M. H. J., Nelson, J. I., and Bullier, J. A. C. (1995). Structural basis of cortical synchronization. I. Three types of interhemispheric coupling. *Journal of Neurophysiology* 74: 2379–2400.

Ojakangas, C. L., Hatsopoulos, N. G., and Donoghue, J. P. (1997). Reorganization of neuronal synchrony in

M1 during visuomotor adaptation. *Society for Neuroscience Abstracts* 23: 1399.

Palm, G. (1990). Cell assemblies as a guideline for brain research. *Concepts in Neuroscience* 1: 133–147.

Riehle, A., Grün, S., Diesmann, M., and Aertsen, A. (1997). Spike synchronization and rate modulation differentially involved in motor cortical function. *Science* 278: 1950–1953

Rodriguez, E., George, N., Lachaux, J.-P., Martinerie, J., Renault, B., and Varela, F. J. (1999). Perception's shadow: long-distance synchronization of human brain activity. *Nature* 397: 430–433.

Roelfsema, P. R., Engel, A. K., König, P., and Singer, W. (1996). The role of neuronal synchronization in response selection: a biologically plausible theory of structured representation in the visual cortex. *Journal of Cognitive Neuroscience* 8: 603–625.

Roelfsema, P. R., Engel, A. K., König, P., and Singer, W. (1997). Visuomotor integration is associated with zero time-lag synchronization among cortical areas. *Nature* 385: 157–161.

Roelfsema, P. R., König, P., Engel, A. K., Sireteanu, R., and Singer, W. (1994). Reduced synchronization in the visual cortex of cats with strabismic amblyopia. *European Journal of Neuroscience* 6: 1645–1655.

Sanes, J. N., and Donoghue, J. P. (1993). Oscillations in local field potentials of the primate motor cortex during voluntary movement. *Proceedings of the National Academy of Sciences of the USA* 90: 4470–4474.

Schmidt, K. E., Goebel, R., Löwel, S., and Singer, W. (1997). The perceptual grouping criterion of colinearity is reflected by anisotropies of connections in the primary visual cortex. *European Journal of Neuroscience* 9: 1083–1089.

Shadlen, M. N., and Newsome W. T. (1994). Noise, neural codes and cortical organization. *Current Opinion in Neurobiology* 4: 569–579.

Singer, W. (1995). Development and plasticity of cortical processing architectures. *Science* 270: 758–764.

Singer, W. (1999). Neuronal synchrony: A versatile code for the definition of relations? *Neuron* 24: 49–65; references for review 111–125.

Singer, W., Engel, A. K., Kreiter, A. K., Munk, M. H. J., Neuenschwander, S., and Roelfsema, P. R. (1997). Neuronal assemblies: Necessity, signature and detectability. *Trends in Cognitive Sciences* 1: 252–261.

Singer, W., and Gray, C. M. (1995). Visual feature integration and the temporal correlation hypothesis. *Annual Review of Neuroscience* 18: 555–586.

Softky, W. (1994). Sub-millisecond coincidence detection in active dendritic trees. *Neuroscience* 58: 13–41.

Steriade, M., Amzica, F., and Contreras, D. (1996). Synchronization of fast (30–40 Hz) spontaneous cortical rhythms during brain activtion. *Journal of Neuroscience* 16: 392–417.

Tallon-Baudry, C., Bertrand, O., Delpuech, C., and Pernier, J. (1996). Stimulus specificity of phase-locked and non-phase-locked 40 Hz visual responses in human. *Journal of Neuroscience* 16: 4240–4249.

Tallon-Baudry, C., Bertrand, O., Delpuech, C., and Pernier, J. (1997). Oscillatory γ-band (30–70 Hz) activity induced by a visual search task in humans. *Journal of Neuroscience* 17: 722–734.

Tallon-Baudry, C., Bertrand, O., Peronnet, F., and Pernier, J. (1998). Induced γ-band activity during the delay of a visual short-term memory task in humans. *Journal of Neuroscience* 18: 4244–4254.

Usher, M., and Donnelly, N. (1998). Visual synchrony affects binding and segmentation in perception. *Nature* 394: 179–182.

Vaadia, E., Haalman, I., Abeles, M., Bergman, H., Prut, Y., Slovin, H., and Aertsen, A. (1995). Dynamics of neuronal interactions in monkey cortex in relation to behavioural events. *Nature* 373: 515–518.

Volgushev, M., Chistiakova, M., and Singer, W. (1998). Modification of discharge patterns of neocortical neurons by induced oscillations of the membrane potential. *Neuroscience* 83: 15–25.

Von der Malsburg, C. (1985). Nervous structures with dynamical links. *Berichte der Bunsengesellschaft für Physikalische Chemie* 89: 703–710.

9

Reentry and the Dynamic Core: Neural Correlates of Conscious Experience

Gerald M. Edelman and Giulio Tononi

Consciousness has been looked on as both a mystery and a source of mystery. It is one of the main targets of philosophical inquiry, but only recently has it been accepted into the family of scientific objects that are worthy of experimental investigation. The reasons for this late acceptance are clear enough: While all scientific theories assume consciousness, and while conscious sensation and perception are necessary for their application, the means to carry out objective scientific investigations of consciousness itself have only recently become available. Recent studies in neurobiology and cognitive psychology have made it possible to address a series of questions the answers to which should help resolve some of the mysteries associated with consciousness. In this article, we will focus on two of these questions: (1) What are the neural mechanisms that can account for the emergence of consciousness? (2) How can such neural processes account for key properties of conscious experience—that each conscious state is an indivisible whole and, at the same time, that each person can choose among an immense number of different conscious states?

The Specialness of Consciousness: Some Assumptions

To avoid confusion, it is necessary to be quite clear about the assumptions one makes in investigating consciousness as a scientific object. We have proposed three such assumptions: the physics assumption, the evolutionary assumption, and the qualia assumption (Edelman 1989; Edelman and Tononi 2000). The physics assumption states that only conventional physical processes are required for a satisfactory explanation of consciousness—no dualism is allowed. In particular, we assume that consciousness is a process which arises in the structure and dy-

namics of certain brains. As a physical process, conscious experience can be characterized by certain general or fundamental properties or states (Tononi and Edelman 1998a). One such property is that conscious experience is integrated—conscious states cannot be subdivided into independent components. Another property is that at the same time it is highly differentiated—one can experience billions of different conscious states. The scientific task is, then, to describe what particular kinds of neural processes can simultaneously account for these properties.

The evolutionary assumption states that consciousness evolved during natural selection in the animal kingdom. This implies that consciousness is associated with certain biological structures—it depends on dynamic processes generated by a certain morphology. Insofar as that morphology is the product of evolutionary selection, consciousness not only is such a product but also influences various behaviors that are subject both to natural selection and to selective events within an individual animal lifetime—consciousness is efficacious. The evolutionary assumption also implies that, as a result of relatively recent morphological developments, consciousness is not a process shared by all animal species. If taken seriously, this assumption about the evolutionary origin of consciousness helps us to avoid fruitless efforts, such as attempting to characterize consciousness as a by-product of computation or applying bizarre or exotic scientific notions, such as quantum gravity, while ignoring neurology.

Finally, the qualia assumption states that the subjective, qualitative aspects of consciousness, being private, cannot be communicated directly through a scientific theory, which by its nature is public and intersubjective. Accepting this assumption does not mean that the necessary and sufficient conditions for consciousness cannot be described. It implies only that describing them is not the same as generating and experiencing them. Qualia can be considered scientifically as forms of multidimensional discrimination carried out by a complex brain. We can analyze them and give a prescription for how they emerge, but obviously we cannot give rise to them without first giving rise to appropriate brain structures and their dynamics within the body of an individual organism. This assumption helps us to avoid the notion that a successful scientific theory of consciousness can act as a surrogate for conscious experience itself or can allow one to grasp the *experience* of any quale simply on the basis of scientific descriptions and hypotheses, however pertinent they may be.

In addressing the mechanisms and principles of consciousness, it is also helpful to keep in mind the distinction between primary consciousness and higher-order consciousness (Edelman 1989). Primary consciousness is seen in animals with certain brain structures similar to ours (e.g., dogs). These animals appear able to construct a mental scene but seem to have very limited semantic or symbolic capabilities, and no true language. Higher-order consciousness (which is seen to flourish in humans and which presupposes the coexistence of primary consciousness) is accompanied by a sense of self and the ability in the waking state to explicitly construct past and future scenes. Higher-order consciousness requires, at the minimum, a semantic capability, and in its most developed form, a linguistic capability. In this article, we will not explicitly discuss higher-order consciousness.

We believe that, at the present state of our knowledge, it is essential to focus on those properties of consciousness which are fundamental, and resist the temptation of providing a specific account of the many different forms it can take (Tononi and Edelman 1998b). As we are all aware, conscious states manifest themselves as sensory percepts, images, thought, inner speech, emotional feelings, and feelings of will, of self, of familiarity, and so on. These can occur in any conceivable subdivision and combination. Sensory percepts—the paradigmatic constituents of conscious experience—come in many different modalities, such as sight, hearing, touch, olfaction and taste, proprioception, kinesthesia, pleasure, and pain. Furthermore, each modality comprises many different submodalities. Visual experience, for example, includes color, form, movement, depth, and so on. Though less vivid and less rich in detail than sensory percepts, thought, inner speech, and conscious imagery are all powerful reminders that a conscious scene can be constructed even in the absence of external inputs. Dreams provide perhaps the most striking demonstration of this fact.

As interesting as the rich phenomenology of consciousness may be, however, we have chosen not to indulge in a discussion of its multitudinous aspects. We will simply acknowledge that the possible modalities and contents of conscious experience, while not arbitrary, are exceedingly numerous, and move on to a consideration of its fundamental properties.

The Unity and Informativeness of Conscious Experience

We will concentrate here on a few principles that, like the three unities of classical drama—time, place, and action—are shared by every conscious experience. By deliberate choice, our focus will therefore be on those fundamental aspects of conscious experience which are common to all of its phenomenological manifestations. These properties include privateness, unity, and informativeness (Tononi and Edelman 1998a).

Some of the most striking indications of the inescapable unity of conscious experience come from the examination of certain pathological phenomena. Many neuropsychological disorders demonstrate that consciousness can bend or shrink, and at times even split, but it does not tolerate breaks of coherence. For example, a stroke in the right hemisphere leaves many patients with their left side paralyzed and affected with complete sensory loss. As was noticed by Anton at the turn of the century, many of these patients deny their paralysis, a phenomenon called anosognosia. If confronted with the evidence that their limb does not move, some patients may even deny that it belongs to them, and may treat it like an extraneous object. Some patients with massive bilateral occipital damage cannot see anything, yet do not recognize that they are blind. Split-brain patients provide another demonstration that consciousness abhors holes or discontinuities. After surgery, the visual field of each hemisphere is split in two at the middle. However, split-brain patients typically do not report any halving of their vision, or any sharp boundary between vision and blindness on the midline. In fact, if the left hemisphere is shown only the right half of a face, the patient reports seeing an entire face.

If a fundamental property of conscious experience is that it is inherently private, unified, and coherent (in other words, integrated), it is just as important to recognize that an equally fundamental property is what we have called its extraordinary degree of differentiation or informativeness (Tononi and Edelman 1998a). What makes a conscious state informative is not how many "chunks" of information it appears to contain, but the fact that its occurrence discriminates among billions of different states of affairs, each of which would potentially lead to different behavioral outputs. While the content of a conscious state is not arbitrary, the number of possible conscious states is certainly enormous. Think of the number of different people one has seen during a lifetime, or the number of different paintings, or the number of different frames from different movies. The range of possible conscious states is such that there is no fear that experiences of life, art, poetry, and music will ever be exhausted. Yet, despite the enormous number of different conscious states that we can experience or imagine, we can easily discriminate among them, whether or not we can easily describe in words how they differ. It is important to realize what this means. The ability to differentiate

among a large repertoire of possibilities constitutes information—in the precise sense of "reduction of uncertainty." Furthermore, conscious discrimination represents information *that makes a difference*, in the sense that the occurrence of a given conscious state can lead to consequences which are different, in terms of both thought and action, from those which might ensue from other conscious states.

Before considering how integration and differentiation can be accounted for, a brief review of actual observations and experiments is useful.

Some Empirical Evidence

A series of neuropsychological and neurophysiological observations are relevant to the phenomenological issues we have already discussed. They lead to a number of key conclusions. First, conscious experience is associated with the activation and deactivation of distributed populations of neurons. Second, conscious experience requires strong and rapid reentrant interactions among distributed neural populations. Third, conscious experience requires patterns of neural activity that are highly differentiated. We shall briefly review some evidence supporting these conclusions.

Neuroimaging studies demonstrate that changes in specific aspects of conscious experience correlate with changes in activity in specific brain areas, whether the experience is driven by external stimuli, by memory, or by imagery and dreams. Conscious experience as such involves the activation or deactivation of widely distributed brain areas, although what should count as the appropriate baseline related to the absence of consciousness is not clear. In subjects who are comatose or deeply anesthetized, unconsciousness is associated with a profound depression of neural activity in both the cerebral cortex and the thalamus. During slow-wave sleep, in which consciousness is severely reduced or lost, cerebral blood flow is globally reduced, compared with both waking and REM sleep, two brain states associated with vivid conscious reports. Neural activity in slow-wave sleep is reduced in both anterior neocortical regions (most of prefrontal cortex) and posterior cortical regions (especially parietal association areas), in paralimbic structures (anterior cingulate cortex and anterior insula), and in centrencephalic structures (reticular activating system, thalamus, and basal ganglia). In contrast, it is not depressed in unimodal sensory areas (primary visual, auditory, and somatosensory cortex (Braun et al. 1997; Maquet et al. 1996, 1997).

Lesion studies indicate that consciousness is abolished by widely distributed damage and not by localized cortical damage. The only localized brain lesions resulting in loss of consciousness typically affect the reticular core in the upper brain stem and hypothalamus or its rostral extensions in the reticular and intralaminar thalamic nuclei (Plum 1991). While it has been suggested that the reticular core may have a privileged connection to conscious experience, its activity may simply be required to sustain distributed activity patterns in the cortex.

What about the waking state? The transition between conscious, controlled performance and unconscious, automated performance may be accompanied by a change in the degree to which neural signals are distributed in the brain. When tasks are novel, brain activation related to a task is widely distributed; when the task has become automatic, activation is more localized and may shift to a different set of areas (Petersen et al. 1998). In animal studies, neural activity related to sensory stimuli can be recorded in many brain regions before habituation. After habituation sets in (a time when humans report that stimuli tend to fade from consciousness), the same stimuli evoke neural activity exclusively along their specific sensory pathways (Horel et al. 1967). These observations suggest that when tasks are automatized and require less or no conscious control, the spread of signals that influence the performance of a task involves a more restricted

and dedicated set of circuits that become "functionally insulated." This produces a gain in speed and precision, but a loss in context-sensitivity, accessibility, and flexibility (Baars 1988).

Activation and deactivation of distributed neural populations in the thalamocortical system are not sufficient bases for conscious experience unless the activity of the neuronal groups involved is integrated rapidly and effectively. We have suggested that such rapid integration is achieved through the process of reentry—the ongoing, recursive, highly parallel signaling within and among brain areas (Edelman 1987, 1989; Tononi et al. 1992). An indication comes from the study of patients with disconnection syndromes, in which one or more brain areas are anatomically or functionally disconnected from the rest of the brain due to some pathological process. In the paradigmatic disconnection syndrome, the split brain, visual or somatosensory stimuli can activate the nondominant hemisphere and lead to behavioral responses, but the dominant, verbal hemisphere is not aware of them (Gazzaniga 1995). Although the two hemispheres can still communicate through indirect, subcortical routes, rapid and effective neural interactions mediated by direct reentrant connections are abolished by the lesion of the corpus callosum.

Modeling studies suggest that a telltale sign of effective reentrant interactions is the occurrence of short-term temporal correlations between the neuronal groups involved (Sporns et al. 1991). Experiments on cats show that short-term temporal correlations between the activity of neuronal groups responding to the same stimulus, but located in different hemispheres, are abolished by callosal transections (Engel et al. 1991). Other studies indicate that various kinds of cognitive tasks are accompanied by the occurrence of short-term temporal correlations among distributed populations of neurons in the thalamocortical system (Bressler et al. 1993; Gevins et al. 1996; Joliot et al. 1994; Singer and Gray 1995).

The requirement for fast, strong, and distributed neural interactions may explain why stimuli that are feeble, degraded, or short-lasting often fail to be consciously perceived. Although such stimuli may produce a behavioral response (perception without awareness [Marcel 1983]), they are unlikely to ignite neural activity of sufficient strength or duration to support fast-distributed interactions. Conversely, attention may increase the conscious salience of certain stimuli by boosting the corresponding neural responses as well as the strength of neural interactions (Friston 1998; Maunsell 1995). Neural activity is also more likely to contribute effectively to distributed neural interactions if it is sustained for hundreds of msec. This would lead to the functional closure of longer reentrant loops and thereby support reentrant interactions among more distant regions. Experimental findings are consistent with this idea. High-frequency somatosensory stimuli delivered to the thalamus require about 500 msec for the production of a conscious sensory experience, while less than 150 msec is sufficient for sensory detection without awareness (Libet 1993). The sustained evoked potentials associated with a conscious somatosensory sensation are apparently generated by the excitation of pyramidal neurons of primary somatosensory cortex through reentrant interactions with higher cortical areas (Cauller 1995).

Evidence for a correlation between conscious experience and sustained neural activity also comes from tasks involving visuospatial working memory, that is, the ability to rehearse or "keep in mind" a spatial location. Working memory is used to bring or keep some item in consciousness or close to conscious access. In working memory tasks, sustained neural activity is invariably found in prefrontal cortex of monkeys, and it is apparently maintained by reentrant interactions between frontal and parietal regions (Fuster et al. 1985; Goldman-Rakic and Chafee 1994). Sustained neural activity may facilitate the integration of the activity of spatially segregated brain regions into a coherent, multimodal neural process that is stable enough to permit decision making and planning.

Although strong and fast reentrant interactions among distributed groups of neurons are necessary for conscious experience, in themselves they are not sufficient. This is strikingly demonstrated by the unconsciousness accompanying generalized seizures and slow-wave sleep. During generalized seizures, the brain not only is extremely active, but most neurons fire in a highly synchronous manner. For example, the electroencephalogram (EEG) during petit mal absences indicates that groups of neurons over the whole brain are either all firing together or all silent together, and these two states alternate every third of a second. Although such hypersynchronous firing is indicative of strong and distributed interactions, a subject who experiences such a seizure is unconscious. Similarly, during slow-wave sleep, neurons in the thalamocortical system are both active and remarkably interactive, as shown by their synchronous firing in a stereotyped, burst-pause pattern. During this stage of sleep, however, it is rare to obtain vivid and extensive conscious reports. By contrast, during REM sleep, when neural activity is not globally synchronous but resembles the rapid and complex patterns of waking, subjects typically report vivid dreams if awakened. We suggest that the low-voltage, fast-activity EEG characteristic of waking and REM sleep reflects the availability of a rich and diverse repertoire of neural activity patterns. If the repertoire of differentiated neural states is large, consciousness is possible. Conversely, if this repertoire is reduced, as when most groups of neurons in the cortex discharge synchronously and functional discriminations among them are obliterated, consciousness is curtailed or lost.

Mechanisms and Models

Considering the mechanisms by which consciousness arises in the brain, we have suggested that reentry plays an essential role (Edelman 1987, 1989). Reentry is a process of ongoing parallel and recursive signaling between separate brain maps along massively parallel anatomical connections, most of which are reciprocal. Reentry involves selection and is not feedback, which proceeds along only two connected lines and involves an explicit and instructive error signal. It is reentry acting by neuronal group selection that assures the integration so essential to the creation of a scene in primary consciousness.

How reentry leads to integration can best be illustrated by considering in a large-scale model exactly how functionally segregated maps in the cerebral cortex might operate coherently together even though there is no superordinate map or logically determined program (Tononi et al. 1992). The organization of the cerebral cortex is such that even within a single modality—for example, vision—there is a multitude of specialized or functionally segregated maps devoted to different submodalities—color, movement, and form. Despite this diversity, we are aware of a coherent perceptual scene. Our ability to act coherently in the presence of diverse, often conflicting, sensory stimuli requires a process of neural interaction across many levels of organization without any superordinate map to guide the process. This is the so-called binding problem (Damasio 1989).

Within a single area, linking must occur among various neuronal groups in the same feature domain or submodality. Examples are perceptual groupings within a map sensing color or within another map sensing movement. At a higher level, binding must take place among different distributed maps, each of which is functionally segregated or specialized. Binding, for example, requires the integration of the neuronal responses to a particular object contour with its color, position, and direction of movement. The question is: How does binding actually take place?

Large-scale simulations based on key anatomical and physiological properties of the visual

system (Tononi et al. 1992) provide a powerful indication of the dynamics of the simultaneous interactions among tens of thousands of neuronal groups. The model contains no units that are directly selective for arbitrary conjunctions of object properties, such as a "red cross located in the upper-left quadrant." Instead, in these simulations reentrant interactions rapidly establish a pattern of short-term temporal correlations among widely spaced neuronal groups in different maps. Selection of those circuits which are temporally correlated leads to a coherent output. In this way, integration is achieved not in any place but by a coherent *process*. Furthermore, integration occurs rapidly, within 100–250 msec after the presentation of the stimulus. The model therefore illustrates how reentry can solve the binding problem by coupling neuronal responses in distributed cortical areas to achieve synchronization and global coherency.

In a different and much more detailed model of cortical areas, which included interconnected thalamic regions, we further examined the dynamics of reentrant interactions within the thalamocortical system (Lumer et al. 1997a, 1997b). The results obtained from these simulations indicate that reentrant signaling within the cortex and between the cortex and the thalamus, bolstered by fast changes in synaptic efficacy and spontaneous activity within the network, can serve to rapidly establish a transient, globally coherent process. This process is characterized by strong and rapid interactions among the participating neuronal groups in the cortex and the thalamus, and it emerges at a well-defined threshold of activity. What is remarkable is that this coherent process is quite stable, being capable of sustaining itself continuously while at the same time changing its precise composition. This process includes a large number of neurons both in the cortex and in the thalamus, although by no means does it include all of them nor even all of those which are active at a given time. That such a self-perpetuating dynamic process, characterized by the strength and speed of reentrant neural interactions, can originate from the connectivity of the thalamocortical system is of considerable significance for understanding the actual neural events that underlie the unity of consciousness. Against this background, we have suggested that consciousness arose in evolution as a result of new reentrant connections between posterior thalamocortical systems mediating perceptual categorization, and more anterior systems mediating categorical memory (Edelman 1987).

Principles: The Dynamic Core

The previous considerations indicate that reentry is the key mechanism for the generation of an integrated and yet differentiated neural process that appears to be necessary for consciousness to emerge. But what is meant, precisely, when we say that a neural process is integrated? How can integration be measured, and how can one determine the extent and boundaries of an integrated neural process? And how is one to conceptualize and measure the degree to which such a neural process can be differentiated?

A useful intuitive criterion for integration is the following: A subset of elements within a system will constitute an integrated process if, on a given time scale, these elements interact much more strongly among themselves than with the rest of the system. Such a subset of strongly interacting elements that is functionally demarcated from the rest of the system can be called a "functional cluster." It is important to be able to make this criterion explicit and to possess an actual measure of functional clustering that is theoretically satisfactory and empirically useful. Unfortunately, no universally accepted definition of "cluster" exists in the statistical literature, although it is generally agreed that a cluster should be defined in terms of internal cohesion and external isolation. With this in mind, we have developed a measure of functional clustering designed to evaluate whether within a neural system there are subsets of elements that strongly

interact among themselves but interact much less strongly with the rest of the system (Tononi et al. 1998b). This functional *cluster index* reflects the relative strength of the interactions within a subset of elements (measured by their integration) compared with the interactions between that subset and the rest of the system (measured by their mutual information; for an exposition of these measures, see Tononi et al. 1998a). Thus, the cluster index allows us to identify a neural process that is highly integrated.

In order to evaluate the degree to which a neural process is differentiated, and therefore informative, we have introduced a measure called complexity (Tononi et al. 1994), which reflects the number of different states that a neural process can take on by virtue of its intrinsic interactions. Complexity is a function of the average mutual information between each subset and the rest of the system, and it reflects the number of states of a system that result from interactions among its elements. It can be shown that high values of complexity reflect the coexistence of a high degree of functional specialization and functional integration within a system, as appears to be the case for systems such as the brain. For example, the dynamic behavior of a simulated cortical area containing thousands of spontaneously active neuronal groups resembled the low-voltage, fast-activity EEG of waking and had high complexity. Such a system, whose connections were organized according to the rules found in the cortex, visited a large repertoire of different activity patterns that were the result of interactions among its elements. If the density of the connections was reduced, the dynamic behavior of the model resembled that of a noisy TV screen and had minimal complexity. A large number of activity patterns were visited, but they were merely the result of the independent fluctuations of the model's elements. If the connections within the cortical area were instead distributed at random, the system yielded a hypersynchronous EEG that resembled the high-voltage waves of slow-wave sleep or of generalized epilepsy.

The system visited a very limited repertoire of activity patterns and its complexity was low.

The Dynamic Core Hypothesis

The approach we have pursued here has been to focus on the fundamental properties of conscious experience such as integration and differentiation, and to provide an adequate explanation for them in terms of neural processes. If one takes such an approach, it appears that an adequate explanation is unlikely to come from the assumption that certain local properties of neurons may sooner or later hold the key to the mystery of consciousness. How could having a specific location in the brain, firing in a particular mode or at a particular frequency, or expressing a particular biochemical compound or gene, endow a neuron with the remarkable property of giving rise to conscious experience? The logical and philosophical problems of hypostatization associated with such assumptions are all too obvious, as has been remarked upon many times by both philosophers and scientists.

By contrast, if integration and differentiation are indeed fundamental features of consciousness, they can be explained only by a distributed neural process rather than by specific local properties of neurons. In fact, it is possible to formulate a hypothesis that explicitly states what, if anything, is special about the particular subset of neuronal groups which sustain conscious experience, and how they can be identified. To do so, we have proposed the dynamic core hypothesis (Tononi and Edelman, 1998a), which states that:

1. A group of neurons can contribute directly to conscious experience only if it is part of a distributed functional cluster that, through reentrant interactions in the thalamocortical system, achieves high integration in hundreds of milliseconds.

2. To sustain conscious experience, it is essential that this functional cluster be highly differentiated, as indicated by high values of complexity.

We call such a cluster of neuronal groups that strongly interact among themselves and have distinct functional borders with the rest of the brain at the time scale of fractions of a second a "dynamic core," in order to emphasize both its integration and its constantly changing composition. A dynamic core is a process rather than a thing or a place, and it is defined in terms of neural interactions rather than in terms of neural location, connectivity, or activity. While a dynamic core can have a spatial range or extension, it is in general spatially distributed and thus cannot be localized to a single place in the brain. Furthermore, even if a functional cluster with such properties is identified, we predict that it will be associated with conscious experience only if the reentrant interactions within the core are sufficiently differentiated, as indicated by its complexity. Finally, the dynamic core is neither coextensive with the entire brain nor restricted to any special subset of neurons. The term "dynamic core" deliberately does not refer to a unique, invariant set of brain areas (be they prefrontal, extrastriate, or striate cortex), and the core may change in composition over time. The core would typically include posterior corticothalamic regions involved in perceptual categorization interacting reentrantly with anterior regions involved in concept formation, value-related memory, and planning, although it would not necessarily be restricted to the thalamocortical system.

Since our hypothesis highlights the role of the functional interactions among distributed groups of neurons rather than their local properties (Crick and Koch 1995; Zeki and Bartels 1998), the same group of neurons may at times be part of the dynamic core and underlie conscious experience, and at other times it may not be part of it and thus may be involved in unconscious processes. Furthermore, since participation in the dynamic core depends on the rapidly shifting functional connectivity among groups of neurons rather than on anatomical proximity, the composition of the core can transcend traditional anatomical boundaries. Finally, as suggested by imaging studies (Tononi et al. 1998c), the exact composition of the core related to particular conscious states is expected to vary significantly across individuals.

The dynamic core hypothesis avoids the category error of assuming that certain local, intrinsic properties of neurons have, in some mysterious way, a privileged correlation with consciousness. Instead, it accounts for fundamental properties of conscious experience by linking them to global properties of particular neural processes. We have seen that conscious experience itself is a process that is unified and private, that is extremely differentiated, and that evolves on the time scale of hundreds of msec. The dynamic core is a process, since it is characterized in terms of time-varying neural interactions, not as a thing or a location. It is unified and private, since its integration must be high at the same time its mutual information with what surrounds is low, thus creating a functional boundary between what is part of it and what is not. The requirement for high complexity means that the dynamic core must be highly differentiated—it must be able to select, based on its intrinsic interactions, among a large repertoire of different activity patterns. Finally, the selection among its integrated states must be achieved within hundreds of msec, reflecting the time course of conscious experience.

Conscious and Unconscious Neural Processes

The dynamic core hypothesis is heuristically useful not only because it specifies the kinds of neural processes that underlie conscious experience but also because it provides a rationale for distinguishing them from those which remain unconscious (Tononi and Edelman 1998a, 1998b). For example, neural processes involved in the regulation of blood pressure normally do not contribute to conscious experience. Why is this the case? According to our hypothesis, this is because the neurons dealing with the regulation

of blood pressure are not part of the dynamic core, and in any event they do not by themselves generate an integrated neural process of sufficient dimensionality and complexity.

In a similar vein, the dynamic core hypothesis suggests that the neural substrate of many well-learned, automatic neural routines in both the motor and the cognitive domains, which allow us to carry out complicated motor acts as well as to read and to speak, and which remain largely unconscious, should be quite different dynamically from the core processes that are responsible for conscious experience. Such unconscious routines, which are both motor and cognitive, involve long, parallel neural loops running through cortical appendages such as the basal ganglia, the cerebellum, and the hippocampus. According to the dynamic core hypothesis, such motor and cognitive routines should be carried out by dedicated, polysynaptic circuits that are functionally insulated from each other and from the core except for their input and output stages. Instead of involving changes in the state of the entire core, such routines would be carried out by rapid state changes that are local and remain confined to a relatively small number of neurons.

Finally, the core hypothesis suggests the possibility that the thalamocortical system may support, at any one time, more than one large functional cluster. Because of an anatomical or functional disconnection, certain ongoing neural processes in the thalamocortical system may not become incorporated into the dominant dynamic core and thus may remain functionally insulated from it. Functional or anatomical disconnections of this kind may underlie several of the pathological dissociations encountered in psychiatry (e.g., dissociative disorders and conversion disorders) and in neuropsychology, notably the split-brain syndrome (Tononi and Edelman 2000). For example, in hysterical blindness a subject is capable of avoiding obstacles and yet denies seeing anything. An interesting possibility would be that in such patients, a small functional cluster including certain visual areas is autonomously active, may not fuse with the dominant functional cluster, and yet still be capable of accessing motor routines in the basal ganglia and elsewhere. This may very well be the case in split-brain patients, in whom at least two functional clusters appear to coexist in the brain because of the callosal disconnection. It is also conceivable that splinter cores may exist alongside a dominant core in normal subjects. Such splinter cores may underlie cognitive activities that remain unconscious despite the fact that they share many of the hallmarks of the "mental" and that they can powerfully influence our actions (Edelman and Tononi 2000).

Neural Correlates: Pointing to the Core

The core hypothesis has the important feature that it is possible to design experiments to test its predictions, especially if one takes advantage of imaging techniques that offer high temporal resolution. Indeed, we have performed some initial experiments in this direction using whole-head magnetoencephalography (Tononi et al. 1998c). A specific reference state for consciousness would be the response to a simple sensory input when a subject is unaware of it versus when the subject is aware of it. In a study in our laboratory, we attempted to capture that difference and thus measure some neural correlates of consciousness. Our experiments were carried out under conditions of binocular rivalry. In binocular rivalry, a subject views two incongruent stimuli through each eye but consciously perceives only one stimulus at a time, with a switch in perceptual dominance every few seconds without specific voluntary attention. For example, a subject may see a red vertical grating with his left eye through a red lens, and a blue horizontal grating with his right eye through a blue lens. Although both stimuli are presented, he will alternately report only one or the other. Somehow, while the visual system receives signals from both stimuli, only one at a time makes it to conscious experience.

We used magnetoencephalography (MEG) to measure electrical brain responses to rivalrous visual stimuli. A key to the success of this study was to have a way to know which brain responses corresponded to blue and which to red. This was achieved by causing each stimulus to flicker in intensity at a specific frequency. It turned out that the MEG potentials from the brain—the so-called steady-state evoked responses—show a sharp response to that frequency, which can thus be used as a tag for that particular stimulus.

In this study, each stimulus was flickered at a different tag frequency in the range of 7–12 oscillations per second; for example, red vertical at 7.4 Hz and blue horizontal at 9.5 Hz. Steady-state evoked responses at either tag frequency specific to each stimulus could be detected in many MEG channels. When we analyzed the data, a first important observation was that neural electrical responses to rivalrous visual stimuli occurred in a large number of cortical regions both when the subject consciously perceived the stimuli and when he did not. The second striking finding of this study was, however, that the neuromagnetic responses evoked by a stimulus were stronger by 50–85 percent when the subjects were conscious of it than when they were not. These increased neural responses to a stimulus associated with its conscious perception were simultaneously distributed to a large subset of different brain regions, including occipital, temporal, and frontal areas, although by no means were they seen in all the regions showing stimulus-related activity. Finally, a particularly striking finding was that the specific subsets of different brain regions showing such modulation by conscious perception varied significantly from subject to subject. Thus, the results of this study provided a clear indication that the set of brain regions whose activity correlates with conscious experience is a widely distributed one and, equally important, that the distribution differs in different subjects.

Perhaps most important of all, more recent investigations have shown that various kinds of cognitive tasks which require awareness are accompanied by short-term *temporal* correlations among distributed populations of neurons in the thalamocortical system (Srinivasan et al. 1999). When we examined binocular rivalry with MEG to look for signs of interactions among brain areas, for example, we found a remarkable result. An index of how much the activity of distant brain regions is synchronized or in phase is provided by their so-called coherence. Coherence values between brain regions can be taken as a reflection of the strength of the reentrant interactions among them. In striking agreement with our predictions, coherence between distant brain regions responding to the stimulus was always higher when a subject was aware of the stimulus than when he was not. Taken together with the findings mentioned above, these results provide strong evidence that for conscious experience to occur, the rapid integration of the activity of distributed brain regions through reentrant interactions is required.

This position is open to further experimentation in which the refinement of qualitative discriminations in any modality can be investigated via improved imaging technology. The ability to define functional clustering and to estimate neural complexity over short periods of time will be particularly useful in designing experiments to test this hypothesis directly. We have already seen, for example, that by exploiting frequency tagging in MEG studies of binocular rivalry, relatively direct approaches to the neural substrates of consciousness can be designed. Whether all aspects of the dynamic core hypothesis are correct or not, the criteria outlined here should facilitate the design of similar experiments using imaging methodologies that offer wide spatial coverage as well as high temporal resolution. These include fMRI, topographic EEG, and MEG. Such experiments might answer several relevant questions about brain dynamics: Is there, whenever a subject is conscious, a set of brain regions that interact much more strongly among themselves than with the rest of the brain over fractions of a second (i.e., can we directly show the existence of a dynamic core)? Does its composition change, depending upon the conscious activity the subject is engaged in? Are certain brain regions always included or always excluded? Is it the case that cognitive or motor activities which remain unconscious are mediated by neural circuits that are functionally insulated? Can the core split, or can multiple dynamic cores coexist in a normal subject? Are there pathological conditions that reflect such multiple cores, or are there abnormalities of a single core? Finally, what is the complexity of the dynamic core itself, and how can this complexity be correlated with the ability to differentiate that is such a fundamental property of conscious experience? These questions, and their associated predictions prompted by our hypotheses, set an agenda that is amenable to direct experimental tests.

Success in such experimentation and confirmation of the existence of a dynamic core should go a long way toward providing a sound scientific description of conscious experience, an experience that is obviously based upon morphology in an individual body. While being is not describing, an appropriate scientific description should allow us to expand our understanding of the physical base of mental experience.

Acknowledgments

This work was carried out as part of the theoretical neurobiology program at The Neurosciences Institute, which is supported by Neurosciences Research Foundation. The Foundation receives major support for this program from Novartis and the W. M. Keck Foundation. Part of this material is based on a previously published article (Tononi and Edelman 1998a) and on a forthcoming book (Edelman and Tononi 2000).

References

Baars, B. J. (1988). *A Cognitive Theory of Consciousness.* New York: Cambridge University Press.

Braun, A. R., Balkin, T. J., Wesenten, N. J., Carson, R. E., Varga, M., Baldwin, P., Selbie, S., Belenky, G., and Herscovitch, P. (1997). Regional cerebral blood flow throughout the sleep-wake cycle. An $H_2(^{15}O)$O PET study. *Brain* 120: 1173–1197.

Bressler, S. L., Coppola, R., and Nakamura, R. (1993). Episodic multiregional cortical coherence at multiple frequencies during visual task performance. *Nature* 366: 153–156.

Cauller, L. (1995). Layer I of primary sensory neocortex: Where top-down converges upon bottom-up. *Behavioural Brain Research* 71: 163–180.

Crick, F., and Koch, C. (1995). Are we aware of neural activity in primary visual cortex? *Nature* 375: 121–123.

Damasio, A. R. (1989). Time-locked multiregional retroactivation—a systems-level proposal for the neural substrates of recall and recognition. *Cognition* 33: 25–62.

Edelman, G. M. (1987). *Neural Darwinism: The Theory of Neuronal Group Selection.* New York: Basic Books.

Edelman, G. M. (1989). *The Remembered Present: A Biological Theory of Consciousness.* New York: Basic Books.

Edelman, G. M., and Tononi, G. (2000). *A Universe of Consciousness.* New York: Basic Books.

Engel, A. K., Konig, P., Kreiter, A. K., and Singer, W. (1991). Interhemispheric synchronization of oscillatory neuronal responses in cat visual cortex. *Science* 252: 1177–1179.

Friston, K. J. (1998). Imaging neuroscience: Principles or maps? *Proceedings of the National Academy of Sciences of the United States of America* 95: 796–802.

Fuster, J. M., Bauer, R. H., Jervey, J. P. (1985). Functional interactions between inferotemporal and prefrontal cortex in a cognitive task. *Brain Research* 330: 299–307.

Gazzaniga, M. S. (1995). Principles of human brain organization derived from split-brain studies. *Neuron* 14: 217–228.

Gevins, A., Smith, M. E., Le, J., Leong, H., Bennett, J., Martin, N., McEvoy, L., Du, R., and Whitfield, S. (1996). High resolution evoked potential imaging of the cortical dynamics of human working memory. *Electroencephalography and Clinical Neurophysiology* 98: 327–348.

Goldman-Rakic, P. S., and Chafee, M. (1994). Feedback processing in prefronto-parietal circuits during memory-guided saccades. *Society for Neuroscience Abstracts* 20: 808.

Horel, J. A., Vierck, C. J., Jr., Pribram, K. H., Spinelli, D. N., John, E. R., and Ruchkin, D. S. (1967). Average evoked responses and learning. *Science* 158: 394–395.

Joliot, M., Ribary, U., and Llinás, R. (1994). Human oscillatory brain activity near 40 Hz coexists with cognitive temporal binding. *Proceedings of the National Academy of Sciences of the United States of America* 91: 11748–11751.

Libet, B. (1993). The neural time factor in conscious and unconscious events. *CIBA Foundation Symposium* 174: 123–137.

Lumer, E. D., Edelman, G. M., and Tononi, G. (1997a). Neural dynamics in a model of the thalamo-cortical system. 1. Layers, loops and the emergence of fast synchronous rhythms. *Cerebral Cortex* 7: 207–227.

Lumer, E. D., Edelman, G. M., and Tononi, G. (1997b). Neural dynamics in a model of the thalamo-cortical system. 2. The role of neural synchrony tested through perturbations of spike timing. *Cerebral Cortex* 7: 228–236.

Maquet, P., Degueldre, C., Delfiore, G., Aerts, J., Péters, J. M., Luxen, A., and Franck, G. (1997). Functional neuroanatomy of human slow wave sleep. *Journal of Neuroscience* 17: 2807–2812.

Maquet, P., Péters, J., Aerts, J., Delfiore, G., Degueldre, C., Luxen, A., and Franck, G. (1996). Functional neuroanatomy of human rapid-eye-movement sleep and dreaming. *Nature* 383: 163–166.

Marcel, A. J. (1983). Conscious and unconscious perception: An approach to the relations between phenomenal experience and perceptual processes. *Cognitive Psychology* 15: 238–300.

Maunsell, J. H. (1995). The brain's visual world: Representation of visual targets in cerebral cortex. *Science* 270: 764–769.

Petersen, S. E., van Mier, H., Fiez, J. A., and Raichle, M. E. (1998). The effects of practice on the functional anatomy of task performance. *Proceedings of the National Academy of Sciences of the United States of America* 95: 853–860.

Plum, F. (1991). Coma and related global disturbances of the human conscious state. In A. Peters and

E. G. Jones, eds., *Normal and Altered States of Function*, Vol. 9, 359–425. New York: Plenum Press.

Singer, W., and Gray, C. M. (1995). Visual feature integration and the temporal correlation hypothesis. *Annual Review of Neuroscience* 18: 555–586.

Sporns, O., Tononi, G., and Edelman, G. M. (1991). Modeling perceptual grouping and figure-ground segregation by means of active reentrant connections. *Proceedings of the National Academy of Sciences of the United States of America* 88: 129–133.

Srinivasan, R., Russell, D. P., Edelman, G. M., and Tononi, G. (1999). Increased synchronization of magnetic responses during conscious perception. *Journal of Neuroscience* 19: 5435–5448.

Tononi, G., and Edelman, G. M. (1998a). Consciousness and complexity. *Science* 282: 1846–1851.

Tononi, G., and Edelman, G. M. (1998b). Consciousness and the integration of information in the brain. In H. H. Jasper et al., eds., *Consciousness: At the Frontiers of neuroscience*. New York: Plenum Press.

Tononi, G., and Edelman, G. M. (2000). Schizophrenia and the mechanisms of conscious integration. *Brain Research Reviews* 31: 391–400.

Tononi, G., Edelman, G. M., and Sporns, O. (1998a). Complexity and the integration of information in the brain. *Trends in Cognitive Sciences* 2: 44–52.

Tononi, G., McIntosh, A. R., Russell, D. P., and Edelman, G. M. (1998b). Functional clustering: Identifying strongly interactive brain regions in neuroimaging data. *Neuroimage* 7: 133–149.

Tononi, G., Sporns, O., and Edelman, G. M. (1992). Reentry and the problem of integrating multiple cortical areas: Simulation of dynamic integration in the visual system. *Cerebral Cortex* 2: 310–335.

Tononi, G., Sporns, O., and Edelman, G. M. (1994). A measure for brain complexity: Relating functional segregation and integration in the nervous system. *Proceedings of the National Academy of Sciences of the United States of America* 91: 5033–5038.

Tononi, G., Srinivasan, R., Russell, D. P., and Edelman, G. M. (1998c). Investigating neural correlates of conscious perception by frequency-tagged neuromagnetic responses. *Proceedings of the National Academy of Sciences of the United States of America* 95: 3198–3203.

Zeki, S., and Bartels, A. (1998). The asynchrony of consciousness. *Proceedings of the Royal Society of London* ser. B, 265: 1583–1585.

III CANDIDATES FOR THE NCC II: VISION

For human beings, visual experience clearly occupies the dominant portion of their phenomenal space. A considerable part of the philosophical discussion on qualia is centered around the issue of color qualia, and many researchers on the empirical frontier of consciousness research have chosen to focus first on vision, since the visual system is obviously the one part of the brain of which we presently have the best understanding. For a number of reasons, heuristically the visual modality is the best place to start an investigation of the sensory aspects of phenomenal experience. There is no doubt that in the future this situation will change and we will see a lot of rigorous research trying to reveal the neural underpinnings of conscious auditory experience, of phenomenal gustation and olfaction, and of other highly interesting yet too much neglected aspects of consciousness, such as tactile and visceral sensitivity, proprioception, pain, or the phenomenal representation of vestibular information. This third part of the book, however, will start to introduce readers to some examples of current research on the conscious experience of seeing.

Based on work by Vorberg et al. (in prep.), Thomas Schmidt presents data that demonstrate the possibility of color processing without awareness. He shows the existence of response priming by color, which implies that response control is not functionally isolated from the flow of color information in the human brain. On the other hand, it is not critical whether or not the primes used are phenomenally available, if they actually form the content of visual awareness. The functional profile of our cognitive architecture sets limits to what is accessible to conscious experience. This has interesting methodological implications, but simultaneously generates questions possessing a typically philosophical flavor, such as: Could something like "invisible colors" actually exist?

Phenomenal experience plays an important role in the processing of social stimuli because it makes implicit information about conspecifics

globally available for attention, the generation of motor behavior and social cognition. The conscious experience of faces is a highly specific and particularly compelling example. In our own case, face perception acts like a sensory window into the emotional state and intentions of fellow human beings. Jonathan Cole (1997, 193) introduced the notion of "facial embodiment," pointing out how crucial facial animation is for our own emotional existence as well. Faces are "embodied communication areas." How much of this highly specialized type of information processing is actually independent of conscious experience?

What are the neuroanatomical substrates of phenomenal face representation? In her contribution Beena Khurana presents visual priming findings which suggest that the visual system is capable of creating representations of human faces "on the fly" in the absence of focused attention. The results are largely in accord with response profiles of "face" cells in the superior temporal sulcus, and it is suggested that these cells are involved in the implicit, nonconscious processing of faces. Explicit face representation, however, may require the additional involvement of the face cells in the inferior prefrontal cortex that receive direct input from the superior temporal sulcus. This leads to the conclusion that the activity of these cells either alone or in conjunction with face-sensitive cells in the superior temporal sulcus renders representations that correspond to the phenomenal experience of seeing someone.

Melvyn Goodale and Kelly Murphy continue by presenting evidence that the visuospatial information processing which helps us to control our visually guided actions directed at certain objects in our environment is functionally separate from the kind of information processing which eventually leads to our conscious *perception* of these objects. In their essay, based on a substantial amount of neuropsychological data and contrary to commonly held assumptions, they argue that the way our visual system codes space is not unitary. For instance, some neurological patients are able to carry out successful visually guided movements like grasping objects, despite not having any conscious visual experience of the location, size, shape, or orientation of these objects whatsoever. In other words, visual information about object features can be successfully exploited by the systems mediating visually guided action, but remains unavailable at the level of phenomenal representation.

This, and a number of other recent findings, contradict the classical "what" versus "where" distinction for visual processing in the dorsal and ventral streams introduced by Ungerleider and Mishkin in 1982. The new interpretation of the division of labor between the two streams now emerging differentiates between allocentric and egocentric spatial information: The ventral stream, which mediates conscious experience, computes allocentric spatial information about the layout of objects in the visual scene, whereas dorsal stream mechanisms, subserving mainly the automatic visual control of action, generate precise egocentric spatial information about the location of objects with regard to a body-centered frame of reference. The ventral stream mechanisms deliver conscious percepts, whereas dorsal stream mechanisms provide the unconscious visual control of action.

One of the phenomenal primitives of conscious vision is the perception of motion. Obviously, if conscious vision is supposed to help us in successfully getting around in the world, it should represent moving objects in a way that allows us to, for instance, grasp them at their current position in the external world. However, the mechanisms that lead to the phenomenal experience of motion are themselves time-consuming—there will be different representations of the actual position of a moving object at different times and at different levels of the visual system. Immediately a question about the veridicality of the phenomenal level of representation arises: Does conscious experience depict the instantaneous position of a moving object correctly, or does the percept lag behind the actual location? Romi Nijhawan and Beena Khurana offer experimental support and a number of very interesting theoretical considerations for the "no lag" conjecture, which claims that the phenomenal position of a moving object agrees with its actual position. In the end this leads to a number of valuable insights not only about the possible neural correlates of phenomenal motion experience, but also about a feature of phenomenal content that philosophers sometimes call its "transparency": In standard situations the illusion of direct and "instantaneous" contact with the external world created by the internal structures subserving the process of conscious experience is so perfect that we "look through" these structures and do not recognize them as representational structures any more. We don't see the window, but only the bird flying by.

Dominic ffytche begins by offering theoretical considerations concerning different possible research strategies utilizing neuroimaging studies to pin down the neural correlate(s) of consciousness: Are we looking for the correlates of different types of phenomenal content, like conscious face perception, the conscious experience of color, or motor planning, or are we trying to correlate one unified, highest-order phenomenon —"the whole of consciousness as such"—with its physical basis? Holism and modularism as methodological background assumptions yield different research strategies, and, as ffytche shows, both look back to long historical traditions in neurobiology. He then goes on to relate two recent fMRI studies to this historical background. The first study looked for the correlates of visual hallucinations and found that hallucinated phenomenal content correlated with activity within specialized visual areas, following a simple "additive logic" for the relationship between active correlate and consciously available content. The second study, done with the now famous blindsight subject GY, directly related the amount of activity in the motion area to the conscious experience of "seeing" motion, suggesting that the difference between conscious and unconscious visual representation is not coded by the location of activity but by the *type of processing* it realizes. And this leads us back to the theoretical issues outlined by ffytche at the beginning of his paper.

In the last essay of this section, Erik Lumer reviews recent research exploiting the phenomenon of binocular rivalry for the project of delineating the neural correlates of conscious vision. Binocular rivalry is a particularly interesting phenomenon, because changes in the content of conscious representations take place without any changes in the stimulus itself (see also ffytche, chapter 14). While the actual input on the retina is held stable, phenomenal content varies. This makes it possible to search for covarying elements in concomitant brain activity, looking for those functional aspects and those levels of processing which exhibit the greatest strength of correlation. A number of findings demonstrate that activity in multiple, functionally distinct, visual and prefrontal regions of human cortex is correlated with conscious perception during binocular rivalry. The picture that emerges from the imaging studies described by Lumer is that the ventral pathway is not sufficient to produce conscious visual perception; rather, these studies suggest that awareness of a visual stimulus is accomplished by the coactivation of neurons distributed over multiple brain regions, including cortical areas in both ventral and dorsal visual pathways, and in the prefrontal lobe. The functional properties of these areas further suggest that their coactivation combines three distinct capacities that appear crucial for the formation of conscious perceptual states: to extract higher-order features of the visual input, to select among countless alternative interpretations of how these features make up a visual scene, and to integrate the selected scene in the broader temporal and behavioral context in which it occurs.

Further Reading

Barbur, J. L., Watson, J. D. G., Frackowiak, R. S. J., and Zeki, S. (1993). Conscious visual perception without V1. *Brain* 116: 1293–1302.

Berry, M. J., Brivanlou, I. H., Jordan, T. A., and Meister, M. (1999). Anticipation of moving stimuli by the retina. *Nature* 398: 334–338.

Cole, J. (1997). *On Face.* Cambridge, MA: MIT Press.

DeSchepper, B., and Treisman, A. (1995). Visual memory for novel shapes: Implicit coding without attention. *Journal of Experimental Psychology: Learning, Memory, & Cognition* 22: 27–47.

ffytche, D. H., Howard, R. J., Brammer, M. J., David, A., Woodruff, P., and Williams, S. (1998). The anatomy of conscious vision: An fMRI study of visual hallucinations. *Nature Neuroscience* 1: 738–742.

Frith, C., Perry, R., and Lumer, E. D. (1999). The neural correlates of conscious experience: An experimental framework. *Trends in Cognitive Sciences* 3: 105–114.

Goodale, M. A., and Humphrey, G. K. (1998). The objects of action and perception. *Cognition* 67: 179–205.

Khurana, B. (2000). Not to be and then to be: Visual representation of ignored unfamiliar faces. *Journal of Experimental Psychology: Human Perception & Performance* 26: 246–263.

Leopold, D. A., and Logothetis, N. K. (1999). Multistable phenomena: Changing views in perception. *Trends in Cognitive Sciences* 7: 254–264.

Lumer, E. D., Friston, K. J., and Rees, G. (1998). Neural correlates of perceptual rivalry in the human brain. *Science* 280: 1930–1934.

Lumer, E. D., and Rees, G. (1999). Covariation of activity in visual and prefrontal cortex associated with subjective visual perception. *Proceedings of the National Academy of Sciences of the United States of America,* 96: 1669–1673.

Macknik, S. L., and Livingstone, M. S. (1998). Neuronal correlates of visibility and invisibility in the primate visual system. *Nature Neuroscience* 1: 144–149.

Milner, A. D., and Goodale, M. A. (1995). *The Visual Brain in Action.* Oxford: Oxford University Press.

Nijhawan, R. (1994). Motion extrapolation in catching. *Nature* 370: 256–257.

Nijhawan, R. (1997). Visual decomposition of color through motion extrapolation. *Nature* 386: 66–69.

Schmidt, T. (in prep.). Online-control of speeded pointing movements: Isoluminant color stimuli can specify motor responses.

Tipper, S. P., Weaver, B., and Houghton, G. (1994). Behavioural goals determine inhibitory mechanisms of selective attention. *Quarterly Journal of Experimental Psychology* 47A: 809–840.

Ungerleider, L. G., and Mishkin, M. (1982). Two cortical visual systems. In D. J. Ingle, M. A. Goodale, and R. J. W. Mansfield (eds.), *Analysis of Visual Behavior*. Cambridge, MA: MIT Press.

Weiskrantz, L. (1997). *Consciousness Lost and Found: A Neuropsychological Exploration*. Oxford: Oxford University Press.

Zeki, S., and ffytche, D. H. (1998). The Riddoch syndrome: Insights into the neurobiology of conscious vision. *Brain* 121: 25–45.

10

Visual Perception Without Awareness: Priming Responses by Color

Thomas Schmidt

Priming and Visual Awareness

Invisible Colors?

In vision science, the term "color" refers to conscious experience, as opposed to terms like "wavelength," which describe physical properties of the stimulus. Therefore, a notion like "nonconscious perception of color" seems self-contradictory. However, there is some evidence that conscious perception of a color can be dissociated from other aspects of color processing. For example, Cowey and Heywood (1997) describe a patient with achromatopsia (a selective disturbance of color vision following brain damage) who is not able to discriminate isoluminant color signals but can still detect color boundaries. There are similar observations in some blindsight patients who can make discriminative responses to stimuli of different wavelengths appearing within their scotoma (Stoerig and Cowey 1989, 1992). These data suggest that the processing of spectral information does not inevitably lead to what these patients would call "seeing color."

Nonconscious influences of color stimuli are particularly interesting for biological theories of visual awareness. For instance, Milner and Goodale (1995) have linked visual awareness and color processing to a common visual pathway. In this view, the visual area V4—often regarded as the "color center" of the primate brain (e.g., Zeki 1993; but see Hadjikhani et al. 1998)—is part of a *ventral stream* of visual computation that is assumed to be the sole basis of visual awareness of color. It is not, however, the assumed basis of visually guided motor responses, which are controlled by a second, *dorsal stream*.

How can nonconscious influences of color stimuli be demonstrated? Most psychological experiments on nonconscious perception (e.g., Draine and Greenwald 1998) have used a variant of the *task dissociation procedure* (Reingold and Merikle 1988). In this procedure, two properties of the critical stimulus (referred to here as the "prime") must be demonstrated. First, the prime must influence the response to another stimulus (e.g., by slowing or speeding performance). Such a *priming effect* is an *indirect measure* of visual processing of the prime because it implies that the prime must have been sufficiently analyzed. Second, one must show that the prime cannot be consciously perceived, usually by establishing near-chance performance in a forced-choice discrimination or detection task. This is taken as a *direct measure* of visual awareness of the prime. Although it is usually easy to demonstrate indirect effects in the first part of the procedure, many experiments have been criticized for imperfections in the second part, namely, convincingly establishing that the prime was really not consciously identified at the time of presentation (for critical reviews, see Eriksen 1960; Holender 1986).

Using the task dissociation procedure, Marcel (1983) used masked color words to prime responses to color patches. When the prime word was inconsistent with the color of the patch, responses were slowed, even when identification performance for the prime word did not exceed a preset critical value (60 percent correct discriminations). However, Cheesman and Merikle (1984), using a stricter and more reliable procedure of threshold estimation, found that the amount of priming simply covaried with identifiability of the prime. When prime–mask intervals were so short that the prime words became indiscriminable, the priming effect disappeared. They concluded that presenting primes with above-chance discriminability was a necessary precondition for obtaining a priming effect.

Both studies investigated semantic influences of the prime, which may not be the most powerful effects that it can have. I will present evidence for nonsemantic features of the prime having large effects on motor responses assigned to them in the context of the experimental task. Moreover, the priming effect seems to depend primarily on temporal properties of the stimuli and to be independent of visual awareness.

Studies in Response Priming

Neumann and Klotz (1994; Klotz and Wolff 1995) used *metacontrast*, a form of visual backward masking, to reduce the visibility of the primes to a point where they could not be discriminated. In metacontrast, the visibility of a briefly flashed stimulus is reduced when it is followed by a masking stimulus with adjacent but nonoverlapping contours (Francis 1997; Macknik and Livingstone 1998). The critical feature of the task was that prime and mask were similar in shape, so that they shared features relevant for either the correct or the alternative response. The authors found that unidentifiable primes still affected response time (RT) to the masking stimulus, showing facilitatory effects from response-consistent primes and interference effects from inconsistent primes.

We extended these findings to study the time course of the priming effect (Vorberg et al. submitted). We used arrow stimuli as masks that could point either to the left or to the right, and participants made a speeded 2-alternative keypress response to the direction of the mask. Priming stimuli also were arrows, presented in a central cutout of the mask so that their visibility was strongly reduced by metacontrast. Varying the stimulus onset asynchrony (SOA) between prime and mask, we found that a prime pointing in the same direction as the mask speeded responses to the mask, whereas a prime pointing in the opposite direction slowed responses. The *priming effect* (the response time difference between inconsistent and consistent cases) increased linearly with SOA, yielding a *priming function* with nearly constant slope. On the other hand, there was no indication of visual awareness of

the prime in any condition: Despite extended practice and a highly reliable measurement procedure, participants were not able to discriminate the primes in a forced-choice test.

In another experiment, varying the relative durations of prime and mask presentations yielded qualitatively different time courses of prime identification performance. However, the shape of the priming function was unchanged, regardless of whether the prime could be identified, or whether prime identifiability was an increasing or decreasing function of SOA. These data suggest *independence* of the time courses of priming and visual awareness, so that the time course of the priming effect depends on the prime–mask SOA only. Since then, these results have proven extremely reliable and have been replicated with different stimuli and types of response.

Schlaghecken and Eimer (1997; Eimer and Schlaghecken 1998) used both event-related potentials and response times to study the physiological dynamics of the priming effect in a task similar to ours. They found that magnitude and direction of the priming effect were paralleled by shifts in lateralized potentials above motor cortex. This strongly suggests that the prime does affect motor responses rather than only visual or semantic aspects of processing.

In short, it seems that the prime directly affects motor performance by activating an assigned response, with the activation level depending only on the time course of visual availability of the prime (the prime–mask SOA). For this reason, I will use the term *response priming* for this type of priming task with a unique and consistent mapping of primes to responses.

Response Priming—Dorsal vs. Ventral?

One possible explanation for the dissociation of visual awareness and response priming is in terms of the Milner and Goodale (1995) framework: Perhaps the priming effect originates in visuomotor transformation processes within the dorsal stream, while awareness of the prime is constructed within the ventral stream. This would allow for a dissociation between direct and indirect measures. However, response priming by color would defy this explanation.

For the sake of argument, let's use a simplified (and surely somewhat distorted) version of Milner and Goodale's framework to make predictions about response priming by color:

1. Color processing and visual awareness are confined to the ventral stream.

2. Response priming is confined to the dorsal stream.

3. Color information is not transmitted from the ventral to the dorsal stream and therefore cannot control motor responses directly.

In this view, the division of the visual system into two separate streams also produces a demarcation line between nonconscious (dorsal) and possibly conscious (ventral) visual processing. However, any processing of color signals (conscious or not) could occur only in the ventral stream.

This set of hypotheses is simplistic and is not meant as a paraphrase of the original theory, but it can be evaluated in a single experiment. If all three assertions were correct, response priming by color would be impossible, because there would be no way for color information to directly prime motor behavior. So, if response priming occurs with stimuli that differ in their color signal only, this implies that response control is not isolated from color information. As a consequence, if response priming by color occurs without awareness, this cannot be explained by a dissociation between ventral and dorsal streams.

Method

Each participant performed two tasks: a speeded choice response to the color of the mask (*mask identification task*) and an unspeeded choice re-

sponse to the color of the prime (*prime identification task*). Both tasks provided measures of color processing of the prime, but only the prime identification task was a measure of visual awareness (Reingold and Merikle 1988).

Participants

Six right-handed undergraduate psychology students (5 female, 1 male, with a mean age of 27.7 years) from the Technical University of Braunschweig, Germany, participated for course credit in 4 hour-long sessions. All participants had normal or corrected-to-normal vision. One subject reported a general problem with red–green discrimination but did not exhibit a discrimination deficit in any of the experimental tasks. All participants were unfamiliar with the task.

Apparatus and Stimuli

Participants sat in a dim room in front of a 60 Hz computer monitor controlled by a 80386 PC. Viewing distance was 90 cm. Displays consisted of a central fixation point ($0.13°$), a prime, and a mask. The prime was a red or green dot ($0.38°$) that could appear either above or below the fixation point, with an eccentricity of $2.42°$. The mask was a red or green annulus ($0.83°$) at the same position, with a central cutout that was exactly the size of the prime. All stimuli were presented against a dark background. In this particular experiment, red and green stimuli were not exactly isoluminant, with green stimuli appearing brighter than red ones; however, this factor did not interact with the major findings.[1] Saturation was low; colors departed only slightly from a common gray level.

Procedure

The procedure is described in figure 10.1. Each trial started with the presentation of the fixation point. Participants were instructed to look at this

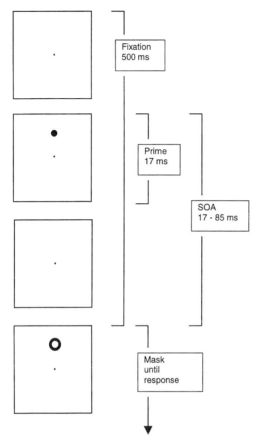

Figure 10.1
Time course of a single trial. Stimuli could appear either above or below the fixation point. Prime and mask color were independent; both stimuli could be either red or green.

point and not move their eyes during the presentation of stimuli. After presentation of a fixation point, the prime appeared for 17 msec either above or below the fixation point. After a prime–mask SOA of 17, 34, 51, 68, or 85 msec, the mask appeared at the same position as the prime and remained on the screen until the participant pressed one of two response keys on the computer keyboard, using the left or right index

finger, respectively. The interval between the onset of the fixation point and the onset of the mask was constant at 500 msec. After a constant intertrial interval (ITI) of 500 msec, the next trial started. Prime color, mask color, stimulus position, and prime–mask SOA were varied randomly and independently. Stimulus conditions were identical for the mask and prime identification tasks.

Two Tasks: Mask and Prime Identification

In the mask identification task, participants had to indicate the color of the mask by pressing the appropriate key (left or right). They were instructed to respond as quickly and accurately as possible. After an incorrect response, a tone (100 Hz, 500 msec) was sounded and the following ITI was prolonged to 1000 msec. At the end of the block, participants received visual feedback about their average response time and number of errors.

The prime identification task was similar, but participants had to identify the prime rather than the mask. However, to diminish possible nonconscious influences from the prime, responses were slightly delayed. A warning signal (1000 Hz, 200 msec) was sounded when the response time was shorter than 600 msec, and the following ITI was prolonged to 1000 msec. There was no feedback about the accuracy of the response. At the end of the block, however, participants received visual feedback about the number of errors.

In both tasks, the same keys on the computer keyboard were used (either "y" or "-" on a European-style QWERTZ keyboard). The mapping of colors to responses was constant across tasks for each participant and counterbalanced across participants.

Sessions

Each participant took part in 4 sessions. Each session started with 6 blocks of mask identification, followed by 6 blocks of prime identification, another 6 blocks of mask identification, and another 6 blocks of prime identification, with 40 trials per block. The first block in each new task was excluded from data analysis. The computer program announced every change in task and repeated the most important parts of the instructions. Participants could take a short break after each block.

At the beginning of the first session, participants were carefully instructed and practiced both tasks in a demonstration program. In the first block of this program, participants performed the mask identification task, with stimuli in the same temporal sequence as in the main experiment. In the second and third blocks, they performed the prime identification task with prolonged prime–mask SOAs so that the primes were clearly visible. All prime–mask combinations were used, so that participants had full information about stimulus combinations except the variation in SOAs.

At the beginning of each subsequent session, the most important parts of the instructions were repeated. After the final session, participants were informed about the purpose of the experiment and could examine their data patterns.

Analyses and Results

For all analyses of variance (ANOVAs) reported in this chapter, repeated observations from a single combination of participant and treatment were modeled as conditionally independent, due to randomization of treatments. To combine individual data, participants were introduced as a random factor, forming a higher-way classification. For analyses of individual participants, the participant factor was fixed and restricted to a single level, using the same dataset. For simplicity, I generally will not report effects associated with the participant factor.

Priming Effects in Mask Identification

Only correct responses were used for the analysis of response times in this task. Responses times shorter than 100 msec or longer than 999 msec (0.4 percent of the data) were excluded.

Figure 10.2a shows the response times in the mask identification task.[2] A three-way ANOVA (consistency × SOA × participant) revealed that responses to the mask were faster when preceded by a consistent rather than an inconsistent prime: $F(1, 5) = 731.17$, $MSE = 5,096,623.00$, $p < .001$. There was also an effect of SOA: $F(4, 20) = 3.30$, $MSE = 5,434.78$, $p < .05$. Most important, there was an interaction of consistency with SOA, showing that response times in inconsistent trials increased with SOA, whereas response times in consistent trials decreased: $F(4, 20) = 9.44$, $MSE = 23,261.31$, $p < .001$.

Sensitivity to the Prime

Signal detection theory (SDT) provides standard procedures for separating sensitivity and bias effects (Macmillan and Creelman 1991). The prime identification task was modeled as a yes–no detection task, with bias reflecting a tendency to respond "green" more often than "red" (or vice versa).

No data were excluded from this analysis. Tests of the hypothesis that participants had no sensitivity to the prime were based on Pearson's χ^2. Hits and false alarms were arbitrarily defined as correct and incorrect responses to red primes, respectively, while misses and correct rejections were analogously assigned to green primes. Two-by-two tables consisting of hits, false alarms, misses, and correct rejections were analyzed separately for each combination of participant and SOA, based on 360 observations each. To combine analyses, χ^2 statistics and associated degrees of freedom were summed across participants (Agresti 1996).

Figure 10.2b shows the mean response accuracy in the prime identification task. For the shortest prime–mask SOA, discrimination performance was not significantly different from chance: $\chi^2(6, N = 2160) = 7.01$, $p > .25$, uncorrected. For the remaining SOAs, performance

All participants:
Mask vs. prime identification

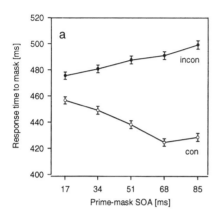

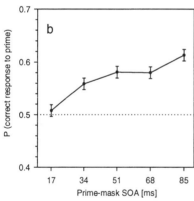

Figure 10.2
(a) Response times in the mask identification task, for primes with consistent vs. inconsistent color. (b) Mean response accuracy in the prime identification task. Error bars denote the standard error of the mean.

was better than chance: $26.88 \leq \chi^2(6, N = 2160) \leq 149.46$, all $p < .001$, uncorrected.

Error Rates in Mask Identification

Figure 10.3 shows that error rate in the mask identification task was low when prime and mask

All participants:
Error rates in mask identification

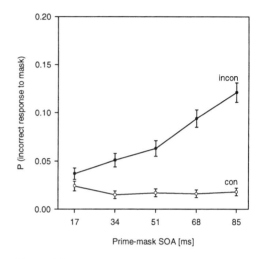

Figure 10.3
Error rates in the mask identification task, for primes with consistent vs. inconsistent color. Error bars denote the standard error of the mean.

were consistent. However, error rate was an increasing function of SOA when prime and mask were inconsistent. In accordance with this, a three-way ANOVA (consistency × SOA × participant) revealed a significant main effect of consistency: $F(1, 5) = 12.48$, $MSE = 0.58$, $p < .05$, as well as a main effect of SOA: $F(4, 20) = 5.32$, $MSE = 0.10$, $p < .005$. Most important, there was an interaction of consistency with SOA, $F(4, 20) = 6.90$, $MSE = 0.09$, $p < .01$.

Response Strategies

Figure 10.4 contains the same data as figure 10.2b, but they are split into groups of consistent and inconsistent cases. The figure reveals that response selection depended not only on prime color but also on mask color. A three-

All participants:
Response biases in prime identification

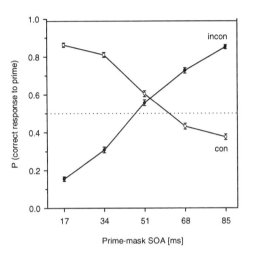

Figure 10.4
Response accuracy in the prime identification task, for masks with consistent vs. inconsistent color. Error bars denote the standard error of the mean.

way ANOVA (consistency × SOA × participant) revealed a significant main effect of SOA: $F(4, 20) = 6.75$, $MSE = 0.43$, $p < .001$. However, for inconsistent cases, accuracy was an increasing function of SOA, whereas it decreased for consistent cases, which is reflected in a strong interaction of consistency with SOA: $F(4, 20) = 27.54$, $MSE = 4.45$, $p < .001$. However, these departures from mean accuracy were largely symmetric, as indicated by a nonsignificant main effect of consistency: $F(1, 5) = 2.80$, $MSE = 8.19$, $p > .10$.

My interpretation of this reversing pattern of consistency effects is that participants employed a response strategy based on some residual visual qualities of the prime, like flicker or apparent motion. Several participants reported that they had used these residual cues to infer whether the prime had been consistent with the mask,

assuming that a prime would be masked more effectively by a mask of the same rather than of the opposite color. At shorter SOAs, detecting little flicker or apparent motion, they therefore assumed that the prime was consistent with the mask, and were biased to respond with the mask color. At longer SOAs, however, detecting stronger flicker or motion, they inferred that the prime had the color opposite to that of the mask. Without sensitivity at any SOA, this reversing bias would cause an X-shaped response pattern symmetrical about the line of chance performance. Here, increasing sensitivity distorts the symmetry and raises overall performance level at longer SOAs. This is evident when the data are plotted in terms of the SDT sensitivity and bias measures d' and c, respectively (not shown here).

Two Predictors of the Priming Effect

Figure 10.5a shows the priming function, defined as the difference between the RT means in consistent and inconsistent trials ($RT_{incons} - RT_{cons}$) plotted against SOA. Linear regression of the mean priming effects on SOA was used to estimate parameters of a linear priming function. There was no significant intercept parameter ($b_0 = 5.90$, $t(3) = 1.32$, $p > .25$), but the slope was significantly different from zero ($b_1 = 0.81$, $t(3) = 10.27$, $p < .005$). Linear regression accounted for a high proportion of variance ($R = 0.986$, $R = 0.972$).

For comparison, figure 10.5b plots the priming effect against response accuracy in the prime identification task. At least in the present sample of participants, indirect effects of the prime are not easily predicted by direct discrimination performance.[3] There are two features in the figure that make this evident. First, there was a clear priming effect at the shortest SOA, as confirmed by planned comparisons (Bonferroni-adjusted F tests of the main effect of consistency in 2-way ANOVAs [consistency × participant]) performed at each of the 5 SOAs: at a prime–

All participants: Predictors of the priming effect

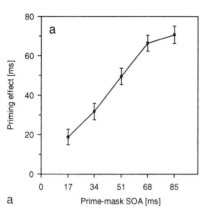

a

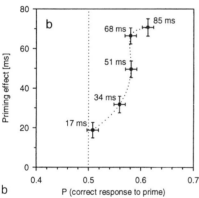

b

Figure 10.5
(a) Priming effects in the mask identification task, plotted against prime–mask SOA. The priming effect is defined as the difference of response times in the presence of consistent vs. inconsistent primes. Error bars denote the standard error of this difference, assuming additive variances. (b) Same priming effects plotted against response accuracy in the corresponding SOA conditions (indicated by numbers). Bivariate error bars denote standard errors of the mean along the corresponding axes of the diagram. The curved line serves only to connect consecutive data points.

mask SOA of 17 msec, $F(1, 5) = 18.79$, $MSE = 152,437.80$, $p < .05$. There was no evidence of prime discriminability in this condition (see "Sensitivity to the Prime"). Second, SOAs between 34 and 68 msec produced similar accuracy but dissimilar priming effects, suggesting that the priming measure was more sensitive to slight changes in the time course of stimuli.

Participant AN: Dissociated Time Courses of Sensitivity and Priming

Data from one participant, AN, show that the priming function can be perfectly dissociated from visual awareness. AN was 38 years old, was right-handed, and had reportedly normal, uncorrected vision. She had no significant sensitivity to the prime at any prime–mask SOA: $0.005 \leq \chi^2(1, N = 320) \leq 2.97$, all $p > .05$, uncorrected (figure 10.6b). However, the time course of the response times in the mask identification task was similar to that of the total sample (figure 10.6a), with a monotonously rising priming function up to an SOA of 68 msec (figure 10.7a). A two-way ANOVA (consistency × SOA) revealed a significant effect of prime consistency: $F(1, 1510) = 60.05$, $MSE = 8,654.64$, $p < .001$, and a prime consistency by SOA interaction: $F(4, 1510) = 5.90$, $MSE = 8,654.64$, $p < .001$. It is more obvious than in the total sample of participants that sensitivity in the prime identification task is not a good predictor of the priming effect (figure 10.7b), because given priming effects are not predicted by unique accuracy values.

Discussion

Dissociation of Priming and Awareness

In the present dataset, there is clearly some evidence for color processing without awareness. At each prime–mask SOA, there is a substantial priming effect when participants perform a

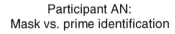

Participant AN:
Mask vs. prime identification

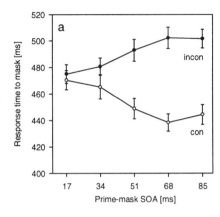

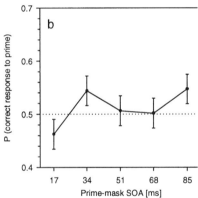

Participant AN:
Predictors of the priming effect

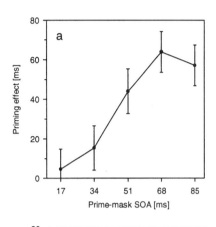

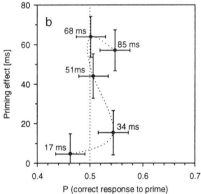

Figure 10.6
(a) Response times from participant AN in the mask identification task, for primes with consistent vs. inconsistent color. (b) AN's mean response accuracy in the prime identification task. Error bars denote the standard error of the mean.

Figure 10.7
(a) Priming effects from participant AN in the mask identification task, plotted against prime–mask SOA. (b) Same priming effects plotted against response accuracy in the corresponding SOA conditions (indicated by numbers). See the caption to figure 10.5 for further details.

speeded response to the color of the mask in the presence of a consistent vs. inconsistent prime. This priming effect increases with SOA, forming a priming function with nearly constant slope. The shape of the priming function and the pattern of errors are very similar to previous findings (Vorberg et al. in prep.).

Although prime discriminability and priming effect covary here, there is a substantial priming effect even at the shortest prime–mask SOA, a condition where no participant had any detectable sensitivity to the prime. Analysis of data from participant AN shows that the shape of the priming function can be perfectly dissociated from sensitivity to the prime, consistent with previous findings (Vorberg et al. in prep.). This suggests that visibility of the prime is correlated with, but not causally connected to, the magnitude of the priming effect. Moreover, response behavior in the prime identification task seems governed more by response biases than by sensitivity, leading to suboptimal performance for mask-consistent primes at long SOAs. One might therefore speculate that prime color has remained below a subjective threshold (Reingold and Merikle 1988), because participants would be expected to give up these response biases if they had unambiguous visual awareness of the prime.

Analogous to our previous findings, response priming by color is clearly possible, and there is also evidence that it can be dissociated from visual awareness. In any event, the speeded mask discrimination task seems more sensitive to the SOA manipulation: Response times group into segregated clusters up to an SOA of 68 msec, whereas the response accuracies at SOAs between 34 and 68 msec are very similar.

"Perception" Versus "Action": How Can Color Control Responses?

Response priming by nondiscriminable colors is what Milner and Goodale (1995) would probably call a dissociation between "perception" (a perceptual judgment based on visual awareness) and "action" (a visually guided motor response that might occur without visual awareness). In their framework, such dissociations are explained by different properties of the ventral and dorsal streams of visual processing. Applying this scheme to the present dataset, the ventral stream would be responsible for constructing visual awareness of the prime, while the dorsal stream would control speeded motor responses to the mask but also be influenced by the prime. Because of their clustering into different anatomical structures, the two streams could occasionally produce dissociated results, like priming without awareness.

At the beginning of this chapter, I used a simplification of this theory to make predictions about the possibility of response priming by color as clear and pointed as possible: If (a) color processing and visual awareness are confined to the ventral stream, and (b) response priming is confined to the dorsal stream, and (c) the streams are functionally separate with respect to immediate response control, then response priming by color should be impossible. The present data, especially those from participant AN, falsify the logical conjunction of these three premises. The existence of response priming by color implies that response control is not isolated from color information. Furthermore, this means that the evidence for priming without awareness could not be explained by a dissociation of dorsal and ventral streams. How can color affect response control, and how is color processing without awareness possible?

Solution 1:   Cross Talk

A radical solution to this problem would be to discard the idea of functionally separate streams altogether. A brief glance at an elaborated chart of the visual areas (e.g., Van Essen and Deyoe 1995) shows that there are many anatomical connections between the principal areas. On the other hand, this does not mean that there is enough cross talk to destroy the postulated division of labor between the streams, which is functional rather than anatomical.

It is nevertheless possible that color signals might reach the dorsal stream, and there are several plausible sources. Apart from direct connections between the principal areas (including V4 and V5; Merigan and Maunsell 1993; Felleman and Van Essen 1991), there is always the possibility that backward projections to early visual areas could be used to transmit a signal to areas downstream, so that a feature detected in one stream could be used in another, traveling via V1–V3. For example, there is evidence that second-order motion boundaries are topologically represented in V1 (Reppas et al. 1997), which seems an unexpected region for the computation of this kind of signal.

Finally, the assignment of specialized areas to distinct networks still leaves room for speculation, even with areas whose connectivity and function seemed clear enough for some time. For example, it is still debated whether a human "color center" (i.e., a human homologue of macaque area V4) does exist, and if it does, where it is located. Work by Hadjikhani et al. (1998) suggests a large area located more anteriorly than previously thought.

Solution 2: Response Selection Mechanisms Independent of the Visual Streams

One different solution to the problem of how responses can come under the control of color information is not restricted to color processing. I propose that the relevant control processes are decoupled from the visual streams, so that motor responses in the mask identification task are not directly controlled by the dorsal stream.

One argument for this is that response priming effects seem very general (Vorberg et al. in prep.). We have obtained comparable priming functions with different kinds of stimuli, like arrows and color patches. We also found them in different motor tasks, like keypress responses, manual pointing, and eye movements. Therefore,

the mechanism generating the priming function seems to be independent of particular stimuli as well as motor systems. This has led us to speculate that motor responses can come under any kind of visual control, provided there is an appropriate task context.

So this is also a matter of cognitive control. Many models of cognitive control assume that people sometimes submit response control to the stimulus input, given a task with a clearly defined stimulus–response mapping (for a review, see Monsell 1996). For example, Neumann's (1990; Neumann and Klotz 1994) theory of *direct parameter specification* proposes that people can prepare several alternative responses, waiting only for that unique stimulus parameter which will trigger the response assigned to it.

We have developed a stochastic model that quantitatively predicts the observed linear priming functions as well as the pattern of errors in the mask identification task, assuming competitive response selection processes (Vorberg et al. in prep.). The data presented in this chapter suggest that this mechanism can be programmed in a task-specific manner, even with the perfectly arbitrary stimulus–response mappings used here. If the required visual input to the response selection process is really arbitrary and task-specific, it cannot be confined to any of the visual streams but must be functionally independent of both of them.

Invisible Colors Revisited

For a demonstration of response priming by color, it is not critical whether or not the primes are consciously perceived. However, it is fascinating that color processing can be dissociated from visual awareness. Although this is consistent with Milner and Goodale's (1995) framework, which allows for dissociations within the streams, I think it is counterintuitive that a ventral-stream feature like color should be isolated from other ventral-stream processing but easily accessible by the dorsal stream. One might expect visual awareness, compared with visuomotor transformations, to have more direct access to color information.

So, what if there really are "invisible colors"? Many areas of visual psychophysics depend on what observers express about their subjective experience (e.g., whether or not a stimulus was present, whether it was red or green, and similar judgments about phenomenal qualities). On the basis of these experiential data, theories about quite early perceptual processes can be formed. Although this is obviously valid in many areas of vision (like color matching; see Wandell 1995), functional dissociations in our cognitive architecture set limits to what is accessible for conscious report. This is why we cannot expect to get uniform answers when posing our questions to different parts of the system.

Acknowledgments

The data presented here are from my master's thesis, which was supervised by Dirk Vorberg and Klaus Nippert. I thank Dirk, Klaus, Armin Heinecke, Jens Schwarzbach, and Uwe Mattler for their great support. The present experiment is based upon and subsequent to our common work, which is to appear in a future article. Thanks to Michael Blum-Kalagin for his work on the graphical art in this chapter. Thanks also to Alan Allport and Gisa Aschersleben for stimulating discussions and helpful comments.

Notes

1. By now, all major findings (including the time course and size of the priming effects) have been replicated several times, using isoluminant stimuli, as determined by heterochromatic flicker photometry.

2. Here and in all further figures depicting data from more than one participant, between-subjects variance has been removed from the error bars because it does not contribute to error variance in the statistical tests.

3. There are statistical procedures for evaluating indirect effects in the absence of direct effects, provided that the two measures covary, using linear regression (see Draine and Greenwald 1998). This approach is elegant because the statement of no indirect effects, given no direct effects, becomes a null hypothesis that can be rejected by testing the intercept parameter. However, along with other problems with the procedure, there is no point in fitting a linear (or a particular nonlinear) model to data like those in figure 10.7b. Therefore, the approach is used here for descriptive purposes only.

References

Agresti, A. (1996). *An Introduction to Categorical Data Analysis.* New York: John Wiley and Sons.

Cheesman, J., and Merikle, P. M. (1984). Priming with and without awareness. *Perception and Psychophysics* 36: 387–395.

Cowey, A., and Heywood, C. A. (1997). Cerebral achromatopsia: Colour blindness despite wavelength processing. *Trends in Cognitive Sciences* 1, no. 4: 133–139.

Draine, S. C., and Greenwald, A. G. (1998). Replicable unconscious semantic priming. *Journal of Experimental Psychology: General*, 127, no. 3: 286–303.

Eimer, M., and Schlaghecken, F. (1998). Effects of masked stimuli on motor activation: Behavioral and electrophysiological evidence. *Journal of Experimental Psychology: Human Perception & Performance* 24: 1737–1747.

Eriksen, C. W. (1960). Discrimination and learning without awareness: A methodological survey and evaluation. *Psychological Review* 67: 279–300.

Felleman, D. J., and Van Essen, D. C. (1991). Distributed hierarchical processing in the primate cerebral cortex. *Cerebral Cortex* 1: 1–47.

Francis, G. (1997). Cortical dynamics of lateral inhibition: Metacontrast masking. *Psychological Review* 104: 572–594.

Hadjikhani, N., Liu, A. K., Dale, A. M., Cavanagh, P., and Tootell, R. B. H. (1998). Retinotopy and color sensitivity in human visual cortical area V8. *Nature Neuroscience* 1, no. 3: 235–241.

Holender, D. (1986). Semantic activation without conscious identification in dichotic listening, parafoveal vision, and visual masking: A survey and appraisal. *Behavioral and Brain Sciences* 9: 1–66.

Klotz, W., and Wolff, P. (1995). The effect of a masked stimulus on the response to the masking stimulus. *Psychological Research* 58: 92–101.

Macknik, S. L., and Livingstone, M. S. (1998). Neuronal correlates of visibility and invisibility in the primate visual system. *Nature Neuroscience* 1, no. 2: 144–149.

Macmillan, N. A., and Creelman, C. D. (1991). *Detection Theory: A User's Guide.* Cambridge: Cambridge University Press.

Marcel, A. J. (1983). Conscious and unconscious perception: Experiments on visual masking and word recognition. *Cognitive Psychology* 15: 197–237.

Merigan, W. H., and Maunsell, J. H. R. (1993). How parallel are the primate visual pathways? *Annual Review of Neuroscience* 16: 369–402.

Milner, A. D., and Goodale, M. A. (1995). *The Visual Brain in Action.* Oxford: Oxford University Press.

Monsell, S. (1996). Control of mental processes. In V. Bruce, ed., *Unsolved Mysteries of the Mind: Tutorial Essays in Cognition*, 93–148. East Sussex: UK: Lawrence Erlbaum Associates.

Neumann, O. (1990). Direct parameter specification and the concept of perception. *Psychological Research* 52: 207–215.

Neumann, O., and Klotz, W. (1994). Motor responses to nonreportable, masked stimuli: Where is the limit of direct parameter specification? In C. Umiltà and M. Moscovitch, eds., *Attention and Performance XV: Conscious and nonconscious information processing*, 124–150. Cambridge, MA: MIT Press.

Reingold, E. M., and Merikle, P. M. (1988). Using direct and indirect measures to study perception without awareness. *Perception and Psychophysics* 44, no. 6: 563–575.

Reppas, J. B., Niyogi, S., Dale, A. M., Sereno, M. I., and Tootell, R. B. H. (1997). Representation of motion boundaries in retinotopic human visual cortical areas. *Nature* 388: 175–179.

Schlaghecken, F., and Eimer, M. (1997). The influence of subliminally presented primes on response preparation. *Sprache und Kognition* 16: 166–175.

Stoerig, P., and Cowey, A. (1989). Wavelength sensitivity in blindsight. *Nature* 342: 916–918.

Stoerig, P., and Cowey, A. (1992). Wavelength discrimination in blindsight. *Brain* 115: 425–444.

Van Essen, D. C., and Deyoe, E. A. (1995). Concurrent processing in the primate visual cortex. In M. S. Gazzaniga, ed., *The Cognitive Neurosciences*, 383–400. Cambridge, MA: MIT Press.

Vorberg, D., Mattler, U., Heinecke, A., Schmidt, T., and Schwarzbach, J. (in prep.). Invariant time course of priming with and without awareness.

Wandell, B. (1995). *Foundations of Vision.* Sunderland, MA: Sinauer Associates.

Zeki, S. (1993). *A Vision of the Brain.* Cambridge, MA: Blackwell Scientific Publications.

11 Face Representation Without Conscious Processing

Beena Khurana

Faces are notably abundant in our visual world. Their accurate and timely perception is important for such biologically significant functions as social communication and recognition of individual members of one's species (Desimone 1991). A great many social interactions rely critically on one's ability to process the visual information in human faces. Developmentally, it has been shown that faces are salient stimuli for infants. Face versus nonface patterns are discriminated very early on (Meltzoff and Moore 1977; Sackett 1966). For example, infants look longer at facelike stimuli (Kleiner and Banks 1987), and are more accurate at tracking a moving face pattern as opposed to a scrambled face pattern (Goren et al. 1975; Morton and Johnson 1991).

In terms of evolutionary significance, it has been suggested that faces and facial expressions in higher primates have replaced the role played by olfaction in communication. Such alteration of function has resulted in selective pressure to evolve neural mechanisms for face processing (Allman and McGuinness 1988). Neurally distinct face-processing mechanisms have been posited since the early 1970s (Gross et al. 1972). Over almost 30 years, evidence for neural tissue in the brain selective to face stimuli has accumulated (Desimone 1991; Perrett et al. 1987; Perrett et al. 1982; Rolls et al. 1993; Rolls et al. 1989; Rolls et al. 1985). These single-cell electrophysiological findings have been further buttressed by data from patients in which brain injury compromises face recognition abilities while sparing the perception of other objects (Damasio et al. 1982; Meadows 1974; Whiteley and Warrington 1977; Yin 1970; but see Farah 1990 for a less ecologically privileged perspective on face processing) or the reverse (Moscovitch et al. 1997). Thus, given its critical role in mental life, it is hypothesized that face processing is likely to have substantial com-

ponents that are computed independent of conscious intervention.

Explicit face recognition and face categorization are automatic and effortless (for a review, see Young and Bruce 1991). In both instances, face perception is considered a function of matching input to previously existing representations. Though this research has led to a greater understanding of the cognitive process in the identification and retrieval of familiar faces (Ellis et al. 1987; Hay and Young 1982; Bruce and Young 1986; Burton et al. 1990), we lack considerably in our understanding of the nature of basic perceptual processes that subserve face representation (Bruce et al. 1994; Young and Bruce 1991).

To better specify the processes that underlie automatic face coding, unfamiliar faces were processed in the absence of focused attention. Human faces were presented as targets and distractors in a selective attention task. It has been suggested that sensory systems are capable of processing, and actually perceptually process, entire input arrays up to the level of object recognition (Deutsch and Deutsch 1963; Duncan 1980). On this view, selection takes place further upstream, where perceptual and motor decisions about pertinent objects are made. These decisions entail the inhibition of distractor representations that compete for the control of attention and action (Neill 1977; Neill and Westberry 1987; Tipper 1985; Tipper and Cranston 1985).

Critical evidence for this view of selection essentially comes from a procedure in which the processing of the distractors on a given trial is ascertained on a subsequent trial. Tipper and Cranston (1985) presented observers with partially overlapping red and green letters (figure 11.1) with instructions to name the target red letter (say) as quickly as possible. Naming latencies were impaired when the ignored distractor

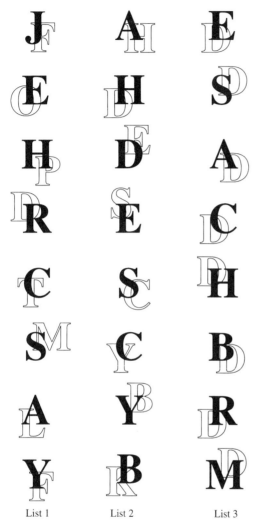

List 1   List 2   List 3

Figure 11.1
Each column of letters depicts different trial sequences. Observers are instructed to name the black letter and ignore the outline one. In list 1 the distractors on the previous trial bear no relationship to the target on the subsequent trial. In list 2 the distractor from the previous trial becomes the target in the subsequent trial. In list 3 the distractor remains constant throughout. Response times are fastest on list 3, followed by list 1, with list 2 being the slowest. (From Tipper and Cranston 1985; modified.)

letter on the previous trial became the target letter on the next trial (see list 2). It was proposed that *all* the letters in the display—whether relevant to the task or not—are automatically processed, but that the irrelevant letter is inhibited from accessing response systems (Tipper and Cranston 1985). If the irrelevant letter became the relevant letter on the subsequent trial, the inhibition previously applied would have to be overcome, resulting in delayed response times. The phenomenon is referred to as *negative priming* because a prior encounter with an object in the role of a distractor retards future performance with it when it becomes the target of action.

Despite the abundance and variety of empirical findings using negative priming (e.g., Tipper and Driver 1988; Tipper et al. 1990; Tipper et al. 1992), the locus of the inhibition remains an open question. In other words, does the inhibition measured act at the level of internal representations, the level of responses, or both?

Neill et al. (1990) investigated this issue by decoupling the overt response of the observer from the identity of the targets and distractors. They developed a same–different matching procedure to distinguish between inhibitory tags that disallow communication between distractor representations and response systems from tags that are associated with a particular identification response. On each trial, observers were shown a row of five letters (figure 11.2) in which the second and fourth letters (from left to right) were targets, and the first, third, and fifth letters were distractors. Observers were instructed to indicate via a keypress whether the targets in a given trial were the *same* letter or *different* letters. On the "related" trials, one or both of the target letters were the distractor letter from the preceding trial. On the "unrelated" trials, the target letter or letters in a given trial did not match the distractor letter on the previous trial. Response times to the targets on related trials were longer relative to the unrelated trials. Moreover, the response times were independent of the nature of the responses on successive trials. Thus

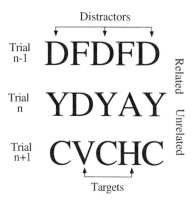

Figure 11.2
When asked to decide whether the second and the fourth letter in a five-letter string, e.g. ABABA are "the same" or "different," observers are slower if one or both of the current targets are identical to the distractors on the previous trial. (Adapted from Neill et al. 1990.)

the inhibition was not associated with the particular "same" or "different" response made, but operated at a level prior to the computation of the exact response to be made. This matching procedure is also sensitive to the nature of perceptual coding. Neill (1991) reported that negative priming occurred for same-case sequences (e.g., ABABA–DADAD, or ababa—dadad) but did not occur for opposite-case sequences (ABABA–dadad).

It is obvious that the internal representations of these overlearned stimuli are well-formed. Treisman and DeSchepper (1996) altered the same–different matching procedure to study whether the inhibition in negative priming *requires* preestablished representations. In other words, can inhibition act on a single instance—a token—in the way it has been shown to act on a stored abstract representation—a type? Observers were presented two novel overlapping shapes, one red and the other green, and a comparison shape (figure 11.3). They were instructed to report whether the green shape (black in the figure)

matched the comparison white shape (striped border in the figure). The overlapping red shape (gray in the figure) was to be ignored. Response times to target green shapes were significantly longer if they had previously been presented as to-be-ignored red shapes. Treisman and DeSchepper (1996) concluded that the visual system was capable of setting up "on the fly" representations without attention based on a single exposure. Used this way, the negative priming procedure can provide an indirect measure of the automatic and involuntary aspects of perceptual representation.

Though humans are remarkably adept at recognizing faces after extremely limited exposures (Diamond and Carey 1986), logically they cannot have preformed representations of faces they have not yet seen. The first question, then, is whether observers even represent unfamiliar faces when given instructions to ignore them. To gauge the ability of the visual system to represent token faces without focused attention, observers compared target faces in the presence of distractor faces. Evidence was found for the representation and inhibition of never-before-seen distractor faces, thus establishing that the negative priming paradigm can be used for the study of face perception without conscious processing. Negative priming for physically identical faces in the role of distractors and targets having been established, the visual information in distractor faces was perturbed in further experiments to specify (1) the aspects of a face that are represented in an involuntary fashion, (2) the aspects that are inhibited, and (3) the relationship between (1) and (2).

Experiment 1: Negative Priming of Faces

Experiment 1 was designed to investigate whether an ignored unfamiliar face generates a representation that has to be actively inhibited in order to act upon the attended target face (Khurana et al. 1994; Khurana 2000). Since

KEY:
■■■■ GREEN
▒▒▒▒ RED
||||||| WHITE

PRIME:

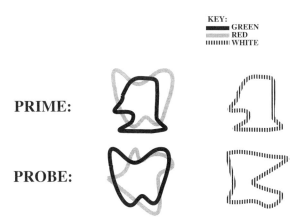

PROBE:

Figure 11.3
Example of the prime–probe trial sequence using novel shapes. Observers were asked to match the green shape with the white comparison shape while ignoring the red shape. When the ignored red shape became the target green shape in a probe trial, observers were significantly slower in their response. (Adapted from DeSchepper and Treisman 1996.)

the target faces were unfamiliar, observers could not be asked to name them. Therefore a same–different matching task was employed in which observers viewed a row of five unfamiliar faces (figure 11.4) on each trial, in order to judge whether or not the target faces in positions 2 and 4 were identical or not. A face irrelevant to the observer's matching task (the distractor face) appeared in the middle and outermost positions. Unbeknownst to observers, on half the trials, the distractor face from the previous trial matched one or both of the targets in the succeeding trial. In the control condition, the targets did not match the previous trial's distractor face.

Method

Eighteen Cornell undergraduates with normal or corrected-to-normal vision participated in the experiment. All were naive with respect to the hypotheses. The stimuli were black-and-white frontal photographic stills frame-grabbed from videotape of Ithaca College undergraduates wearing a neutral expression. Clothing, jewelry,

and any hair below ear height were deleted from the images. For a more complete description of the methods and stimulus details, see Khurana (2000).

A given trial n was either related or unrelated to the previous trial $n - 1$. On a related trial n, at least one of the target faces (or both target instances of the same face) had been presented as the distractor on trial $n - 1$. On an unrelated trial, both the target faces were distinct from the distractor presented on the previous trial. Within any one trial, the distractor face was always different from both of the target faces; across trials, the distractor face changed (figure 11.4).

Observers were instructed to compare the faces in the second and fourth positions. They were told that faces in the other three positions were irrelevant and were presented to make their task more realistic. Furthermore, they were told to respond as quickly as possible without making errors. It was pointed out that same faces would be identical images and that different faces would be faces of different individuals—not different views of the same individual. All observers

Targets

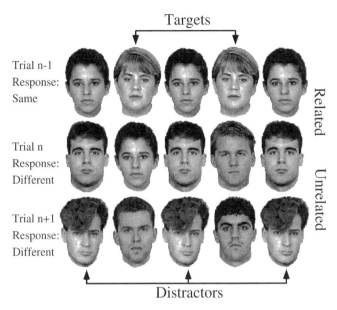

Trial n-1
Response:
Same

Trial n
Response:
Different

Trial n+1
Response:
Different

Related

Unrelated

Distractors

Figure 11.4
A row of five unfamiliar faces was presented to observers on each trial. Faces in positions 2 and 4 were targets that observers were instructed to compare to decide if they were the same or different. Two types of trial sequences were presented: related—distractor faces in trial $n - 1$ were the same as one or both of the target faces in trial n; unrelated—distractor faces in trial n were different from the target faces in trial $n + 1$.

were interviewed after completion of the 100 trials to determine whether they had noticed any relationship between the distractors and targets of adjacent trials.

Results and Discussion

Observers were slower in comparing the target faces on related trials than on unrelated trials. No consistent patterns of performance were found for same versus different trials; hence the data were analyzed with respect to related and unrelated trials. The difference in reaction times to the related versus the unrelated trials of 24 msec was significant: $t(17) = 2.57$; $p < .01$. There was an average of 3.0 percent errors on the unrelated trials and 2.4 percent errors on the related trials. Although the difference in errors

is consistent with a speed-accuracy trade-off, it was not significant: $t(17) = .67$; ns. These findings have been replicated with a different set of observers who were not told anything about the distractors. The results of the replication were not different from those reported here.

Performance being slower and just as accurate on the related trials relative to the unrelated trials confirms that the to-be-ignored distractor faces were processed and inhibited. Thus, it is suggested that the visual system is capable of representing unfamiliar faces without focused attention. The results of experiment 1 indicate that the representational by-products of the unattended faces render sufficient competition that they must be inhibited to successfully execute the task of comparing the target faces. Thus, meaningful stimuli that are structurally rich yet unfamiliar to the observer, and irrelevant to the task, are automatically represented. These attention-free representations are then inhibited in order to act upon target stimuli.

When considering the status of unattended stimuli (Deutsch and Deutsch 1963; Duncan 1980), it has been asserted that object identification and recognition take place prior to selective attention. One rather straightforward consequence would be that the representations of the distractor faces in experiment 1 are as complete and detailed as those of the target faces. However, one must establish the truth of the previous statement empirically, because inhibition need not imply that the representations of the distractors and the target are of comparable detail. For example, the representations of unattended distractors could differ from those of the attended targets in more ways than their mere accessibility via explicit memory. DeSchepper and Treisman (1996) raise the possibility that the unattended distractor representations could be kept at a less articulated level than target representations, and yet be detailed enough to match the subsequent target representation.

Faces are information-rich stimuli that allow a great deal of manipulation. The subsequent experiments took advantage of this fact by altering the visual content of the distractors. Alteration of the visual content of faces is an approach that has been highly successful in understanding the perception of faces and their physiological underpinnings.

Experiment 2:   Priming by Noise-Added Distractors

Experiment 2 investigated (1) the level of representation achieved by the unattended distractor and (2) whether the inhibition found in experiment 1 is applied to the representations of distractors per se or to their access to response systems. To understand how distractors may compete with target faces for responses, let us consider the nature of the task. Target faces are processed in order to decide whether they are the same individual or not. In order to determine whether two faces are the same or different, it is suggested that observers use fine-scale structural information present in the eyes, nose, and mouth. Information about these differences is specified by the contents of the high-spatial-frequency end of the spectrum (Fiorentini et al. 1983; Lehmkule et al. 1980). In experiment 2 the fine facial features of the distractors were obscured by a checkerboard pattern (figure 11.5).

Three logical possibilities exist: (1) If obscuring the high-spatial-frequency information of the distractors renders a sufficiently detailed internal representation to match that of the complete target face on the subsequent trial, then an equivalent inhibitory effect is expected. (2) However, the significant reduction in physical overlap between distractors and targets could render a poorer match between distractor and target representations, thus reducing the inhibitory effect. (3) The inhibition found in experiment 1 is very specific to the visual information required by the task. Thus one might predict a complete lack of inhibition because the distractors do not contain the information that is being used to compare the targets (Tipper et al. 1994).

Method

Methods were identical to those used in experiment 1 except for the following changes. The distractor faces were obscured with a white, high-frequency checkerboard consisting of squares that were 2 pixels on a side. In order to make the presence of the checkerboard easily perceptible, the faces were surrounded with a gray border. The distractors were referred to as "tile" distractors. Another group of eighteen undergraduates at Cornell University participated in this experiment.

Targets

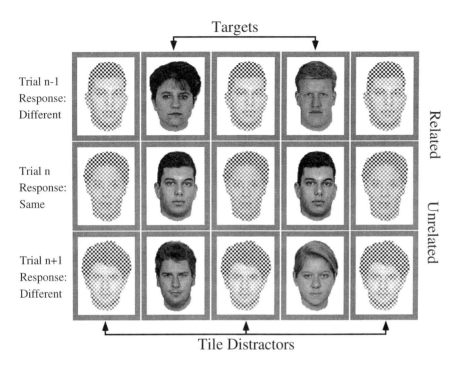

Figure 11.5
Distractor faces were obscrured with a white high-frequency checkerboard consisting of squares that were two pixels on a side. The two types of trial sequences—related and unrelated—are shown.

Results and Discussion

The empirical outcomes did not agree with any of the above predictions. Intriguingly, the preview of a tile distractor led to a speeding up of response times on the related trials! The difference in response times between unrelated and related trials was 18 msec: $t(17) = -2.41$, $p < .025$. There was no speed-accuracy trade-off, since there was an equivalent error rate, 3 percent in both conditions: $t(17) = 0.0$, $p = 1.0$, *ns*.

How can one account for these polar results? Inhibition may be a function of the internal representation of the distractors when the distractor representations vie for response selection in a task. Facilitation is to be expected if it is assumed that the distractors activate processing mechanisms to set up representations that remain in a state of activation. The results of experiment 2 can be explained by noting that the tile distractors do not offer strong competition to the targets in the process of selection; thus the lack of inhibition. However, the tile distractors do activate face-processing mechanisms sufficiently to render facilitation in future encounters.

One may now ask how this facilitation came about. Disrupting faces by high-spatial-frequency noise can be considered similar to rendering a block image of a face through coarse quantization (figure 11.6). While fine facial features of the face are obscured its recognition is still possible (Harmon and Julesz 1973; Hayes 1991; Hayes

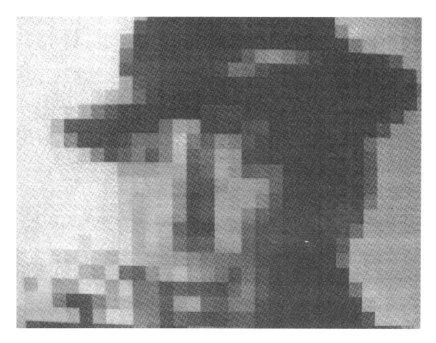

Figure 11.6
Coarse-quantized (blocked) image of a well-known actor. Each square is set to the average intensity of the image in that region (Sekular and Blake 1994).

and Ross 1995; Morrone et al. 1983) by presenting just the information in the low spatial frequencies (Harmon and Julesz 1973). High-spatial-frequency noise can be filtered by blurring the image (e.g., inspect figure 11.7 while squinting) or otherwise interfering with the spurious edges (Hayes 1991; Morrone et al. 1983), thus allowing recognition. Natural images such as faces are processed by recovering low-spatial-frequency structure and progressively aligning it with the high-spatial-frequency structure. The structure at the fine scales in fact determines perception (Hayes 1991; Hayes and Ross 1995). For tile distractors the outlined progression aligns the low-spatial-frequency structure with the high-spatial-frequency structure of the tiles rather than the facial features.

It is proposed that the tile distractors were not inhibited because they did not offer strong competition to the target faces. In accordance with previous research (Harmon and Julesz 1973; Hayes 1991; Hayes and Ross 1995; Morrone et al. 1983), however, the noise-corrupted distractors contain sufficient information to stimulate face-processing mechanisms. The overlap in the coarse-scale structure (Hayes and Ross 1995) of the tile distractor and subsequent target faces on the related trials can be held accountable for the observed facilitation. Thus, inhibition precludes action being taken on distractor faces, but does not suppress the activation of encoding mechanisms or the formation of perceptual representations.

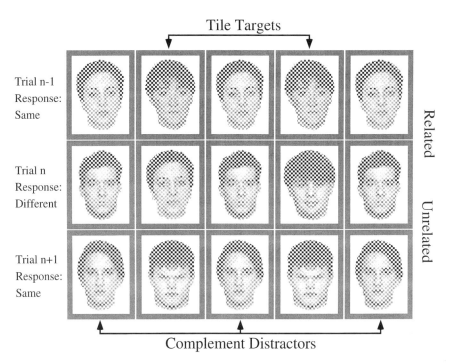

Figure 11.7
Checkerboard-obscured faces were presented on every trial in either a related or unrelated sequence.

Experiment 3: Priming by Complement Noise-Added Distractor Faces

The facilitation observed in experiment 2 could be due to the partial physical overlap between distractor and target faces in the related trials, as opposed to an equivalence in their coarse-scale structural content (Harmon and Julesz 1973; Hayes and Ross 1995; Morrone et al. 1983; Rolls et al. 1985). To test these alternatives, two mutually exclusive, complementary sets of faces were constructed in which the distractor and target versions of a face had virtually no pixel-to-pixel correspondence. Thus, the two versions of each face shared *only* their low-spatial-frequency content. If the facilitation in experiment 2 was caused by the physical overlap

between distractors and targets, then none is predicted for the complement distractors. But if the equivalence in the coarse-scale structural content of the faces caused the facilitation, then there should also be facilitation for the complement distractors.

Method

A new set of eighteen observers from the Cornell undergraduate population participated in the experiment. Complement versions of each face were constructed by placing two complementary, nonoverlapping grids on the image. In figure 11.7, one tiled version of a female face is presented as the distractor in trial $n - 1$ and its complement is presented as one of the targets in trial *n*. It is difficult, if not impossible, to spontaneously tell the difference between these complementary versions of a face. But upon careful scrutiny one can confirm that there is no physical overlap between them. Though the task became highly artificial, observers succeeded by devoting more time to it.

Results and Discussion

The tile distractors facilitated the processing of the complement tile targets on the subsequent trial. Related trials were responded to faster by 29.8 msec: $t(17) = 4.16$, $p < .001$. Accuracy was also greater on related trials, with only 3 percent errors, compared with 5.6 percent on the unrelated: $t(17) = -2.51$, $p < .025$. While the coarse-scale structure of the distractors did not compete in target-directed action, it was sufficient to produce a faster responses on a subsequent encounter. This facilitation between distractor and target faces is present even in the absence of any low-level pixel overlap between stimuli.

The data of experiments 2 and 3 concur with what is known about the activity of cells in superior temporal sulcus that selectively respond to the low spatial frequencies present in faces (Rolls et al. 1985). These cells in the macaque monkey respond to low-pass-filtered images of monkey faces that include frequencies of up to 8 cycles/face. A considerable amount of information is missing from these images, and perceptually they appeared rather blurred to humans. Despite being blurred, however, these images do permit recognition of individuals (Fiorentini et al. 1983).

It may seem curious that the tile distractors did not compete with the targets in this experiment, given that the distractors and targets had the same degraded featural information. If observers had based their decisions on just the coarse-scale structure of the target faces, then distractor faces would have to be inhibited because their representations contain the information being used in the target comparison task

(Khurana 2000; Tipper et al. 1994). The target faces with checkerboard noise added couldn't easily be compared because the most natural solution to deciding whether two faces are the same or different calls for a comparison of feature information. It is also known that if viewing distances are small, such as those used in experiments 2 and 3, the fine-scale structure dominates or perceptually masks the coarse-scale structure (Hayes and Ross 1995). In the postexperiment interview observers told experimenters that they painstakingly worked at recovering the facial features from the degraded tiled complement targets in order to do the task. Despite the efficacy of using coarse-scale structure in this experiment, it is not a strategy that observers adopt. The longer reaction times in experiment 3 agree with observers' self-reports of what they did.

Establishing the identity of the target faces in experiment 3 was not automatic, and called for additional resources. The distractors were not competitors in the time-consuming task of piecemeal comparison of target faces. In experiment 4 the targets and distractors were identical in all respects but one. This difference alone did not allow the automatic establishment of the identity of the individual.

Experiment 4: Priming by Contrast-Inverted Distractor Faces

Prior research shows that contrast-inverted faces impair both perceptual discrimination and explicit recognition (Galper 1970; Phillips 1972; Luria and Strauss 1978; Hayes et al. 1986; Hayes 1988; Kemp et al. 1990; Johnston et al. 1992; Bruce and Langton 1994). Recognition deficits cannot be explained by any two-dimensional descriptions because negatives do not differ from positives in terms of zero-crossings and the spatial location of features.

Studies using contrast-inverted faces generally elicit explicit responses from observers. There

Targets

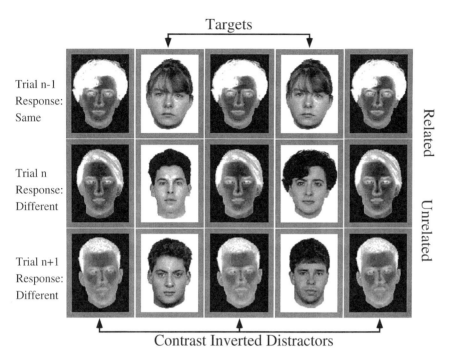

Trial n-1
Response:
Same

Trial n
Response:
Different

Trial n+1
Response:
Different

Related

Unrelated

Contrast Inverted Distractors

Figure 11.8
Observers viewed a row of five faces that consisted of contrast-inverted distractors and positive-contrast targets.

is now substantial evidence that conscious and implicit processes may be independent (Jacoby 1991; Schacter et al. 1993; Treisman and DeSchepper 1996; Tulving and Schacter 1990). The processing of contrast-inverted faces may be similar in that explicit responses may not be adequate predictors of underlying processing mechanisms. One hint at the validity of this point of view comes from physiological recordings in the superior temporal sulcus of macaque monkeys. Little decrement is measured in the responses of cells as a function of contrast inversion of face stimuli (Rolls and Baylis 1986). One may now ask whether the representations established by the contrast-inverted distractors provide any priming of their positive-contrast target counterparts.

Method

Contrast-inverted versions of faces were constructed. Observers viewed a row of five faces that consisted of negative-contrast distractors and positive-contrast targets (figure 11.8). Eighteen different observers participated.

Results and Discussion

Observers were significantly faster (15.4 msec) on related trials compared with unrelated trials: $t(17) = 2.41$, $p < .025$. They were also significantly more accurate on the related trials, committing 2.8 percent errors, compared with 4.4 percent on unrelated trials: $t(17) = -2.41$, $p < .025$. Contrast-inverted faces did not compete for response selection of positive-contrast targets, as predicted by the behavioral studies of recognition; rather, in consonance with physiological recordings, they facilitated processing of their positive-contrast counterpart in the role of a target.

Experiment 5:   Priming by Upside-down Distractor Faces: Humans, Monkeys, and Sheep

Given the agreement of the results of experiments 2, 3, and 4 with physiological recordings of the primate visual system, one further experiment was conducted. Upside-down faces pose a rather serious challenge to recognition (Arnheim 1954; Kohler 1940; Scapinello and Yarmey 1970; Valentine and Bruce 1986; Yarmey 1971; Yin 1969; Young et al. 1987). These recognition decrements are generally accounted for by the inability of the visual system to recover configural information from these faces (Diamond and Carey 1986; Rhodes et al. 1993; Rock 1973, 1974; Tanaka and Farah 1993; Thompson 1980; Young et al. 1987). The single-cell recordings using upside-down faces give mixed results, depending upon the species involved. Perrett et al. (1982) found cells in the fundus of the superior temporal sulcus of rhesus monkeys that exhibit an equal magnitude of response to faces rotated 90° or to an inverted position. They argued that while inversion leads to impaired recognition in humans, the arboreal existence of monkeys might justify cells that code faces independent of rotation and inversion. The response latencies of these cells are, however, longer for inverted, compared with upright, faces (Perrett et al. 1988), a finding thought to reflect the underpinnings of longer response latencies of humans when processing inverted faces (Morton and Johnson 1989). Behaviorally, however, monkeys, like humans, have difficulty when dealing with upside-down faces (Perrett et al. 1988; Phelps and Roberts 1994).

It is important to note that these response measures are based on explicit processing of upside-down faces. Thus, there appears to be some discrepancy in the processing of upside-down faces between the properties of single cells, on the one hand, and behavioral responses, on the other hand. Recordings in sheep from an area homologous to the superior temporal sulcus in monkeys indicate that face-selective cells, which respond vigorously to upright sheep faces, are more or less quiescent in the presence of upside-down faces (Kendrick and Baldwin 1987).

Do the implicit representations set up by unattended upside-down distractors give rise to priming of upright attended targets in humans? In the light of our primate ancestry, it seems plausible that priming of upright human faces could be based on face-selective cells that are activated by a face regardless of its orientation. But our predominant experience with upright faces (Goldstein and Chance 1980) provides compelling grounds for humans to be like sheep, such that implicit and explicit measures of upside-down face processing are equivalent.

Method

Upside-down versions of faces were created. Observers viewed rows of faces that consisted of upside-down distractors and upright targets (figure 11.9).

Results and Discussion

Observers did not significantly differ on the related trials compared with the unrelated trials: $t(17) = 0.41$, *ns*. Error rates on the two sets of trials also did not differ: related error rate = 2.8 percent; unrelated error rate = 1.9 percent; $t(17) = .78$, *ns*. The lack of positive priming suggests two possibilities. First, the visual system does not use the same neural mechanisms to automatically code upright and upside-down

Targets

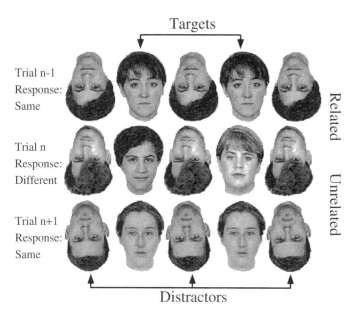

Trial n-1
Response:
Same

Trial n
Response:
Different

Trial n+1
Response:
Same

Related

Unrelated

Distractors

Figure 11.9
Upside-down distractor faces were presented along with upright targets.

faces. These findings agree with the physiological recordings of face-selective cells in sheep (Kendrick and Baldwin 1987). Second, time (Cochran et al. 1983; Perrett et al. 1988; Rock 1973; Valentine and Bruce 1988) or attentive processing is necessary to transform a representation of an upside-down face into its upright counterpart. In either case automatic face processing of upside-down faces without attention does not result in representations that match upright versions of the same face.

General Discussion

In sum, a negative priming procedure showed that response latencies were longer when one or both target faces had appeared as distractors on the immediately preceding trial. Thus, never-before-seen faces are represented and require inhibition. Response latencies were shorter when

target faces had appeared as distractors with high-frequency noise or were contrast-inverted. Thus, underlying representations may in fact be facilitated. Response latencies were unaltered when target faces had appeared as upside-down distractors; not all distractor representations afford response priming (negative or positive). It is proposed that the visual system indeed represents unfamiliar faces without focused attention, but blocks them only if they vie with targets for the control of action (Khurana 2000).

At the simplest level of analysis, the above experiments show that neither negative nor positive priming of human faces requires a network of preexisting face representations. The present findings suggest that the visual system creates representations of human faces "on the fly" in the absence of focused attention. It is possible that all the perceptual mechanisms which process objects present in a negative priming display are activated and primed, regardless of whether they are used to process distractors or targets. If the distractors compete with the targets in the selection of a response, their representations must be suppressed. Whether a distractor competes with targets depends upon the nature of the representations that task performance relies upon (Khurana 2000; Tipper et al. 1994). In the absence of inhibition, if the pathways that rendered the internal representations are accessed again, they will result in faster or more accurate task performance.

Finally, the priming results reported here are largely in accord with response profiles of "face" cells (Desimone 1991; Kendrick and Baldwin 1987; Perrett et al. 1982; Perrett et al. 1987; Rolls et al. 1993; Rolls et al. 1989; Rolls et al. 1985; Rolls and Baylis 1986). This form of face priming could specify the structural descriptions achieved by gnostic cells (Konorski 1967) selectively tuned to faces in humans. However, the present priming results make it unlikely that these cells are the neural correlates of the explicit representations of faces (Crick and Koch 1998). If anything, the present findings suggest that the cells in the superior temporal sulcus are involved in the implicit processing of faces. Explicit face representation may require the involvement of the recently reported face cells in the inferior prefrontal cortex that receive direct input from the superior temporal sulcus (Scalaidhe et al. 1997). The activity of these cells either alone or in conjunction with face-sensitive cells in the superior temporal sulcus might render representations that correspond to the experience of seeing someone.

Acknowledgments

This research was partially supported by the Pew Science Education Research Program at Cornell University and NSF Grant BCS-9727841. Portions of this research were reported at the Association for Research in Vision and Ophthalmology meeting at Sarasota, Florida; the Second Annual Meeting of the Cognitive Neuroscience Society, San Francisco; and the Neural Correlates of Consciousness Meeting, Bremen, Germany. I thank Christof Koch and Romi Nijhawan for discussions regarding the issues raised in this paper.

References

Allman, J., and McGuinness, E. (1988). Visual cortex in primates. In H. D. Steklis and J. Erwin, eds., *Comparative Primate Biology*. Vol. 4, 279–326. New York: Alan R. Liss.

Arnheim, R. (1954). *Art and Visual Perception: A Psychology of the Eye*. Berkeley: University of California Press.

Bruce, V., Burton, M., Carson, D., Hanna, E., and Mason, O. (1994). Repetition priming of face recognition. In C. Umilta and M. Moscovitch, eds., *Attention and Performance XV: Conscious and Nonconscious Information Processing*. Cambridge, MA: MIT Press.

Bruce, V., and Langton, S. (1994). The use of pigmentation and shading information in recognizing the sex and identities of faces. *Perception* 23: 803–822.

Bruce, V., and Young, A. W. (1986). Understanding face recognition. *British Journal of Psychology* 77: 305–327.

Burton, A. M., Bruce, V., and Johnston, R. A. (1990). Understanding face recognition with an interactive activation model. *British Journal of Psychology* 18: 45–60.

Cochran, E. L., Pick, A. D., and Pick, H. L. (1983). Task-specific strategies of mental "rotation" of facial representations. *Memory and Cognition* 11: 41–48.

Crick, F., and Koch, C. (1998). Consciousness and neuroscience. *Cerebral Cortex* 8: 97–107.

Damasio, A. R., Damasio, H., and van Hoesen, G. W. (1982). Prosopagnosia: Anatomic basis and behavioral mechanisms. *Neurology* 32: 331–341.

DeSchepper, B., and Treisman, A. (1996). Visual memory for novel shapes: Implicit coding without attention. *Journal of Experimental Psychology: Learning, Memory, and Cognition* 22: 27–47.

Desimone, R. (1991). Face-selective cells in the temporal cortex of monkeys. *Journal of Cognitive Neuroscience* 3: 1–8.

Deutsch, J. A., and Deutsch, D. (1963). Attention: Some theoretical considerations. *Psychological Review* 70: 80–90.

Diamond, R., and Carey, S. (1986). Why faces are and are not special: An effect of expertise. *Journal of Experimental Psychology: General* 115: 107–117.

Duncan, J. (1980). The locus of interference in the perception of simultaneous stimuli. *Psychological Review* 87: 272–300.

Ellis, A. W., Young, A. W., Flude, B. M., and Hay, D. C. (1987). Repetition priming of face recognition. *Quarterly Journal of Experimental Psychology* 39A: 193–210.

Farah, M. J. (1990). *Visual Agnosia.* Cambridge, MA: MIT Press.

Fiorentini, A., Maffei, L., and Sandini, G. (1983). The role of high spatial frequencies in face perception. *Perception* 12: 195–201.

Galper, R. E. (1970). Recognition of faces in photographic negative. *Psychonomic Science* 19: 207–208.

Goldstein, A. G., and Chance, J. E. (1980). Memory for faces and schema theory. *Journal of Psychology* 105: 47–59.

Goren, C., Sarty, M. M., and Wu, P. (1975). Visual following and pattern discrimination of face-like stimuli by newborn infants. *Pediatrics* 56: 544–549.

Gross, C. G., Rocha-Miranda, C. E., and Bender, D. B. (1972). Visual properties of neurons in inferotemporal cortex of the macaque. *Journal of Neurophysiology* 35: 96–111.

Harmon, L. D., and Julesz, B. (1973). Masking in visual recognition: Effects of two-dimensional filtered noise. *Science* 180: 1194–1197.

Hay, D. C., and Young, A. W. (1982). The human face. In A. Ellis, ed., *Normality and Pathology in Cognitive Functions*, 173–202. New York: Academic Press.

Hayes, A. (1988). Identification of two-tone images: Some implications for high- and low-spatial-frequency processes in human vision. *Perception* 17: 429–436.

Hayes, A. (1991). Local phase relationships of image spatial-frequency components at different spatial scales. *McGill Vision Research Centre Memo 9108.* Montreal: McGill University.

Hayes, A., Morrone, M. C., and Burr, D. (1986). Recognition of positive and negative bandpass-filtered images. *Perception* 15: 595–602.

Hayes, A., and Ross, J. (1995). Lines of sight. In R. Gregory, J. Harris, P. Heard, and D. Rose, eds., *The Artful Eye.* Oxford: Oxford University Press.

Jacoby, L. L. (1991). A process-dissociation framework: Separating automatic from intentional uses of memory. *Journal of Memory and Language* 30: 513–541.

Johnston, A., Hill, H., and Carman, N. (1992). Recognizing faces: Effects of lighting direction, inversion, and brightness reversal. *Perception* 21: 365–375.

Kemp, R., McManus, C., and Piggot, T. (1990). Sensitivity to the displacement of facial features in negative and inverted images. *Perception* 19: 531–543.

Kendrick, K. M., and Baldwin, B. A. (1987). Cells in the temporal cortex of conscious sheep can respond preferentially to the sight of faces. *Science*: 236: 448–450.

Khurana, B. (2000). Not to be and then to be: Visual representation of ignored unfamiliar faces. *Journal of Experimental Psychology: Human Perception and Performance* 26: 246–263.

Khurana, B., Smith, W. C., Baker, M. T., and Huang, C. (1994). Face representation under conditions of inattention. *Investigative Ophthalmology and Visual Science* 35: 4135.

Kleiner, K. A., and Banks, M. S. (1987). Stimulus energy does not account for 2-month-olds face preferences. *Journal of Experimental Psychology: Human Perception and Performance* 13: 594–600.

Kohler, W. (1940). *Dynamics in Psychology.* New York: Liveright.

Konorski, J. (1967). *Integrative Activity of the Brain.* Chicago: University of Chicago Press.

Lehmkule, S., Kratz, E., Mangel, S. C., and Sherman, S. M. (1980). Spatial and temporal sensitivity of X- and Y-cells in dorsal lateral geniculate nucleus of the cat. *Journal of Neurophysiology* 43: 520–541.

Luria, S. M., and Strauss, M. S. (1978). Comparison of eye-movements over faces in photographic positives and negatives. *Perception* 7: 349–358.

Meadows, J. C. (1974). The anatomical basis of prosopagnosia. *Journal of Neurology, Neurosurgery and Psychiatry* 37: 489–501.

Meltzoff, A. N., and Moore, M. K. (1977). Imitation of facial and manual gestures by human neonates. *Science* 198: 75–88.

Morrone, M. C., Burr, D. C., and Ross, J. (1983). Added noise restores recognizability of coarse quantized images. *Nature* 305: 226–228.

Morton, J., and Johnson, M. H. (1989). Four ways for faces to be special. In A. W. Young and H. D. Ellis, eds., *Handbook of Research on Face Processing.* Amsterdam: North-Holland.

Morton, J., and Johnson, M. H. (1991). Conspec and conlern: A two-process theory of infant face recognition. *Psychological Review* 98: 164–181.

Moscovitch, M., Winocur, G., and Behrmann, M. (1997). What is special about face recognition? Nineteen experiments on a person with visual object agnosia and dyslexia but normal face recognition. *Journal of Cognitive Neuroscience* 9: 555–604.

Neill, W. T. (1977). Inhibitory and facilitory processes in selective attention. *Journal of Experimental Psychology: Human Perception and Performance* 3: 444–450.

Neill, W. T. (1991). *Consciousness and the Inhibitory Control of Cognition.* Invited address to the meeting of the American Psychological Association, San Francisco.

Neill, W. T., Lissner, L. S., and Beck, J. L. (1990). Negative priming in same–different matching: Further evidence for a central locus of inhibition. *Perception and Psychophysics* 48: 398–400.

Neill, W. T., and Westberry, R. L. (1987). Selective attention and the suppression of cognitive noise. *Journal of Experimental Psychology: Learning, Memory, and Cognition* 13: 327–334.

Perrett, D. I., Mistlin, A. J., and Chitty, A. J. (1987). Visual neurons responsive to faces. *Trends in Neuroscience* 10: 358–364.

Perrett, D. I., Mistlin, A. J., Chitty, A. J., Smith, P. A., Potter, D. D., Broennimann R., and Harries, M. (1988). Specialized face processing and hemispheric asymmetry in man and monkey: Evidence from single unit and reaction time studies. *Behaviour and Brain Research* 29: 245–258.

Perrett, D. I., Rolls, E. T., and Caan, W. (1982). Visual neurons responsive to faces in the monkey temporal cortex. *Experimental Brain Research* 47: 329–342.

Phelps, M. T., and Roberts, W. A. (1994). Memory for pictures of upright and inverted primate faces in humans (homo sapiens), squirrel monkeys (samiri sciureus), and pigeons (columba livia). *Journal of Comparative Psychology* 108: 114–125.

Phillips, R. J. (1972). Why are faces hard to recognize in photographic negative? *Perception and Psychophysics* 12: 425–426.

Rhodes, G., Brake, S., and Atkinson, A. (1993). What's lost in inverted faces? *Cognition* 47: 25–57.

Rock, I. (1973). *Orientation and Form.* New York: Academic Press.

Rock, I. (1974). The perception of disoriented figures. *Scientific American* 230: 78–85.

Rolls, E. T., and Baylis, G. C. (1986). Size and contrast have only small effects on the responses to faces of neurons in the cortex of the superior temporal sulcus of the monkey. *Experimental Brain Research* 65: 38–48.

Rolls, E. T., Baylis, G. C., Hasselmo, M. E., and Nalwa, V. (1989). The effect of learning on the face selective responses of neurons in the cortex in the superior temporal sulcus of the monkey. *Experimental Brain Research* 76: 153–164.

Rolls, E. T., Baylis, G. C., and Leonard, C. M. (1985). Role of low and high spatial frequencies in the face-selective responses of neurons in the cortex in the superior temporal sulcus in the monkey. *Vision Research* 25: 1021–1035.

Rolls, E. T., Tovee, M. J., and Ramachandran, V. S. (1993). Visual learning reflected in the responses of neurons in the temporal visual cortex of the macaque. *Society for Neuroscience Abstracts* 19: 1910.

Sackett, G. P. (1966). Monkeys reared in isolation with pictures as visual input: Evidence for innate releasing mechanism. *Science* 154: 1470–1473.

Scalaidhe, S. P. O., Wilson, F. A. W., and Goldman-Rakic, P. S. (1997). Areal segregation of face-processing neurons in prefrontal cortex. *Science* 278: 1135–1138.

Scapinello, K. F., and Yarmey, A. D. (1970). The role of familiarity and orientation in immediate and delayed recognition stimuli. *Psychonomic Science* 21: 329–330.

Schacter, D. L., Chui, C. Y. P., and Ochsner, K. N. (1993). Implicit memory: A selective review. *Annual Review of Neuroscience* 16: 159–182.

Sekular, R., and Blake, R. (1994). *Perception*. New York: McGraw-Hill.

Tanaka, J. W., and Farah, M. J. (1993). Parts and wholes in face recognition. *Quarterly Journal of Experimental Psychology* 46A: 225–245.

Thompson, P. (1980). Margaret Thatcher: A new illusion. *Perception* 9: 483–484.

Tipper, S. P. (1985). The negative priming effect: Inhibitory priming by ignored objects. *Quarterly Journal of Experimental Psychology* 37A: 571–590.

Tipper, S. P., Brehaut, J. C., and Driver, J. (1990). Selection of moving and static objects for the control of spatially-directed action. *Journal of Experimental Psychology: Human Perception and Performance* 16: 492–504.

Tipper, S. P., and Cranston, M. (1985). Selective attention and priming: Inhibitory and facilitory effects of ignored primes. *Quarterly Journal of Experimental Psychology* 37A: 591–611.

Tipper, S. P., and Driver, J. (1988). Negative priming between pictures and words: Evidence for semantic analysis of ignored stimuli. *Memory and Cognition* 16: 64–80.

Tipper, S. P., Lortie, C., and Baylis, G. C. (1992). Selective reaching: Evidence for action-centered attention. *Journal of Experimental Psychology: Human Perception and Performance* 18: 891–905.

Tipper, S. P., Weaver, B., and Houghton, G. (1994). Behavioural goals determine inhibitory mechanisms of selective attention. *Quarterly Journal of Experimental Psychology* 47A: 809–840.

Treisman, A., and DeSchepper, B. (1996). Object tokens, attention, and visual memory. In T. Inui and J. McClelland, eds., *Attention and Performance XVI: Information Integration in Perception and Communication*. Cambridge, MA: MIT Press.

Tulving, E., and Schacter, D. L. (1990). Priming and human memory systems. *Science* 247: 301–305.

Valentine, T., and Bruce, V. (1986). The effect of race, inversion and encoding activity upon face recognition. *Acta Psychologica* 61: 259–273.

Valentine, T., and Bruce, V. (1988). Mental rotation of faces. *Memory and Cognition* 16: 556–566.

Whiteley, A. M., and Warrington, E. K. (1977). Prosopagnosia: A clinical, psychological, and anatomical study of three patients. *Journal of Neurology, Neurosurgery and Psychiatry* 40: 394–403.

Yarmey, A. D. (1971). Recognition memory for familiar "public" faces: Effects of orientation and delay. *Psychonomic Science* 24: 286–288.

Yin, R. K. (1969). Looking at upside-down faces. *Journal of Experimental Psychology* 81: 141–145.

Yin, R. K. (1970). Face recognition by brain-injured patients: A dissociable ability? *Neuropsychologia* 8: 395–402.

Young, A. W., and Bruce, V. (1991). Perceptual categories and the computation of "grandmother." *European Journal of Cognitive Psychology* 38: 109–144.

Young, A. W., Hellawell, D., and Hay, D. C. (1987). Configural information in face perception. *Perception* 16: 747–759.

12 Space in the Brain: Different Neural Substrates for Allocentric and Egocentric Frames of Reference

Melvyn A. Goodale and Kelly J. Murphy

Space, like time, is a fundamental dimension of the world in which we live. To understand and interact with the world, we must compute the positions of objects in space, both with respect to one another and with respect our bodies. Although vision clearly plays a preeminent role in these computations, there is considerable debate as to how and where such spatial information is coded in the visual system. In this paper, we will argue that, contrary to popular belief, the coding of space in the visual system is not unitary. We will present evidence which suggests instead that the visuospatial processing that underlies our conscious perception of objects and their spatial relations is quite separate from the visuospatial processing that controls our actions directed at those objects.

Two Visual Systems

Beyond primary visual cortex (V1), visual information is conveyed to a complex array of higher-order visual areas in the cerebral cortex (for review, see Zeki 1993). Nevertheless, as long ago as 1982, Ungerleider and Mishkin were able to identify two broad "streams" of projections arising from V1 in the macaque monkey: a ventral stream projecting eventually to the inferotemporal cortex and a dorsal stream projecting to the posterior parietal cortex (figure 12.1). These regions also receive inputs from a number of other subcortical visual structures, such as the superior colliculus, which sends prominent projections to the dorsal stream (via connections in the thalamus). Evidence from neuropsychological studies and more recently from neuro-imaging suggests that the visual projections from primary visual cortex to the temporal and parietal lobes in the human brain also involve a separation into ventral and dorsal streams (for review, see Goodale and Humphrey 1998; Milner and Goodale 1995).

Ungerleider and Mishkin (1982) originally proposed that the two streams of visual processing play different but complementary roles in the processing of incoming visual information. According to their account, the ventral stream plays a critical role in the identification and recognition of objects, while the dorsal stream mediates the localization of the same objects. Some have referred to this distinction in visual processing as one between object vision and spatial vision—"what" versus "where." Support for this idea came from work with monkeys. Lesions of inferotemporal cortex in monkeys produced deficits in their ability to discriminate between objects on the basis of their visual features but did not affect their performance on a spatially demanding "landmark" task, in which the relative position of a landmark object with respect to two food wells determined which food well contained a food reward (Pohl 1973; Ungerleider and Brody 1977). Conversely, lesions of the posterior parietal cortex produced deficits in performance on the landmark task but did not affect object discrimination learning (for critiques of these studies, see Goodale 1995; Milner and Goodale 1995). Although the evidence for the original Ungerleider and Mishkin proposal initially seemed quite compelling, recent findings from a broad range of studies in both humans and monkeys have necessitated a reinterpretation of the division of labor between the two streams.

Some of the most telling evidence against the "what" versus "where" distinction has come from studies with neurological patients. It has been known for a long time that patients with damage to the human homologue of the dorsal stream have difficulty reaching in the correct direction for objects placed in different positions in the visual field contralateral to their lesion (even though they have no difficulty reaching out and touching parts of their body touched by the

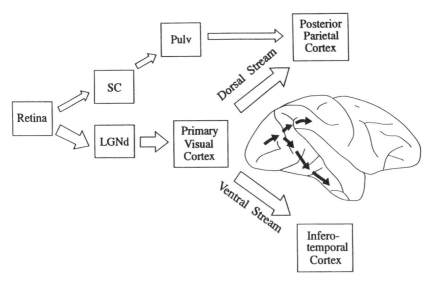

Figure 12.1
The major routes of visual input into the dorsal and ventral streams. The diagram of the macaque brain on the right of the figure shows the approximate routes of the cortico-cortical projections from the primary visual cortex to the posterior parietal and the inferotemporal cortex, respectively. LGNd: lateral geniculate nucleus, pars dorsalis; Pulv: pulvinar; SC: superior colliculus. (Adapted with permission from Goodale et al. 1994).

experimenter). Although this deficit in visually guided behavior, which is known clinically as *optic ataxia* (Bálint 1909), has often been interpreted as a failure of spatial vision, two other sets of observations in these patients suggest a rather different interpretation. First, patients with damage to this region of cortex often show an inability to rotate their hand or open their fingers properly to grasp an object placed in front of them, even when it is always placed in the same location (Goodale et al. 1994; Goodale et al. 1993; Jakobson et al. 1991; Perenin and Vighetto 1988). Second, these same patients are able to describe the orientation, size, shape, and even the relative spatial location of the very objects they are unable to grasp correctly (Jeannerod 1988; Perenin and Vighetto 1988, Goodale et al. 1994). Clearly, this pattern of deficits and spared abilities cannot be explained by appealing to a general deficit in spatial vision.

Other patients, in whom the brain damage appears to involve ventral rather than dorsal stream structures, show the complementary pattern of deficits and spared visual abilities. Such patients have great difficulty recognizing common objects on the basis of their visual appearance, but have no problem grasping objects placed in front of them or moving through the world without bumping into things. Consider, for example, the patient DF, a young woman who suffered damage to her ventral stream pathways from anoxia that was the result of carbon monoxide poisoning. As a result of the brain damage, DF shows *visual form agnosia* and is unable to recognize objects visually on the basis of their shape. Even though DF cannot indicate the size, shape, and orientation of an object, either verbally or manually, she shows normal preshaping and rotation of her hand when reaching out to grasp it (Goodale et al.

1991; Goodale et al. 1994). Appealing to a general deficit in "object vision" does not help us to understand her problem. She is able to use visual information about the location, size, shape, and orientation of objects to control her grasping movements (and other visually guided movements) despite the fact that she has no conscious perception of those object features.

On the basis of these neuropsychological findings and a number of related behavioral and electrophysiological observations in the monkey, Goodale and Milner (1992) set out a new account of the division of labor between the dorsal and ventral streams of processing. In contrast to Ungerleider and Mishkin (1982), they argued that *both* streams process information about object features and about their spatial relations —but each stream uses this visual information in different ways. According to Goodale and Milner, the ventral stream is primarily concerned with the enduring characteristics of objects and their relations, permitting the formation of long-term perceptual representations. Such representations play an essential role in the identification of objects and enable us to classify objects and events, attach meaning and significance to them, and establish their causal relations. These are operations that are essential to the accumulation of a knowledge base about the world. The dorsal stream, according to Goodale and Milner, is not involved in this kind of long-term perceptual representation of objects in the world. Instead, the visual networks in the dorsal stream are more concerned with the moment-to-moment control of skilled actions, such as reaching and grasping movements, directed at a particular object in the world.

Thus, the two streams play complementary roles in the production of adaptive behavior. The perceptual representations constructed by the ventral stream interact with various high-level cognitive mechanisms and enable an organism to select a particular course of action with respect to objects in the world, while the visuomotor networks in the dorsal stream (and associated cortical and subcortical pathways) are responsible for the programming and on-line control of the particular movements that action entails (for a detailed discussion of these ideas, see Milner and Goodale 1995). In short, the ventral stream mechanisms deliver conscious visual percepts; the dorsal stream provides the unconscious visual control of action.

Different Conceptions of Space

The role of the dorsal stream in visuomotor control is now well established, and even those scientists who subscribe to the spatial vision theory of dorsal stream function acknowledge the contributions of the dorsal stream to sensorimotor control (e.g., Boussaoud et al. 1990; Haxby et al. 1993). Nevertheless, proponents of the spatial vision story view visuomotor behavior as a component of dorsal stream function that is subsumed under the broader function of spatial vision. From their point of view, the primary function of the dorsal pathway is the *perception* of the spatial relations between, and locations of, objects in the environment (for review, see Milner and Goodale 1995). Thus, optic ataxia (disordered reaching to visual targets that the subject can "see") is regarded not as a visuomotor deficit but as a visual disorientation—a problem in the perception of space.

In Goodale and Milner's (1992; Milner and Goodale 1993, 1995) original interpretation of ventral stream function, the term "perception" is used in a restricted sense to refer to phenomenological visual experience. This use of "perception" is different from the more general meaning of perception as sensory processing. As we emphasized earlier, it is the ventral stream that mediates our conscious perception of the world. In this context, the processing of the spatial relations of objects (or the parts of objects) is as central to perception as the processing of the intrinsic features of the objects, such as their shape and surface properties. Indeed, without perception of the relative position of objects in a scene, we could make little sense of our visual world.

In contrast to the conscious perception of spatial layout provided by the ventral stream, the computation of spatial location carried out by the dorsal stream is entirely related to the guidance of specific visuomotor actions, such as grasping an object, walking around obstacles, or gazing at different objects in a scene. As a consequence, the dorsal stream mechanisms do not compute the "allocentric" location of a target object (i.e., its location relative to the locations of other objects in the scene), but rather the "egocentric" coordinates of the location of the object with respect to the location of the observer. Indeed, the egocentric coordinates are in the particular frame of reference for the action to be performed. For example, to control a grasping movement, the dorsal stream must eventually transform visual information about the object into arm- and hand-centered coordinates. Moreover, we have no conscious access to the visual information that is transformed into the coordinate frames for action. To reiterate, allocentric spatial information about the layout of objects in the visual scene is computed by the ventral stream mechanisms (which mediate conscious perception), while precise egocentric spatial information about the location of an object in a body-centered frame of reference is computed by the dorsal stream mechanisms (which mediate the more automatic visual control of action). This viewpoint represents a marked departure from traditional spatial vision accounts (e.g., Ungerleider and Mishkin 1982), which appear to assume that both kinds of spatial analysis (allocentric and egocentric) are the domain of the dorsal stream.

Consider the following argument. Perceptual systems are biased toward stability: Objects in the world retain their identity and their spatial relations in spite of dramatic changes in the retinal stimuli that are produced when, for example, the observer moves from one viewpoint to another. Thus, the pen lying on our desk, independent of viewpoint, appears to remain in the

same place on the desk in spite of dramatic rotations about the axes of our favorite swiveling chair. Visuomotor systems, on the other hand, must compute the precise location of objects in the environment in a metrically accurate fashion with respect to the effector being used. Information about the pen's relative position with respect to the corner of the desk is not adequate for guiding an accurate and efficient grasping movement toward it. The visuomotor system must have the position of the pen in precise body-centered coordinates. In short, both dorsal and ventral visual systems compute information about spatial location, but in very different ways.

As we reviewed earlier, much of the evidence for the perception-action account of the ventral-dorsal distinction came from work with neurological patients such as DF. This patient, who has ventral stream damage, is able to produce well-calibrated grasping movements toward objects that she cannot visually discriminate. It was this kind of result that led Goodale and Milner (1992) to suggest that object attributes (i.e., dimensions or shape) are processed by two relatively independent visual mechanisms, one specialized for the perception of objects and the other specialized for the control of actions directed at objects. But although these findings provide support for differential processing of object features for perception and action, they say nothing about how spatial information might be handled by perceptual and action systems.

Of course, as we saw earlier, there have been some studies, admittedly few in number, that have examined the ability of patients with damage to the dorsal stream to perform allocentric and egocentric spatial judgments. Thus, Perenin and Vighetto (1988) noted that even though their optic ataxic patients were unable to reach accurately to objects presented in different positions in their contralesional visual field, they could nonetheless make normal judgments about the relative locations of these objects within the same visual field. In other words, Perenin and Vighetto's patients could use spatial information

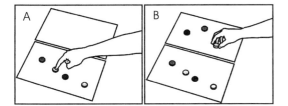

Figure 12.2
The two tasks used to test DF's spatial encoding abilities. Panel A shows the pointing task, in which the subject is required to point to the different colored tokens according to a predetermined order provided by the experimenter. Panel B shows the copying task, in which the subject is required to construct a copy of the arrangement, using an identical set of colored tokens. Subjects are allowed as much time as they need to construct the copy.

for the purposes of making perceptual judgments about the locations of objects in their environment, but they could not use spatial information about object location to make accurate visually guided movements.

A natural question to ask then is this: If patients with dorsal stream damage show preserved allocentric spatial processing in the face of a profound disturbance in egocentric spatial processing, will patients like DF with ventral stream damage show the opposite pattern of behavior? If one subscribes to the "spatial vision" theory of dorsal stream function (Ungerleider and Mishkin 1982), then DF should do well at tasks requiring her to analyze the spatial relations among objects in the environment—her visuomotor abilities indicate that her dorsal stream is intact. In contrast, a strict interpretation of Goodale and Milner's (1992) perception and action story would lead one to expect that DF would show deficits in her ability to perceive the relative location of objects in a visual scene even though she can use information about their location to direct her actions toward them.

Allocentric and Egocentric Spatial Processing in DF

Recently we carried out a set of experiments in which we examined DF's ability to use spatial information about a small group of objects in order to make decisions about where those objects were located relative to her (egocentric) and relative to one another (allocentric) in space (Murphy et al. 1998). For these tasks we presented small groups of differently colored circular tokens that could be easily discriminated on the basis of color but could not be distinguished on the basis of shape or edge-based cues. Thus, relatively pure spatial responses to the group of tokens could be examined. In our egocentric task DF was required to point to all available tokens in the target array in a specified sequence (figure 12.2a). In our allocentric task DF was required to copy the spatial arrangement of tokens in the target array as precisely as possible, using another set of colored tokens (figure 12.2b). Given the fact that DF appears to show normal visually guided movements, which require egocentric spatial processing, we expected that she would show normal sensitivity to the spatial locations of all of the tokens in a given array when she had to point to them. We expected, however, that she would do poorly on the copying task, since to do this, she would have to use an allocentric frame of reference; in other words, she would have to process information about the positions of targets with respect to one another.

As expected, DF showed no difficulty whatsoever in pointing to each of the targets in turn. She pointed acccurately even when she was told

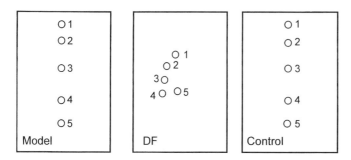

Figure 12.3
Examples of the reproductions of the token arrays made by DF and one of the control subjects. Although DF shows some sensitivity to the relative position of the tokens, her performance is clearly far from normal.

to point to the tokens in a specified order that she was told about just before she began a sequence of pointing movements (e.g., "Point first to the red token, then to the blue, the green, the yellow, and the black, in that order."). Except for the fact that she was slightly slower, her performance was indistinguishable from the control subjects. This means that DF can use egocentric spatial coding of target location to control visuomotor acts such as manual aiming movements. In fact, her normal visuomotor performance on this task is consistent with her past performance on a broad range of visually guided behaviors (for a review, see Milner and Goodale 1995).

DF's normal performance on the pointing task, where egocentric coding was demanded, can be contrasted with her poor performance on the copying task, where allocentric coding had to be used. On the copying task, she showed large displacements of the position of objects with respect to one another when she attempted to reproduce the target arrays. As figure 12.3 illustrates, her copies looked quite different from the actual target patterns she was presented with. The accuracy of all her attempts at copying the token arrays is summarized in figure 12.4, alongside the performance of two control subjects. DF's poor performance in spatial percep-

tion cannot be ascribed to an overarching deficit in "spatial vision," since she had no problem directing her hand to any of the targets. Her problem was with allocentric, not egocentric, coding of spatial position.

It is important to note that DF's poor performance on the copying task cannot be explained by suggesting that this task was more "cognitively challenging" than the other tasks we used. The copying task, for example, did not require much working memory, since the model was always available. In contrast, the pointing task, on which DF did as well as normal subjects, did put a load on working memory, since subjects were required to point to the tokens in a predetermined order. Although DF's copies tended to be displaced slightly toward the top half of the square white background, this shift in placement was unaccompanied by any evidence for a neglect of or inattention to the bottom part of the target display. She always copied the entire array of five tokens. More important, she reproduced the vertical arrangement of the tokens as well (or as poorly) as she did the horizontal.

A recent study by David Milner and his colleagues (Dijkerman et al. 1998) has shown that DF is also unable to use an allocentric frame of reference to guide her grasping movements. When faced with a disk in which two finger holes

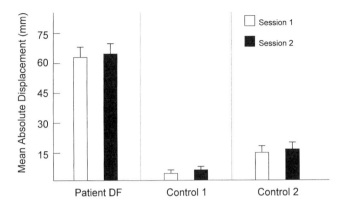

Figure 12.4
Graph summarizing the mean displacements of the positions of the tokens in the reproductions from the positions of corresponding tokens in the sample array for DF and two control subjects. DF is far less accurate than the other two subjects, even in a second session, after she has had more practice.

and a thumb hole had been cut, she was unable to guide her hand successfully so that her two fingers and thumb went into the holes when she reached out to grasp the disk. Thus, when the distance between the forefinger and thumb holes, and the orientation of the line formed by them, were independently varied from trial to trial, she could not adjust either her grip aperture or the orientation of her hand to reflect those variations. She could adjust the orientation of her hand when there were only two holes (one for the thumb and one for the finger), but even here, she could not correctly adjust the aperture between her finger and thumb. This result suggests that DF is unable to use allocentric coding, not just to guide her behavior in "perceptual" tasks such as the copying task described earlier, but also to guide her motor output in an "action" task.

Of course, under other circumstances, DF apparently can locate two or more positions when she is engaged in a motor task. Thus, she can point to two colored tokens simultaneously with her left hand and right hand (Dijkerman et al. 1998). But in this case, each hand is performing a separate act of egocentric localization, and no

allocentric coding is required. Similarly, DF can reach out and pick up objects that vary in outline shape, placing her forefinger and thumb on appropriate "opposition" points on the surface of nonsymmetrical, smoothly contoured objects (Goodale et al. 1994). Clearly, some sort of object-based coding is needed here. It is when the grasping task requires an analysis of the location of separate objects (e.g., holes in a disk) for controlling the posture of one hand that DF's use of allocentric cues for the control of action breaks down. The dorsal stream, by itself, appears unable to perform this analysis.

It is generally believed that patients with a visual agnosia (like DF) have suffered damage to the ventral visual cortical pathway (Milner and Goodale 1995). Typically, such patients have been characterized as having a deficit in the perception of the shape of objects. Rarely has the ability of such patients to perceive the spatial location of objects been investigated. This may be the case for two reasons. First, "spatial vision" is thought by some researchers to be mediated exclusively by the dorsal visual cortical pathway. Second, the severity of the object perception/ recognition deficits overshadows any possible observations of deficits in space perception, particularly when there is an absence of visuomotor disturbance.

Neurological patients who present with spatial perceptual impairments as a primary feature (i.e., patients with hemispatial neglect, dressing dyspraxia, and constructional apraxia) typically have damage in the parietal lobe, in particular the inferior parietal region. We have not observed any of the classically described visuospatial impairments, often reported after parietal lobe damage, in DF's behavior, and this is consistent with the fact that her MRI scan does not show evidence of parietal lobe injury. Nonetheless, we felt it was important to address the issue of constructional apraxia (i.e., the inability to perform familiar movement sequences when engaged in the act of making or preparing something) and to explain why we thought that DF's difficulty in reproducing the allocentric location of an object cannot be accounted for by appealing to some sort of constructional apraxic deficit. First, DF's drawings of objects from memory are remarkably intact and do not show any evidence of constructional apraxia (Servos et al. 1993). Second, DF can perform image construction tasks and is able to use visual imagery to manipulate objects in order to fashion new objects in her mind's eye just as well as normal subjects (Servos and Goodale 1995). In short, DF does not have constructional apraxia; but she does have a fundamental deficit in allocentric spatial coding.

DF's fundamental deficit in allocentric coding cannot be explained in terms of the old idea that all spatial processing resides in the posterior parietal cortex. In fact, regardless of the exact interpretation of the nature of the spatial deficits, DF's perception of spatial relations should be intact if all forms of visuospatial processing, and not just visuomotor control, depended on mechanisms in the dorsal stream. The results of the allocentric spatial tasks demonstrate that this is clearly not the case. Instead, as argued elsewhere (Goodale and Milner 1992; Milner and Goodale

1995), the characterization of dorsal stream function as visuomotor rather than visuospatial predicts the obtained data.

As was discussed earlier, other accounts of single cases support the dissociation of spatial encoding for perceptual representation from spatial encoding for visuomotor control. Recently, Stark et al. (1996) described a patient, with normal visual object recognition abilities, who was impaired at making spatial judgments about the locations of visual (or auditory) targets but could accurately localize these targets with a pointing movement. Bálint's (1909) patient had poor visuomotor control when he used his right hand but not his left, a finding hard to reconcile with the idea of an overarching visuospatial deficit (Harvey and Milner 1995). And as we have already seen, Perenin and Vighetto (1988) have argued that poor manual localization of targets in patients with dorsal stream damage is largely unrelated to the degree of visuospatial dysfunction measured in perceptual tests. In summary, it seems that although the dorsal stream plays a major role in spatial processing, that processing is confined to transforming visual information about a goal into the egocentric frames of reference required for a particular action directed at that goal. Allocentric spatial encoding is not a dorsal stream function, and appears to depend more on perceptual mechanisms in the ventral stream.

Evidence from Monkey Studies

The weight of evidence from single-unit studies of the dorsal stream in monkeys suggests that the spatial coding of visual information is primarily in egocentric coordinates. Although most visually sensitive cells in the posterior parietal cortex show spatial tuning, they are modulated by the concurrent motor behavior of the animal (e.g., Hyvärinen and Poranen 1974; Mountcastle et al. 1975). In reviewing the electrophysiological studies which have been carried out on the posterior parietal cortex, Andersen (1987) concluded that most neurons in these areas "exhibit both sensory-related and movement-related activity." The activity of some visually driven cells in this region has been shown to be linked to saccadic eye movements; the activity of others, to whether or not the animal is fixating a stimulus; and the activity of still other cells, to whether or not the animal is engaged in visual pursuit or is making goal-directed reaching movements (e.g., Snyder et al. 1997).

In other words, as far as spatial coding in the dorsal stream is concerned, the current electrophysiological evidence indicates that egocentric frames of reference predominate. Indeed, there is no clear evidence that allocentric spatial coding —insofar as this refers to the position of an object with respect to other objects—exists in the posterior parietal cortex. Some coding of object size and of configurational properties within single objects is required for guiding actions such as grasping, and evidence is accumulating that subsets of neurons in monkey parietal cortex are able to code some of these object properties (for review, see Sakata et al. 1998). At the same time, there is evidence that cells which are primarily related to limb movements also show subtle modulations by eye and head position (Andersen 1997). But while these mechanisms might permit different levels of abstraction in the coding of location, the coding would nonetheless remain intrinsically egocentric.

Lesion studies of the posterior parietal cortex in monkeys have also revealed deficits in egocentric spatial coding. Misreaching in space is the most immediately obvious visual effect of large lesions of the posterior parietal cortex in monkeys, just as it is in humans with large lesions in the superior regions of the posterior parietal cortex (Ettlinger 1977). And just as is the case in the human patient with optic ataxia, the misreaching in the monkey is a visuomotor, not a purely visuospatial, deficit. For example, after unilateral lesions, the reaching disorder is invariably restricted to the monkey's contralesional arm. In other words, the monkey has no problem reaching to the same visual targets with its ipsilesional arm (Ettlinger and Kalsbeck 1962; Hartje and Ettlinger 1974; Faugier-Grimaud et al. 1978; Lamotte and Acuña 1978). Yet at the same time, a simple motor disorder is ruled out by the fact that the monkey is able, once it has grasped a food object, to bring it efficiently and accurately to its mouth.

Smaller lesions in the posterior parietal cortex can result in more specific deficits. For example, they can result in deficits that are restricted to saccadic eye movements (Lynch and McLaren 1989), ocular pursuit (Dürsteler and Wurtz 1988), or grasping (Gallese et al. 1994). Indeed, except for the well-known landmark studies discussed earlier (Pohl 1973; Ungerleider and Brody 1977), there is little evidence for deficits in the allocentric coding of spatial relations. In fact, the observed deficits in the landmark task (and other maze and route-finding tasks) appear to be more related to deficits in the visual control of eye, hand, or lower limb movements than to a fundamental deficit in allocentric coding of position (for a review, see Goodale 1995; Milner and Goodale 1995).

Evidence from Neuroimaging Studies in Humans

Functional neuroimaging studies also provide some support for the idea that egocentric spatial encoding for action is carried out by mechanisms in the parietal cortex and that different actions depend on spatial encoding in different anatomical sites. Thus, different areas in and around the intraparietal sulcus are activated when subjects make saccadic eye movements as opposed to manual pointing movements toward the same visual targets (e.g., Anderson et al. 1994; Kawashima et al. 1996; Pierrot-Deseilligny and Müri 1997). Similarly, a region in the human brain that appears to correspond to the part of the monkey posterior parietal region where visually sensitive "grasping" cells have been localized shows selective activation during visually guided grasping (Binkofski et al. 1998; Grafton et al. 1996). Finally, a recent study of prism adaptation shows that selective activation of a particular region of the posterior parietal cortex occurs during the remapping of visual and proprioceptive representations of hand position (Clower et al. 1996).

Things are less clear with respect to allocentric spatial encoding. Some studies have found that more superior regions in the vicinity of the intraparietal cortex, similar to those activated with the saccadic and pointing tasks, are also activated in perceptual tasks demanding an allocentric spatial analysis (Courtney et al. 1996; Grady et al. 1994; Haxby et al. 1994). Moreover, this activation is bilateral. Other studies have shown that regions in the inferior parietal lobule, particularly in the right hemisphere, are activated (Jonides et al. 1993; Köhler et al. 1998; Moscovitch et al. 1995). The apparent discrepancy with respect to allocentric coding may be a consequence of the subtraction logic operating in some experiments. In other words, areas that are equally involved in the processing of objects and the processing of spatial relations between those objects may have been overlooked. This is a point we shall return to later. It might also be the case that the tasks requiring relative spatial comparisons may have elicited more eye movements than either the baseline tasks or tasks requiring object or face matching, thus resulting in a pattern of activation which reflects the well-established role of areas in the intraparietal sulcus region in the control of eye movements.

Why Does DF Show a Deficit in Allocentric Spatial Coding?

In addition to her deficits on allocentric spatial tasks, DF has problems in making perceptual estimates of distance. Thus, in unpublished work, we have found that DF's verbal estimates of target distance were quite poor compared with normal control subjects, particularly with monocular vision—although it is important to point out that her estimates were still correlated with the true distance of the target. In other words, DF showed a constant underestimation of the real distance of the targets, and the magnitude of her errors was significantly greater than the magnitude of normal subjects. At the same time, of course, her visuomotor performance with respect to the distance of these objects (as estimated by peak velocity distance scaling) was indistinguishable from that of control subjects. Similar observations have been made with DF using measures of accuracy in various estimation and pointing tasks (Carey et al. 1998). As was the case with DF's performance on the allocentric spatial tasks, the perceptual judgments of distance reveal capacities that appear to fall somewhere between her profound deficits in object perception and her remarkably intact visuomotor performance. Further investigations will be necessary to uncover whether or not these intermediate levels of performance are due to the use of strategies that exploit her spared visuomotor skills (Murphy et al. 1996), or are due to processing in relatively intact brain areas which are responsible for allocentric spatial coding but lie outside the ventral stream itself. If another brain region outside the dorsal or ventral streams is involved, it may not function optimally without appropriate input from object-based mechanisms in the ventral stream.

One region outside the dorsal and ventral streams that might play a role in computing the spatial relations among objects in a scene is the cortical zone between occipitotemporal and superior parietal cortex—the more inferior regions of the posterior parietal cortex. In fact, Milner and Goodale (1995) have suggested that the inferior parietal cortex, near the junction of the parietal, temporal, and occipital lobes, may be a region where the dorsal and ventral streams interact. Lesions to this region, particularly in the right hemisphere, often result in a phenomenon known as visual neglect, in which patients ignore or fail to attend to visual stimuli presented to the side of space contralateral to the lesion. What is seldom appreciated, however, is the fact that the critical region for neglect (Heilman et al. 1983; Vallar and Perani 1986) is several centimeters below the area typically associated with optic ataxia (Perenin and Vighetto 1988). The phenomenon of neglect may reflect the emergence of spatial processing in the human brain that is rather different from that carried out in the dorsal stream, which, as we have argued, is largely concerned with visuomotor control. In fact, the circuitry in humans that corresponds to the dorsal stream in the monkey may be confined largely to the more superior region of the posterior parietal cortex. New systems appear to have emerged in the more inferior parietal cortex of humans for mediating many of the complex visuocognitive abilities (and more "representational" motor acts) that characterize our species. There is considerable evidence, for example, that high-level spatial skills, such as map reading,[1] maze learning, and mental rotation, are particularly sensitive to parietal damage (for a review, see Milner and Goodale 1995; Turnbull et al. 1997).

The circuitry mediating these high-level skills may have co-opted (in the evolutionary sense) some of the transformational algorithms that originally evolved for the control of movement. Thus, some forms of mental rotation and map reading (where one moves from one set of coordinates to another) may make use of egocentric frames of reference that were originally computed only by the dorsal stream. Such mechanisms might also play an important role in the explicit representation of the spatial location of objects in visual scenes with respect to our particular viewpoint. In addition, mechanisms in this new region may be responsible for computing the locations of objects in allocentric frames of reference using input from object-based computations carried out by mechnanisms in the ventral stream. Such perceptual representations would allow us to talk about and cognitively manipulate objects in relation to one another—and to integrate this information about where those objects are with respect to us. It could be the case, therefore, that DF's deficit in allocentric coding arises from a failure of the perceptual mechanisms in her ventral stream to deliver the object representations necessary for these allocentric computations. Of course, as was suggested earlier, it could equally be the case that such allocentric computations take place in the ventral stream itself. But whatever the mechanisms might be that mediate our conscious perception of the spatial relations among objects in a visual scene, it is clear that they do not reside in the dorsal stream, which is primarily concerned with transforming visual information into action using egocentric frames of reference.

Note

1. Route finding using landmarks, however, is not typically associated with damage to the posterior parietal cortex. Patients with topographical agnosia, as this route-finding deficit is sometimes called, typically have lesions in areas corresponding to the ventral stream (Milner and Goodale 1995). Their deficit is more allocentric in nature and is often complicated by a failure to recognize familiar landmarks.

References

Andersen, R. A. (1987). Inferior parietal lobule function in spatial perception and visuomotor integration. In V. B. Mountcastle, F. Plum, and S. R. Geiger, eds., *Handbook of Physiology Section 1: The Nervous System.* Volume V: Higher Functions of the Brain, Part 2, pp. 483–518. Bethesda MD: American Physiology Association.

Andersen, R. A. (1997). Multimodal integration for the representation of space in the posterior parietal cortex. *Philosophical Transactions of the Royal Society of London* B352: 1421–1428.

Anderson, T. J., Jenkins, I. H., Brooks, D. J., Hawken, M. B., Frackowiak, R. S. J., and Kennard, C. (1994).

Cortical control of saccades and fixation in man. A PET study. *Brain* 117: 1073–1084.

Bálint, R. (1909). Seelenlähmung des "Schauens," optische Ataxie, räumliche Störung der Aufmerksamkeit. *Monatschrift für Psychiatrie und Neurologie* 25: 51–81.

Binkofski, F., Dohle, C., Posse, S., Stephan, K. M., Hefter, H., Seitz, R. J., and Freund, H.-J. (1998). Human anterior intraparietal area subserves prehension. *Neurology* 50: 1253–1259.

Boussaoud, D., Ungerleider, L. G., and Desimone, R. (1990). Pathways for motion analysis: Cortical connections of the medial superior temporal and fundus of the superior temporal visual areas in the macaque. *Journal of Comparative Neurology* 296: 462–495.

Carey, D. P., Dijkerman, H. C., and Milner, A. D. (1998). Perception and action in depth. *Consciousness and Cognition* 7: 438–453.

Carey, D. P., Harvey, M., and Milner, A. D. (1996). Visuomotor sensitivity for shape and orientation in a patient with visual form agnosia. *Neuropsychologia* 34: 329–337.

Clower, D. M., Hoffman, J. M., Votaw, J. R., Faber, T. L., Woods, R. P., and Alexander, G. E. (1996). Role of posterior parietal cortex in the calibration of visually guided reaching. *Nature* 383: 618–621.

Courtney, S. M., Ungerleider, L. G., Keil, K., and Haxby, J. V. (1996). Object and spatial visual working memory activate separate neural systems in human cortex. *Cerebral Cortex* 6: 39–49.

Dijkerman, H. C., Milner, A. D., and Carey, D. P. (1998). Grasping spatial relationships: Failure to demonstrate allocentric visual coding in a patient with visual form agnosia. *Consciousness and Cognition* 7: 424–437.

Dürsteler, M. R., and Wurtz, R. H. (1988). Pursuit and optokinetic deficits following chemical lesions of cortical areas MT and MST. *Journal of Neurophysiology* 60: 940–965.

Ettlinger, G. (1977). Parietal cortex in visual orientation. In F. C. Rose, ed., *Physiological Aspects of Clinical Neurology*, pp. 93–100. Oxford: Blackwell.

Ettlinger, G., and Kalsbeck, J. E. (1962). Changes in tactile discrimination and in visual reaching after successive and simultaneous bilateral posterior parietal ablations in the monkey. *Journal of Neurology, Neurosurgery, and Psychiatry* 25: 256–268.

Faugier-Grimaud, S., Frenois, C., and Stein, D. G. (1978). Effects of posterior parietal lesions on visually guided behavior in monkeys. *Neuropsychologia* 16: 151–168.

Gallese, V., Murata, A., Kaseda, M., Niki, N., and Sakata, H. (1994). Deficit of hand preshaping after muscimol injection in monkey parietal cortex. *Neuroreport* 5: 1525–1529.

Goodale, M. A. (1995). The cortical organization of visual perception and visuomotor control. In S. Kosslyn and D. Osherson, eds., *An Invitation to Cognitive Science*. Vol. 2, *Visual Cognition and Action*, 167–213. 2nd ed. Cambridge, MA: MIT Press.

Goodale, M. A., and Humphrey, G. K. (1998). The objects of action and perception. *Cognition* 67: 181–207.

Goodale, M. A., Meenan, J. P., Bulthoff, H. H., Nicolle, D. A., Murphy, K. J., and Racicot, C. I. (1994). Separate neural pathways for the visual analysis of object shape in perception and prehension. *Current Biology* 4: 604–606.

Goodale, M. A., and Milner, A. D. (1992). Separate visual pathways for perception and action. *Trends in Neurosciences* 15: 20–25.

Goodale, M. A., Milner, A. D., Jakobson, L. S., and Carey, D. P. (1991). A neurological dissociation between perceiving objects and grasping them. *Nature* 349: 154–156.

Goodale, M. A., Murphy, K., Meenan, J. P., Racicot, C., and Nicolle, D. A. (1993). Spared object perception but poor object-calibrated grasping in a patient with optic ataxia. *Society for Neuroscience Abstracts* 19: 775.

Grady, C. L., Maisog, J. M., Horwitz, B., Ungerleider, L. G., Mentis, M. J., Salerno, J. A., Pietrini, P., Wagner, E., and Haxby, J. V. (1994). Age-related changes in cortical blood-flow activation during visual processing of faces and location. *Journal of Neuroscience* 14: 1450–1462.

Grafton, S. T., Fagg, A. H., Woods, R. P., and Arbib, M. A. (1996). Functional anatomy of pointing and grasping in humans. *Cerebral Cortex* 6: 226–237.

Hartje, W., and Ettlinger, G. (1974). Reaching in the light and dark after unilateral posterior parietal ablations in the monkey. *Cortex* 9: 346–354.

Harvey, M., and Milner, A. D. (1995). Bálint's patient. *Cognitive Neuropsychology* 12: 261–281.

Haxby, J. V., Grady, C. L., Horwitz, B., Salerno, J., Ungerleider, L. G., and Mishkin, M. (1993). Dissociation of object and spatial visual processing pathways in human extrastriate cortex. In B. Gulyás, D. Ottoson, and P. E. Roland eds., *Functional Organization of the Human Visual Cortex*, 329–340. Oxford: Pergamon Press.

Haxby, J. V., Horwitz, B., Ungerleider, L. G., Maisog, J. M., Pietrini, P., and Grady, C. L. (1994). The functional organization of human extrastriate cortex: A PET-rCBF study of selective attention to faces and location. *Journal of Neuroscience* 14: 6336–6353.

Heilman, K. M., Watson, R. T., Valenstein, E., and Damasio, A. T. (1983). Localization of lesions in neglect. In A. Kertesz, ed., *Localization in Neuropsychology*, 471–492. New York: Academic Press.

Hyvärinen, J., and Poranen, A. (1974). Function of the parietal associative area 7 as revealed from cellular discharges in alert monkeys. *Brain* 97: 673–692.

Jakobson, L. S., Archibald, Y. M., Carey, D. P., and Goodale, M. A. (1991). A kinematic analysis of reaching and grasping movements in a patient recovering from optic ataxia. *Neuropsychologia* 29: 803–809.

Jeannerod, M. (1988). *The Neural and Behavioural Organization of Goal-Directed Movements*. Oxford: Oxford University Press.

Jonides, J., Smith, E. E., Koeppe, R. A., Awh, E., Minoshima., S., and Mintun, M. (1993). Spatial working memory in humans as revealed by PET. *Nature* 363: 623–625.

Kawashima, R., Naitoh, E., Matsumura, M., Itoh, H., Ono, S., Satoh, K., Gotoh, R., Koyama, M., Inoue, K., Yoshioka, S., and Fukuda, H. (1996). Topographic representation in human intraparietal sulcus of reaching and saccade. *NeuroReport* 7: 1253–1256.

Köhler, S., Kapur, S., Moscovitch, M., Winocur, G., Houle, S., and McIntosh, A. R. (1998). Networks of domain-specific and general regions involved in episodic memory for spatial location and object identity. *Neuropsychologia* 36: 129–142.

Lynch, J. C., and McLaren, J. W. (1989). Deficits of visual attention and saccadic eye movements after lesions of parieto-occipital cortex in monkeys. *Journal of Neurophysiology* 61: 74–90.

Lamotte, R. H., and Acuña, C. (1978). Deficits in accuracy of reaching after removal of posterior parietal cortex in monkeys. *Brain Research* 139: 309–326.

Milner, A. D., and Goodale, M. A. (1993). Visual pathways to perception and action. In T. P. Hicks, S. Molotchnikoff, and T. Ono, eds., *Progress in Brain Research*. Vol. 95. Amsterdam: Elsevier.

Milner, A. D., and Goodale, M. A. (1995). *The Visual Brain in Action*. Oxford: Oxford University Press.

Milner, A. D., Perrett, D. I., Johnston, R. S., Benson, P. J., Jordan, T. R., Heeley, D. W., et al. (1991). Perception and action in "visual form agnosia." *Brain* 114: 405–428.

Moscovitch, M., Kapur, S., Köhler, S., and Houle, S. (1996). Distinct neural correlates of visual long-term memory for spatial location and object identity: A positron emission tomography study in humans. *Proceedings of the National Academy of Sciences of the USA* 92: 3721–3725.

Mountcastle, V. B., Lynch, J. C., Georgopoulos, A., Sakata, H., and Acuna, C. (1975). Posterior parietal association cortex of the monkey: command functions for operations within extrapersonal space. *Journal of Neurophysiology* 38: 871–908.

Murphy, K. J., Racicot, C. I., and Goodale, M. A. (1996). The use of visuomotor cues as a strategy for making perceptual judgments in a patient with visual form agnosia. *Neuropsychology* 10: 396–401.

Murphy, K. J., Carey, D. P., and Goodale, M. A. (1998). Perception of allocentric spatial relations in a patient with visual form agnosia. *Cognitive Neuropsychology* 15: 705–822.

Perenin, M. T., and Vighetto, A. (1988). Optic ataxia: A specific disruption in visuomotor mechanisms. I. Different aspects of the deficit in reaching for objects. *Brain* 111: 643–674.

Pierrot-Deseilligny, C., and Müri, R. (1997). Posterior parietal cortex control of saccades in humans. In P. Thier and H. O. Karnath, eds., *Parietal Lobe Contributions to Orientation in 3D Space*, 135–147. Heidelberg: Springer-Verlag.

Pohl, W. (1973). Dissociation of spatial discrimination deficits following frontal and parietal lesions in monkeys. *Journal of Comparative and Physiological Psychology* 82: 227–239.

Sakata, H., Taira, M., Kusunoki, M., Murata, A., Tanaka, Y., and Tsutsui, K. (1998). Neural coding of 3D features of objects for hand action in the parietal cortex of the monkey. *Philosophical Transactions of the Royal Society of London* B353: 1363–1373.

Servos, P., and Goodale, M. A. (1995). Preserved visual imagery in visual form agnosia. *Neuropsychologia* 33: 1383–1394.

Servos, P., Goodale, M. A., and Humphrey, G. K. (1993). The drawing of objects by a visual form agnosic: Contribution of surface properties and memorial representations. *Neuropsychologia* 31: 251–259.

Snyder, L. H., Batista, A. P., and Andersen, R. A. (1997). Coding of intention in the posterior parietal cortex. *Nature* 386: 167–170.

Stark, M., Coslett, H. B., and Saffran, E. M. (1996). Impairment of an egocentric map of locations—implications for perception and action. *Cognitive Neuropsychology* 13: 481–523.

Turnbull, O. H., Carey, D. P., and McCarthy, R. A. (1997). The neuropsychology of object constancy. *Journal of the International Neuropsychological Society* 3: 288–298.

Vallar, G., and Perani, D. (1986). The anatomy of unilateral neglect after right-hemisphere stroke lesions. A clinical/CT-scan correlation study in man. *Neuropsychologia* 24: 609–622.

Ungerleider, L. G., and Brody, B. A. (1977). Extrapersonal spatial orientation: The role of posterior parietal, anterior frontal, and inferotemporal cortex. *Experimental Neurology* 56: 265–280.

Ungerleider, L. G., and Mishkin, M. (1982). Two cortical visual systems. In D. J. Ingle, M. A. Goodale, and R. J. W. Mansfield, eds., *Analysis of Visual Behavior*. Cambridge, MA: MIT Press.

Zeki, S. (1993). *A Vision of the Brain*. Oxford: Blackwell Scientific Publications.

13   Conscious Registration of Continuous and Discrete Visual Events

Romi Nijhawan and Beena Khurana

The facts given by the senses ... are the starting-point and the goal of all the mental adaptations of the physicist [and] the source of every hypothesis and speculation in science.
—Ernst Mach (1890)

Apprehension by the senses supplies ... directly or indirectly, the material of all human knowledge ... there is little hope that he who does not begin at the beginning of knowledge will ever arrive at its end.
—Hermann von Helmholtz (1867)

While the primate visual system is capable of delivering perceived objects in their full glory—color, shape, texture, size, brightness, shadows, highlights, and so on—the sudden appearance of such an object can cost the human observer one-quarter of a precious second in executing a simple, predetermined response. Response times would be much longer if the object features and the exact nature of the response (for example, interception, avoidance, or a rapid switch from interception to avoidance) are unknown prior to the appearance of the object. The tongue-snap response time of animals like toads (*Bufo bufo*) is much shorter, but it is not clear what the visual system of this animal is capable of delivering. These animals respond to only a limited set of objects with relatively small variations in the response. Thus, it would seem that specialized responses to a limited set of objects are capable of being generated faster. Conversely, the adaptability that accompanies the ability of the human visual system to deliver such intricate visual percepts has a cost which is manifested in slower processing.

From the biological point of view, the main function of the human brain, or the brain of any animal, is to provide its owner with valid and reliable information about the outside world. The survival of many animals (and their brains) depends on accurate visual information, in the absence of which accurate action would be impossible. Movement of objects is biologically significant because motion often signifies danger, food, or a mate. It is likely that the structure and physiological properties of the mammalian visual system are, to a large extent, geared toward the efficient and rapid processing of motion. Indeed, the extreme periphery of the primate retina is insensitive to the shape and color of objects, but not to their movement. The eyes of some lower animals can detect objects only when they are in motion. Here we consider a hitherto neglected problem that may further clarify properties of the visual system geared toward the efficient processing of moving objects.

A natural question that arises from our knowledge of neural transmission delays from the retina to higher brain centers is: Are there corresponding delays in our visual experience of the world (Helmholtz 1866)? Given the neural delays, it should not be surprising if our visual experiences are always lagging behind the physical events responsible for those experiences (Cavanagh 1997). One could wonder at length about a static stimulus—for example, a red square—as to whether the stimulus in one's conscious experience is the way the physical object was about 100 msec ago (if one assumes 100 msec transmission delay; see, for example, De Valois and De Valois 1991). But it is certainly possible that once the visual system achieves a description of a given object, it signals only change from then on (MacKay 1958; Koch and Poggio 1999; Rao and Ballard 1999). Thus, if we view the red square for ten seconds, then close to the end of this period, the object of our experience could be based on feedforward input that occurred approximately ten seconds in the past. In our investigation we will primarily use two types of stimuli, continuously changing ones and discretely changing ones, to ask how these stimuli manifest themselves in our visual experience.

Any variable that changes gradually over time, such as the temperature of a body or the weight of an object during the initial upward acceleration of an elevator, may be considered a continuously changing stimulus. Discrete change is a change which is so quick that for all practical purposes, the value of the stimulus variable changes instantaneously for the given sensory modality. In this paper we will consider two types of visual stimuli, one continuous and the other discrete, that have been widely studied by psychologists and neuroscientists alike: continuous movement of an object and a single flash of an object.

In investigating the question of visual delays, one must keep in mind delays in neural signals from the retina to those parts of the visual system whose activation both is necessary for conscious visual experience *and* occurs after the maximum delay from the retinal excitation responsible for those signals. Let us denote the time delay of the maximally delayed response of the necessary brain area by T_m. Consider a single flash of white light localized on a small part of the retina. In this case one may exclude the ganglion cell response to the flash because these delays are shorter than T_m. However, one may not exclude the response of the lateral geniculate nucleus (LGN) to the flash because feedback can modulate activation of LGN cells, after the signals have caused neural activity in many areas of the cortex, well over 100 msec after the flash.

Given the visual delays, the actual instantaneous location of a moving object (or the initial receptor representation based on phototransduction) should be farther along in the trajectory (ahead) of where the moving object is visible to a human observer (figure 13.1). Although at first glance the "obviousness" of this claim seems to leave little room for further investigation, it appears more and more necessary to continue to investigate. We believe the statement concerning the apparent lag of moving objects (Purushothaman et al. 1998; Whitney and Murakami 1998) should be treated as a hypothesis and tested experimentally. It is certainly possible that some visual mechanism, in conjunction with the analysis of motion, samples the retinal input and

performs a visual operation that "corrects" for the expected lag of moving visual objects (Nijhawan 1994). Such a mechanism would restore position correspondence between representations at different levels within the visual system. Therefore, we first address the following question: Is the instantaneous position of a moving object perceived veridically, or is there an illusion in which the percept of a moving object lags behind the actual location of the object by a constant distance?

Conceptual Basis for Why There May Be No Visual Lag for Moving Objects

According to some estimates, neural transmission delays in the visual system should cause an observer to be conscious of physical events that occurred close to 100 msec in the past (DeValois and De Valois 1991). If these neural delays translated directly into visual delays for moving objects, then, for example, a car moving at 30 mph should appear 4.4 feet "behind" in its trajectory. How, then, are ball players able to catch balls traveling at speeds much greater than 30 mph? (It is known that ball players are able to intercept balls that require timing precision of 10–15 msec; Lee and Young 1985). The traditional answer is that the motor plans set up by the observer take these various delays into account, but recently a new possibility has been raised. Several researchers (Ramachandran and Anstis 1990; De Valois and De Valois 1991; P. Cavanagh 1995, personal communication) have suggested that there might be a mechanism within the visual system which compensates for these delays. Thus, a moving object's current actual location and its visual location may be closer to one another than one might expect on the basis of neural delays and pictures like figure 13.1. According to this view, the compensatory motor plans are necessary for overcoming delays due to movement of body parts per se, and that visual delays do not depend on motor plans for

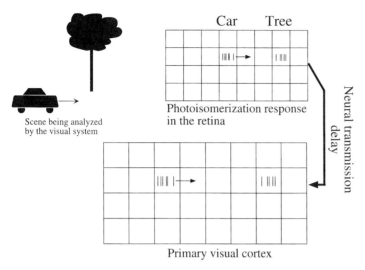

Figure 13.1
A scene depicting a car traveling from left to right. The grids schematically represent the photoreceptor layer and the primary visual cortex. The vertical lines represent neural activity. If perception occurs on the basis of cortical information, then the perceived position of the moving object should lag its actual position.

compensation. This thesis is based on an illusion in which moving elements visible within a window cause the window to appear shifted in the direction of the motion of the elements, that is, in the direction that would most likely be occupied by the moving elements in the immediate future (figure 13.2).

This interpretation of the "movement-based positional bias," however, seems at odds with some other findings. First, the displacement effect has been found to increase rapidly with increased eccentricity, being relatively weak or absent in the fovea (De Valois and De Valois 1991). In interceptive behavior, for which compensation of visual delays would be crucial, the animal attempts to foveate the moving target of interest. Clearly, there are significant delays from the fovea to the cortex, and a mechanism that compensates for peripheral delays, but not foveal delays, is not very plausible. Second, the positional bias occurs only if target (window) boundaries are equiluminous with the background or,

more generally, if sharp luminance-based edges are missing from the stimulus. These conditions are rarely, if ever, satisfied by moving objects in the natural environment.

A fundamental goal of the visual system, unraveled by measurements of retinal ganglion cell responses by Kuffler (1952), is to determine which part of the retina has been stimulated in order to ascertain the visual field location of the object responsible for the stimulation. Might a similar principle hold for objects whose retinal image is in motion? Let us entertain the possibility that this principle holds, and that there is no lag in the visual position of moving objects. The proposal is that the correct instantaneous position of the moving object is determined by the visual system (on the basis of the past trajectory and speed of the object) and given directly in the visual percept of that object (Nijhawan 1994). This implies that the instantaneous visual position of moving objects is already correct, so no further compensation need be postulated.

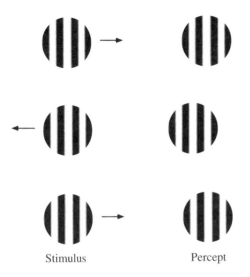

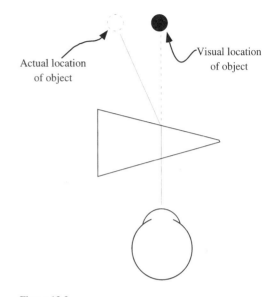

Stimulus   Percept

Figure 13.2
Schematic depiction of the dynamic stimuli used in the study. The patches themselves were stationary within which elements moved. The actual stimulus was (1) a moving sinusoidal grating within a gaussian envelope (DeValois and DeValois 1991) or (2) kinetic edges created by moving random dots in a field of static dots (Ramachandran and Anstis 1990).

Figure 13.3
A wedge prism bends the path of light such that the visible object is displaced toward the wedge.

Let us first tackle a few questions about this "no-lag" conjecture: Is there any conceptual basis for why there may be no lag for a moving item's visual location relative to its actual location? Suppose we do indeed find no lag in the visual position of moving objects. What relevance would this fact have for the study of vision? If a type of "compensation" does occur, what are the possible underlying neural mechanisms that might be responsible for this? Let us consider the first two questions first and defer the consideration of the third to a later section.

The question that must now be faced head-on concerns the meaning of the statement: There is a mismatch between an object's actual location and its perceived location. In this case "actual location" can have at least two different meanings. One meaning becomes apparent when an

observer views a stationary object, say localized directly in front, and then closes his or her eyes before reaching for it. If the reach is successful—that is, if the reach first produces a tactile sensation at the observer's hand, followed by some benefit (e.g., nourishment), then we might say that the object's actual position and its visual position are in agreement. One easy way of causing this mapping between vision and proprioception to temporarily breakdown is to place a wedge prism between the object and the observer's eye (figure 13.3). If the observer now tries to reach for the object with eyes closed, his or her reach will miss the object. We might say this is because the object's actual position and its visual position no longer agree.

A second meaning of "actual location," more relevant to the current topic, is the one associated with the direction in which the light from a given object travels to the eye. Consider light entering the eye at a certain angle from a point source. If the point is seen in the direction of the path of light, then one might say that the point is visible in its "actual location." One common physical situation where the two meanings of the term "actual location" produce different answers is that of the transmission of light from a distant object, such as the sun, to the eye. Neural delays in this case are unimportant because the angle of the sun changes too slowly. It takes light about eight minutes to travel from the sun to Earth; thus one might say that the visual location of the sun is different from its actual location due to Earth's rotation. Therefore, the sun is not seen in its actual location if one considers its material aspects, such as its mass, as representing the term "actual." At the same time one may argue that the sun is visible in its actual position because it is perceived in the direction along which its rays enter the eye, and not in some other direction. Note the association between the material location of a nearby object and the tactile or proprioceptive sensation it has the potential to produce (Cutting and Vishton 1995), and that between the optical location of an object and the retinal image it projects.

Let us call the meaning associated with a given object's material aspects the object's actual (proprioceptive) location, and that involving the path of light, the object's actual (retinal) location. Which of these two meanings of "actual location" does one imply when speaking of neural transmission delays causing a moving object to appear in a position that lags relative to its actual instantaneous position? We believe that if the implied lag were between a moving object's actual (proprioceptive) location and its visual location, then the problem would not be so serious, because there are numerous situations (e.g., figure 13.3) where this can occur. Furthermore, an observer can adapt (within about two weeks for extreme prism distortions, such as retinal image inversion) to a dissociation between the visual and the proprioceptive locations of objects and learn to get around in the world (Stratton 1896, 1897). Examples of dissociation between

an object's actual (retinal) location and its visual location are, however, not easy to find, and there are good indications that this aspect of vision is not modifiable (Harris 1963). Anatomical considerations also suggest that the relationship between a stimulated retinal location (local sign) and the direction in which the stimulus is visually localized is not modifiable (Kaufman 1974). Moreover, findings with congenitally blind children (Schlodtmann 1902) support an innate determination of the connection between the retinal local sign and perceived visual direction. Thus, the connection between the locus of the retina stimulated by an object and the direction in which the object is visible seems innately determined and unmodifiable.

Now consider the implied visual lag for moving objects. In this case not only should the perceived position of the object and the stimulated retinal position disagree, but this disagreement should survive despite the observer's years of experience with the visual environment. Visual lag for moving objects would mean, for example, that an object moving rightward past a vertical line would, during its trajectory close to the line, be visible to the left of the line even after its retinal image has crossed over the retinal image of the line (figure 13.4). It seems simpler to assume that the theory of local sign (Lötze 1971; Rock 1975: 159–183) holds for stationary as well as moving objects, with the "no lag" conjecture a direct consequence of this.

Many experiments have been devoted to the study of adaptations that occur in situations of potential conflict between sensory data, for example, that existing between sound and vision (e.g., ventriloquist effect) or between vision and proprioception. However, the implied dissociation between a moving object's instantaneous visual position and its retinal image position, or the lack there of, has not received adequate attention. This is particularly surprising because the crux of the unresolved debate in the 1960s surrounding the issues of adaptation was between scientists who believed that adaptation

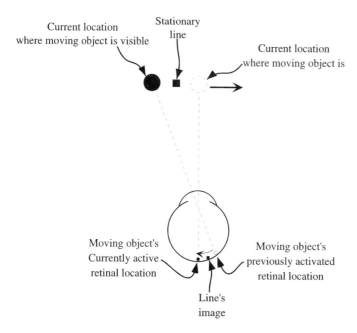

Figure 13.4
Top view of an object moving rightward past a stationary vertical line. The eyeball is stationary. At the instant depicted, the retinal image of the moving object has already crossed the retinal image of the line while the visible moving object has not yet crossed the visible line.

produces a remapping between the retinal image position and the perceived position of objects, and those who opposed such a view (see Harris 1965 for a review).

Suppose it is found that there is no disagreement between a moving object's instantaneous visual location and the local sign. How would this fact be important? First, this would suggest that there is some "corrective" mechanism within the visual system which compensates for the neural transmission delays and establishes a one-to-one correspondence between a moving object's perceived location and its instantaneous local sign. This would certainly have implications for the design of the visual system. Second, this would suggest that smooth motion can essentially be used as an objective "clock" relative to which other visual events can be timed. For

example, it suggests a way of measuring visual delays in the processing of discrete events, such as flashes, which cannot be done with methods like response time measurement. Finally, one could empirically study the consequences of overlap (or lack there of) of two stimuli (one moving and one flashed) in some "high level" representation of space (e.g., V1), while at the same time the two retinal images producing those representations do (or do not) overlap.

Experimental Support for the "No-Lag" Conjecture for Moving Objects

Consider the visual delays involved in the perception of a single flash of white light projected to the observer's fovea. The neural signals generated by the flash must first travel to the ganglion cells and then to the lateral geniculate nucleus on their way to the visual cortex. Suppose, in addition, we now present a moving object that passes the location of the flash at the exact instant of the flash. What observers report in this case is a location mismatch between the two objects, with the flashed object in a lagging position relative to the moving object. One form of this experiment employs a single white rod moving from left to right and two light sources. One of the lights, which illuminates only one section of the rod, is a stroboscopic source capable of producing a 1 microsec flash at a predetermined time. The rest of the rod is continuously illuminated by the other light source, which may be an ordinary lightbulb. A given section of the rod is illuminated by one and only one source. The observer fixates a given location as the moving rod (with some sections continuously illuminated) approaches this location. When the rod is in the neighborhood of the fixation position, the other source briefly illuminates the rest of the rod. What observers see is a rod "broken" into segments, with the flashed segments lagging behind the continuously illuminated segments (figure 13.5a).

In one method of quantitatively measuring this phenomenon, which for simplicity we call the "flash-lag" effect, the observer cancels the effect by positioning the flashed segments physically "ahead" of the continuous segments (Nijhawan 1994). Using rotary motion, it has been found that the flash-lag effect increases monotonically with the speed of the moving item (figure 13.5b). This phenomenon may be explained as follows: The flashed segment of the bar is perceived in the correct location, although after some delay, due to transmission time of neural signals. The continuously visible segments of the moving bar are also seen in the correct location ("no-lag" conjecture). Thus, the flashed segment becomes visible after the moving segments (and their percepts) have passed the location of the flashed segment.

In experiments measuring response time to a flash, it is generally believed that the flash must first produce a visual percept; only then can the observer respond to it (however, see Goodale et al. 1991). However, using response time to measure the time it takes for the flash to become visible is like trying to measure the distance to a mountain surface, on the basis of echoes, without first knowing the speed of sound. In the flash-lag experiment the visual processing delay of the flashed segment is given by the magnitude of the flash-lag effect divided by the object velocity.

There are some additional noteworthy observations concerning the flash-lag phenomenon, of which we would like to mention two. The first has to do with contours that are visible to observers but are not given directly in the retinal image. There is considerable interest in contours that are visible although the conventional features, such as luminance discontinuities, are missing. Among the well-known examples is the Kanizsa triangle (figure 13.6a). We have found that the flash-lag phenomenon produces vivid contours that are not given in the retinal image, and yet these contours are unlike the illusory contours in that observers cannot distinguish them from "real" (luminance-based) contours. The flash-lag-based contours may, in fact, belong to a previously unknown category of contours.

Several experiments have produced these contours, of which the following is a good example. Observers viewed a white ring moving on a gray background while maintaining fixation. A brief flash of a disk "filled" the center of the ring when the ring was in the vicinity of the fixation point. Surprisingly, the perception of a "spurious" edge of a white disk against a gray background accompanied the report of the flash-lag effect (figure 13.6b). This "spurious" edge is treated by the visual system as if it were a real edge (Nijhawan manuscript under review; also see section "Flash-Lag Effect and Visual Attention"), a point that distinguishes it from illusory contours. It would be of interest also to see what

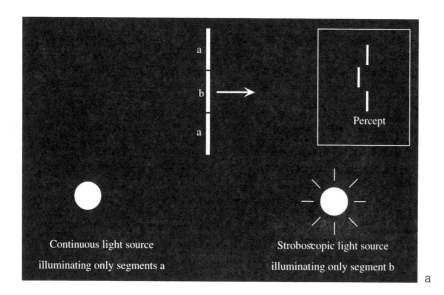

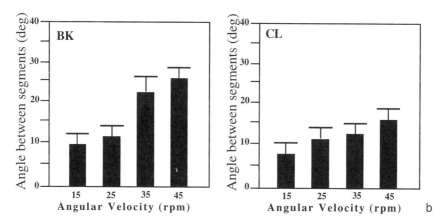

Figure 13.5
(a) A snapshot of the stimulus at the instant of the strobe. (b) Data for two observers at increasing speeds of rotary motion. The vertical axis represents the perceived angle between the flashed and the moving segments.

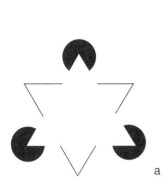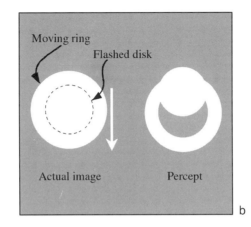

Figure 13.6
(a) The Kanizsa triangle. (b) A snapshot of the ring-disk display at the instant of the flash of the disk (dashed line) centered on the ring. The percept shows contours of the disk visible against the gray background.

characteristics these contours may share with illusory contours. For example, do these contours, like the illusory contours, produce greater activation in area 18 of the monkey cortex than in area 17 (von der Heydt et al. 1984)? Does something special about illusory contours produce the asymmetric responsiveness of neurons between areas 17 and 18, or might the difference reflect a general difference between responses to contours given directly in the image and to those that are not?

A second observation concerns color vision. The connection between space and color vision has been evident since Newton's demonstration with the prism splitting white light into its components. The prism disperses different wavelengths over space (and the retinal surface), each wavelength triggering its own sensation of color. But is there a connection between a neural representation of visual space and color? As first suggested by Hecht (1928), this question is important for theories of color perception. He demonstrated a "binocular fusion of yellow" with an experiment in which a red disk stimulated only one eye while a green disk stimulated

the corresponding retinal region of only the other eye. In these conditions it is not obvious whether observers will see a single fused image or not, but fortunately they do. The fused red-plus-green disks produced the percept of a yellow disk, which is what results when the red and green disks are superimposed (additively mixed) on the retinal surface. Hecht's conclusion was that since neither disk alone can activate a "yellow" mechanism within the retina, the percept of yellow must be a result of cortical processes which are activated by both the disks together, that is, activation of binocular cortical cells stimulated by both disks. This outcome supports the Young-Helmholtz-Maxwell theory of color vision (however, see Hurvich and Jameson 1951).

It would be of interest to see if the reverse is also true, that is, red and green stimuli superimposed on the retinal surface appearing separated in space, and failing to "mix" into yellow. The flash-lag effect was employed to study this issue (Nijhawan 1997). Observers viewed a green bar revolving against a dark background, while a horizontal red line was flashed such that it was

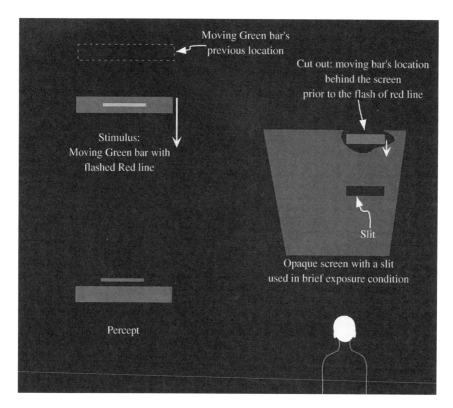

Figure 13.7
The stimulus and the percept are shown at the left. Downward arrows represent the green bar's motion direction. The right side of the figure schematically shows the opaque screen used in the brief exposure condition. At the instant depicted, the downward-moving green bar is invisible to the observer, being occluded by the screen.

optically superimposed on the bar (figure 13.7). There were two viewing conditions: extended exposure and brief exposure. For the brief exposure condition the green bar was briefly flashed such that it elicited no motion signal. (In this condition the bar was exposed only through a narrow slit within an opaque screen that occluded the rest of the bar's motion trajectory.) In this condition observers adjusted the color of the flashed line (by adjusting its intensity) until it appeared yellow. In the extended exposure condition, observers viewed this same stimulus, but now the screen was removed and the bar's motion was visible. In this condition the flashed line appeared to lag the green bar, and against the dark background its color appeared reddish. Thus, despite equal quantal absorption at the photoreceptors, the color of the flashed line was perceived as more greenish in the brief exposure condition and more reddish in the extended exposure condition. This finding adds to Hecht's analysis and suggests that retinal superimposition of red and green is neither necessary nor sufficient for producing the sensation of "yellow."

Possible Neural Mechanisms for Spatial Correction

One prediction of the "no-lag" conjecture is that there should be a mechanism within the visual system that corrects the spatial lag for moving objects. Although the main requirement of this hypothetical "correction" mechanism, lateral connectivity, is a characteristic of the visual system, the exact nature of the mechanism and its location within the visual system are still unknown. The simplest type of mechanism that follows topographic mapping would be based on horizontal interaction between functionally similar cells. One candidate mechanism that employs lateral connections and feedback is the one based on corticothalamic feedback inducing "anticipatory" coordination of firing in a group of lateral geniculate nucleus (LGN) cells in response to a moving bar (Sillito et al. 1994). Such a mechanism seems particularly well suited to explaining the color decomposition effect. Cortical feedback makes contact predominantly with inhibitory interneurons in LGN (Weber et al. 1989), and it is of particular interest that the inhibition might be induced by cortical feedback linked to specific features, such as direction selectivity and color. Such feedback has already been found for features such as direction selectivity and line length (Murphy and Sillito 1987). The color decomposition effect may be explained as follows: Signals from the flashed line and the moving bar arrive in LGN, after the expected delay, at a location that receives inhibition triggered by cortical feedback linked to the moving green bar. Thus, the signal from the line is interpreted by the prestriate color area as emerging from a location devoid of any green signal, which causes the flashed line to appear red.

A second possible mechanism, which is also partially based on lateral connectivity, is related to "predictive remapping" observed in the lateral intraparietal area of monkeys (Duhamel et al. 1992). Although the responses of neurons showing "predictive remapping" require a saccadic eye movement, the purely retinal consequences of image motion that the eye movement causes have been neglected in this study. In localization of continuously visible and flashed stimuli, saccadic eye movements and object motion produce analogous results (MacKay 1970). Consistent with various other studies (Allman et al. 1985), the Duhamel et al. study shows that remote retinal locations, outside a given neuron's fixation (eye stationary) receptive field, can influence that neuron's activity. Assume that for a neuron to contribute to the representation of an object in a specific position, its activity must be raised above a certain value. For such a neuron to participate in the "correction" process, the elevation in its activation produced by a moving stimulus, a given distance from the center of its fixation receptive field, needs to be more than that produced by a flash.

Precisely this type of response has been found in retinal ganglion cells in the salamander (Berry et al. 1997). In these experiments a retinal preparation is stimulated by a moving luminance edge and a multielectrode array measures ganglion cell output. The wave of activity of the cells from which the recording is made leads the luminance edge. In other words, a given cell is activated before the edge passes over the cell's receptive field. Furthermore, this type of "anticipatory" response does not require direction selectivity and "anticipates" motion in all directions. Thus far these findings provide the most direct support for a "correction" process that potentially removes the visual lag for moving objects, as predicted by the "no-lag" conjecture.

Flash-Lag Effect and Visual Attention

Finally, we would like to consider issues related to visual attention and an alternative account of the flash-lag effect. The connection between visual latencies and attention has a long history (Titchener 1908). An account of the flash-lag effect based on attention was proposed by Baldo and Klein (1995), who argued that the perceived lag of a flashed object relative to a moving one is the consequence of the delayed allocation of attention to the flashed object. Though not explicitly stated, this view must assume that moving objects solicit and sustain attentional deployment (Pylyshyn 1989, 1994) prior to the onset of the flashed object. It is known that there are time delays in either the "capture" of attention by the flashed object in a stimulus-driven manner (Hillstrom and Yantis 1994; Jonides and Yantis 1988; Nakayama and Mackeben 1989; Yantis and Hillstrom 1994; Yantis and Jonides, 1984, 1990), or the "shift" of attention from the moving to the flashed object location (Tsal 1983; Weichselgartner and Sperling 1987). On this view, the flash-lag effect is due to some time-dependent process, such as shift time of visual attention, which increases in duration as a function of eccentricity (Baldo and Klein 1995; Tsal 1983; but see Nakayama and Mackeben 1989). These attentional processes act to bring the flashed object to a sufficiently high level of visual awareness that, presumably, is already achieved for the moving object. Consequently, by the time the flashed object is registered, the moving object has traversed some distance and thus the flashed object is perceived as spatially lagging the moving object. The main support for this hypothesis is the increase in the flash-lag effect as a function of the spatial separation between the moving and flashed objects (Baldo and Klein 1995).

We tested the above account by exploring the delays due to a shift in attention (Khurana and Nijhawan 1995). A display was designed in which flashed and moving elements were spatially interleaved. Observers were instructed to *attentively track* (Cavanagh 1992) a rotating line composed of six rectangles. A horizontal line composed of six interleaving circles was flashed for 5 msec (figure 13.8). Since the flashed elements occupied the spaces between the attended rotating elements, we argue that delays due to spatial attention shifts from the moving to the

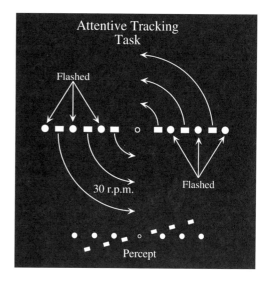

Figure 13.8
Observers were asked to attentively track the rotating line of rectangles. At a given point in its trajectory a static interleaved line of circles was flashed. The stimulus shown in the figure is at the instant of the flash. Observers reported a compelling percept of the flashed line lagging the rotating line (see percept).

flashed items should be negligible. Thus this display should not produce a flash-lag effect. However, we found that this display produced a strong flash-lag effect. Thus, when flashed and moving objects are equated in terms of the shift time of attention, observers continue to report the flash-lag effect.

A still more stringent test of the attention-shift hypothesis is based on the "decomposition" of color (Nijhawan 1997). As noted, when a red line is flashed on a moving green bar, the red line is seen as lagging the bar and appears reddish. In this case the two objects, the moving green bar and the flashed red line, are physically superimposed. It is rather difficult to make a case for a shift of attention under these conditions.

In the above experiments one may reasonably argue that the observer's attention was not

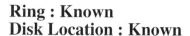

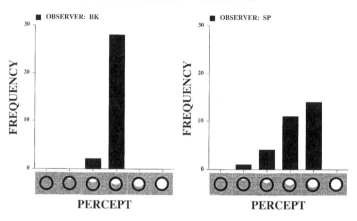

Figure 13.9
Responses of two observers in a multiring display in which the observers were given advance knowledge of both the ring in which the flash was to occur and the location of the flash. Both observers reported sizable flash-lag effects.

manipulated. In order to more fully investigate the role of visual attention in producing the flash-lag effect, we explicitly manipulated attentional allocation. In a series of experiments we explored the relationship between attention and the flash-lag effect by employing two well-established paradigms for manipulating visual attention: (1) spatial indexing (Pylyshyn 1989, 1994) and spatial cuing (Posner 1980; Posner and Cohen 1984), and (2) visual search (Cavanagh et al. 1990; He and Nakayama 1992; Treisman 1986, 1988; Treisman and Gelade 1980; Treisman and Gormican 1988; Treisman and Sato 1990; Wolfe et al. 1989).

Spatial Cuing and the Flash-Lag Effect

A variant of the ring-disk display (figure 13.6b) was created to manipulate the distribution and spatial cuing of attention in the presence of multiple moving objects. On a middle-gray background five equally spaced black rings translated along a circular path (Pylyshyn 1989, 1994). The array rotated around a central dot that the observers fixated. A disk was flashed in one of the rings, and the observers were required to select from a set of stills the one that matched the perceived spatial relation between the ring and the disk. Even when precued as to the ring in which the disk was to be flashed and the exact location of the flash, observers reported a substantial flash-lag effect, shown in figure 13.9 (Khurana et al. 1996). This flash-lag effect was unaltered when both the ring and disk location were unknown (Khurana et al. in press).

Visual Search and the Flash-Lag Effect

One unusual consequence of the perceived spatial lag of the flashed disk relative to the ring is the creation of a "spurious" edge reported by observers that does not exist in the retinal input (see figure 13.6b, percept). We have used visual search to investigate whether these spurious edges are available to preattentive vision. In other words, are these edges present in the early

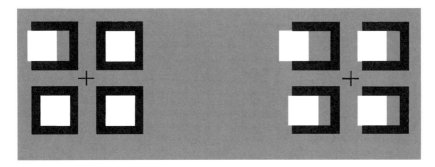

Figure 13.10
Stimulus used in target-present trials in the visual search experiments. The left-hand display shows the physical stimulus for the static and moving conditions. The right-hand display shows the percept of the stimulus in the left-hand side in the moving condition.

surface representations on which search operations are conducted (He and Nakayama 1992)?

On a middle-gray background, outline black squares translated from left to right and solid white squares that completely filled the outline squares were flashed. Two visual search conditions consisting of two, four, six, or eight items were run. On every trial, either all flashed white squares were centered relative to their respective outline squares (target-absent trial), or one of the flashed white squares was displaced 20 percent toward the trailing edge of the moving outline square (target-present trial). Observers indicated the presence (50 percent of trials) or absence (50 percent of trials) of a target with a keypress.

Static Condition All the black outline squares were stationary. Either one of the white squares was misaligned (target present) relative to the outline square, or all of the white squares were centered (target absent) (figure 13.10).

Moving Condition The outline squares translated from left to right. When they reached the middle of the screen, the white squares were flashed with their spatial relationship to the outline squares as described in the static condition.

We (Khurana et al. 1999) found that search for targets in the static condition was relatively easy and accurate (about 80 percent correct). The first question regarding the moving condition is whether all the flashed white squares were seen to lag their respective black outline squares. Observers reported perceiving every physically aligned flashed white square misaligned relative to the outline squares, regardless of the number of items presented (figure 13.10). Performance in the moving condition was significantly poorer than performance in the static condition. We suggest that contours rendered by the flash-lag effect are computed prior to the allocation of attention, thus making the phenomenon not a likely consequence of attentional delays (Khurana and Nijhawan 1995).

Reality of Illusion

In conclusion, the research reported here supports the no-lag conjecture for visual localization of moving objects. Many philosophically minded individuals have raised the following question: Are we conscious of the output of our brains or the "real" world outside? It may be stated that we see (if the modality being considered is visual) the product of our brains and not the "real world" itself. But at the same time this experience is attributed to an "outer world." Thus, if one sees a green square, one's experience is directly linked only to the output of the various areas of one's brain responding concurrently, and yet one sees the object out there in the "real" world. Thus, one suffers from an illusion, although a very persuasive one, that there is really a physical world out there (thus the "illusion of reality").

Based on our findings and conjecture, one might start from the opposite end. This visual system does what it is built for—creating a percept that informs the observer. What is truly interesting is that if the observer uses this visual information to act, then he or she is mostly successful, in that other mechanisms of our body confirm the success of our action, and thus of our percepts. For example, if a tactile or proprioceptive sensation is expected by a certain visually guided action, then this sensation is usually produced by that action. So our percepts appear real because they so frequently produce successful behavior (hence, reality of illusion). This success is what gives our "illusion" the character of reality, and it is the sole reason for the illusion's surviving both ontogenetically and phylogenetically.

Acknowledgments

This work was supported by NSF Grants SBR-9710116 and BCS-9727841.

References

Allman, J., Miezin, F., and McGuinness, E. (1985). Direction- and velocity-specific responses from beyond the classical receptive field in the middle temporal visual area (MT). *Perception* 14: 105–126.

Baldo, M. V. C., and Klein, S. (1995). Extrapolation or attention shift? *Nature* 378: 565–566.

Berry, M. J., Brivanlou, I. H., Smirnakis, S. M., Keat, J. R., and Meister, M. (1997). Anticipation of moving stimuli by the retina. *Society for Neuroscience Abstracts* 23: 763.5.

Cavanagh, P. (1992). Attention-based motion perception. *Science* 257: 1563–1565.

Cavanagh, P. (1997). Predicting the present. *Nature* 386: 19–21.

Cavanagh, P., Arguin, M., and Treisman, A. (1990). Effect of stimulus domain on visual search for orientation and size features. *Journal of Experimental Psychology: Human Perception and Performance* 16: 479–491.

Cutting, J. E., and Vishton, P. M. (1995). Perceiving layout and knowing distances: The integration, relative potency, and contextual use of different information about depth. In J. Hochberg, ed., *Perception of Space and Motion*. San Diego: Academic Press.

De Valois, R. L., and De Valois, K. K. (1991). Vernier acuity with stationary moving gabors. *Vision Research* 31: 1619–1626.

Duhamel, J.-R., Colby, C. L., and Goldberg, M. E. (1992). The updating of the representation of visual space in prietal cortex by intended eye movements. *Science* 255: 90–92.

Goodale, M. A., Milner, A. D., Jakobson, L. S., and Carey, D. P. (1991). A neurological dissociation between perceiving objects and grasping them. *Nature* 349: 154–156.

Harris, C. S. (1963). Adaptation to displaced vision: Visual motor or proprioceptive change? *Science* 140: 812–813.

Harris, C. S. (1965). Perceptual adaptation to inverted, reversed and displaced vision. *Psychological Review* 72: 419–444.

He, Z., and Nakayama, K. (1992). Surfaces versus features in visual search. *Nature* 359: 231–233.

Hecht, S. (1928). On the binocular fusion of colors and its relation to theories of color vision. *Proceedings of the National Academy of Sciences, U.S.A.* 14: 237–241.

Helmholtz, H. (1866; 1968). Concerning the perceptions in general. In R. M. Warren and R. P. Warren, eds., *Helmholtz on Perception*. New York: John Wiley.

Hering, E. (1942). In C. A. Radde, trans., *Spatial Sense and Movements of the Eye*. Maryland: American Academy of Optometry.

Hillstrom, A. P., and Yantis, S. (1994). Visual motion and attentional capture. *Perception and Psychophysics* 55: 399–411.

Hurvich, L. M., and Jameson, D. (1951). The binocular fusion of yellow in relation to color theories. *Science* 114: 199–202.

Jonides, J., and Yantis, S. (1988). Uniqueness of abrupt visual onset in capturing attention. *Perception and Psychophysics* 43: 346–354.

Kaufman, L. (1974). *Sight and Mind: An Introduction to Visual Perception*. New York: Oxford University Press.

Khurana, B., Cavanagh, P., and Nijhawan, R. (1996). Are moving objects "corrected" or flashed objects attentionally delayed? *Investigative Ophthalmology and Visual Science* 36: 2421.

Khurana, B., Gifford, C., and Nijhawan, R. (1999). Flash-lag based contours are available to pre-attentive vision. *Investigative Ophthalmology and Visual Science* 40: 1831.

Khurana, B., and Nijhawan, R. (1995). Extrapolation or attention shift? *Nature* 378: 565–566.

Khurana, B., Watanabe, K., and Nijhawan, R. (in press). The role of attention in motion extrapolation: Are moving objects "corrected" or flashed objects attentionally delayed? *Perception.*

Koch, C., and Poggio, T. (1999). Predicting the visual world: Silence is golden. *Nature Neuroscience.* 2: 9–10.

Kuffler, S. W. (1952). Neurons in the retina: Organization, inhibition and excitation problems. *Cold Spring Harbor Symposia on Quantitative Biology* 17: 281–292.

Lee, D. N., and Young, D. S. (1985). Visual timing of interceptive action. In D. Ingle, M. Jeannerod, and D. N. Lee, eds., *Brain Mechanisms and Spatial Vision*, 1–30. Dordrecht: Martinus Nijhoff.

Lötze. in Pastore, N. (1971). *Selective History of Theories of Visual Perception: 1650–1950*. New York: Oxford University Press.

MacKay, D. M. (1958). Perceptual stability of a stroboscopically lit visual field containing self-luminous objects. *Nature* 181: 507–508.

MacKay, D. M. (1970). Mislocation of test flashes during saccadic image displacements. *Nature* 227: 731–833.

Murphy, P. C., and Sillito, A. M. (1987). Corticofugal feedback influences the generation of length tuning in the visual pathway. *Nature* 329: 727–829.

Nakayama, K., and Mackeben, M. (1989). Sustained and transient components of focal visual attention. *Vision Research* 29: 1631–1647.

Nijhawan, R. (1994). Motion extrapolation in catching. *Nature* 370: 256–257.

Nijhawan, R. (1997). Visual decomposition of color through motion-extrapolation. *Nature* 386: 66–69.

Posner, M. I. (1980). Orienting of attention. *Quarterly Journal of Experimental Psychology* 32: 3–25.

Posner, M. I., and Cohen, Y. (1984). Components of visual orienting. In H. Bouma and D. Bowhuis, eds., *Attention and Performance X*, 531–556. Hillsdale, NJ: Erlbaum.

Purushothaman, G., Patel, S., Bedel, H., and Ogmen, H. (1998). Moving ahead through differential visual latency. *Nature* 396: 424.

Pylyshyn, Z. W. (1989). The role of location indexes in spatial perception: A sketch of the FINST spatial-indexing model. *Cognition* 32: 65–97.

Pylyshyn, Z. W. (1994). Some primitive mechanisms of spatial attention. *Cognition* 50: 363–384.

Ramachandran, V. S., and Anstis, S. M. (1990). Illusory displacement of equiluminous kinetic edges. *Perception* 19: 611–616.

Rao, R. P. N., and Ballard, D. H. (1999). Predictive coding in the visual cortex: A functional interpretation of some extra-classical receptive-field effects. *Nature Neuroscience* 2: 79–87.

Rock, I. (1975). *An Introduction to Perception*. New York: Macmillan.

Schlodtmann, W. (1902). Ein Beitrag zur Lehre von der optischen Lokalisation bei Blindgeborenen. *Archiv fur Ophthalmologic* 54: 256–269.

Sillito, A. M., Jones, H. E., Gerstein, G. L., and West, D. C. (1994). Feature-linked synchronization of thalamic relay cell firing induced by feedback from the visual cortex. *Nature* 369: 479–482.

Stratton, G. (1896). Some preliminary experiments on vision without inversion of the retinal image. *Psychological Review* 3: 611–617.

Stratton, G. (1897). Vision without inversion of the retinal image. *Psychological Review* 4: 341–360.

Titchener, E. B. (1908; 1973). *Lectures on the Elementary Psychology of Feeling and Attention*. New York: Arno Press.

Treisman, A. (1986). Features and objects in visual processing. *Scientific American* 254: 114–125.

Treisman, A. (1988). Features and objects: The fourteenth Bartlett Memorial Lecture. *Quarterly Journal of Experimental Psychology* 40A: 201–237.

Treisman, A., and Gelade, G. (1980). A feature integration theory of attention. *Cognitive Psychology* 12: 97–136.

Treisman, A., and Gormican, S. (1988). Feature analysis in early vision: Evidence from search asymmetries. *Psychological Review* 95: 15–48.

Treisman, A., and Sato, S. (1990). Conjunction search revisited. *Journal of Experimental Psychology: Human Perception and Performance* 16: 459–478.

Tsal, Y. J. (1983). Movement of attention across the visual field. *Journal of Experimental Psychology: Human Perception and Performance* 9: 523–530.

von der Heydt, R., Peterhans, E., and Baumgartner, G. (1984). Illusory contours and cortical neuron responses. *Science* 224: 1260–1262.

Weber, A. J., Kalil, R. E., and Behan, M. (1989). Synaptic connections between corticogeniculate axons and interneurons in the dorsal lateral geniculate nucleus of the cat *Journal Comparative Neurology* 289: 156–164.

Weichselgartner, E., and Sperling, G. (1987). Dynamics of automatic and controlled visual attention. *Science* 238: 778–880.

Whitney, D., and Murakami, I. (1998). Latency difference, not spatial extrapolation. *Nature Neuroscience* 1: 656–657.

Wolfe, J. M., Cave, K. R., and Franzel, S. L. (1989). Guided search: An alternative to the feature integration model for visual search. *Journal of Experimental Psychology: Human Perception and Performance* 15: 419–433.

Yantis, S., and Hillstrom, A. P. (1994). Stimulus-driven attentional capture: Evidence from equiluminant visual objects. *Journal of Experimental Psychology: Human Perception and Performance* 20: 95–107.

Yantis, S., and Jonides, J. (1984). Abrupt visual onsets and selective attention: Evidence from visual search. *Journal of Experimental Psychology: Human Perception and Performance* 10: 601–621.

Yantis, S., and Jonides, J. (1990). Abrupt visual onsets and selective attention: Voluntary versus automatic allocation. *Journal of Experiment Psychology: Human Perception and Performance* 16: 121–134.

Dominic ffytche

The visual mind and the visual brain have been studied for more than a century, yet despite highly detailed neurophysiological and anatomical descriptions of the visual system, a comprehensive psychophysics and a range of cognitive perceptual models, the question of how the two might be related remains unanswered. What follows is an attempt to evaluate the role of neuroimaging in bringing the two realms together. Before presenting the neurobiological background to the imaging evidence, it is worth pausing to consider the sort evidence we are looking for. In Crick and Koch's (1998) terms, the activity being sought is a neural correlate of consciousness. While the "neural" side of the equation is easy to conceive, what do we mean by the consciousness side and the correlation? Here, (visual) consciousness is used as a synonym for "seeing"—for perceptual, phenomenological, or qualia descriptions of visual experience—devoid of linguistic, intentional, or self-referential implications.

Of course, a central question is whether the visual prefix is meaningful in neurobiological terms; this is an issue that will be taken up below. The correlation part of the equation is more complex than it at first appears. In essence, we are looking for activity that is both necessary and sufficient for "seeing"; however, this does not translate into activity that is "on" when we are visually conscious and "off" when we are not, for this simple operational definition includes activity in the very lowest levels of the visual system (retinal photoreceptors, for example) which are unlikely to meet the criteria of sufficiency. Activities that are "on" regardless of whether we are visually conscious or not are not the correlates we are interested in. In practice, these contaminating correlates are controlled for by studying systems in which sensory input and percept are dissociated. In such systems any identified changes in neural activity are related to

conscious perceptual processing rather than to nonconscious afferent sensory signals.

Visual Neurobiology

The monkey visual cortex contains repeated maps of visual space, each specialized for a different visual attribute—one map specialized for color, one for motion, and so forth. Connections between them form overlapping but segregated, parallel, and hierarchical networks (Zeki and Shipp 1988; Van Essen et al. 1992). In man, positron emission tomography (PET) and functional magnetic resonance imaging (fMRI) studies reveal the same mosaic organization (Zeki et al. 1991; Sereno et al. 1995). For example, an area on the lateral surface of the occipital lobe is specialized for motion (Watson et al., 1993), and an area on the ventral surface of the occipital lobe is specialized for color (McKeefry and Zeki 1997). At least twenty primarily visual areas are described in the macaque (see, e.g., Van Essen et al. 1992), and in all likelihood at least as many will be found in man; the specializations of the majority of areas have yet to be determined.

The Perceptual Brain

Some visual neurons seem to correlate with visual consciousness. Zeki (1980) found a subset of neurons in the macaque color area whose activity correlated with the percept of color rather than the spectral properties of light falling on the retina—the two being dissociated under different lighting conditions. More recently, Logothetis et al. have described neurons that correlate with what is "seen" rather than what is presented in experiments on binocular rivalry (Logothetis and Schall 1989; Leopold and Logothetis 1996). Salzman et al. (1992) have influenced the "seen" direction of motion by stimulating macaque motion-specialized visual neurons.

While ethical considerations prohibit such experiments on humans, a similar relationship between the visual brain and visual perception in man can be inferred from studies of patients with acquired cerebral lesions. For example, a lesion in the human color area is associated with a specific deficit of color perception (achromatopsia), and a lesion in the human motion area is associated with a specific deficit of motion perception (akinetopsia; Zeki 1990, 1991).

The evidence for localizing the neural correlate of "seeing" to specialized visual cortex seems convincing. However, it may be criticized on the grounds that neither the lesion evidence (whether based on patients or on experimental lesions in monkeys) nor the single neuron evidence reveals anything about the rest of the brain. In fact, both methods would be blind to a neural correlate of "seeing" localized beyond the visual cortex. A lesion in the color area may simply disrupt a color-related pathway that passes to a visual consciousness area localized elsewhere; similarly, the activity recorded in single neurons may not represent the final destination of the signals.

Neuroimaging techniques such as PET and fMRI record from the whole brain simultaneously and thus overcome these problems of limited sampling. The techniques measure changes in neural activity through regional modulations in blood flow/oxygenation with a spatial resolution of millimeters and a temporal resolution of seconds. From a technical point of view, the existing technology is perfectly adequate to answer the question of whether specialized visual cortex underlies "seeing." In fact, the problem we face is more metaphysical than technical.

Consciousness as Unitary

One model of consciousness is that it is unitary. Visual percepts (whether of colors, objects, faces,

or movement) and other sense modalities (hearing, touching, emotional responses, motor plans, etc.) are all categories of a single thing—"consciousness." The point is that here, consciousness is being used as a high-level descriptor, in the same way that "car" is a high-level descriptor of wheels, chassis, engine, dashboard, and so on. The neurobiological ontology of unitary consciousness is at the level of "car" rather than "wheel." The unitary neural correlate converts different types of neural signals into percepts, remaining indifferent to the type of information it receives (see figure 14.1a). The unitary structure of consciousness has no implications for its neurobiology. The neural correlate could be localized to a single cortical or subcortical region, be distributed across a network, or represent a nonlocalized process, such as the synchronization of neuronal firing. The neural correlate is "on" when we are "conscious" and "off" when we are not "conscious."

Consciousness as Modular

An alternative conception of consciousness is one of multiple, independent, dissociable perceptual modules. Here the neurobiological ontology takes place at the level of "wheel," "chassis," "engine," and "dashboard" rather than "car." In this conception of consciousness, it makes sense to talk of visual consciousness as dissociable from auditory consciousness, for example, and of multiple independent "microconsciousnesses" (Zeki and Bartels 1998)—a consciousness-for-color, a consciousness-for-motion, a consciousness-for-faces, and so forth. Each consciousness-for-category has a separate neural correlate (see Figure 14.1b). Once again, the perceptual modularity has no implications for its neurobiological implementation. Each specialized neural correlate could be colocalized within the relevant functionally specialized cortex, localized elsewhere, be distributed across a network, or represent a nonlocalized process. The neural correlate of consciousness-for-color is

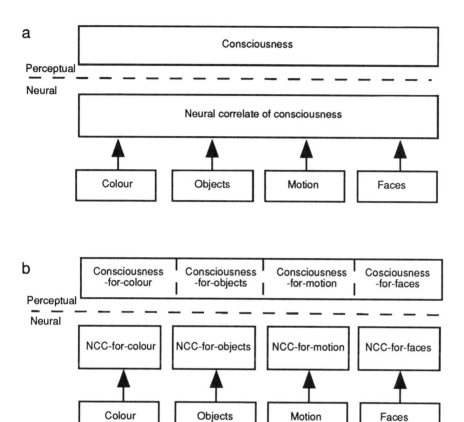

Figure 14.1
Models of visual consciousness. (a) A unitary visual consciousness (top level) arises from a single neural correlate of consciousness (middle level) with inputs from specialized visual areas (lowest level). (b) A modular visual consciousness arises from several neural correlates of consciousness (NCC), each with its own input from specialized visual areas. The dotted line represents the transition between neural (below) to perceptual (above) descriptive levels.

"on" when we are conscious of color and "off" when we are not; the neural correlate of consciousness-for-motion is "on" when we are conscious of motion and "off" when we are not, and so forth.

Historical Perspective

The modular and unitary models presented above are no more than restatements of the positions taken by Gall and Flourens in the nineteenth century (see Young 1970; Clarke and Jacyna 1987). Gall's position was modular. His organology (the term "phrenology" was never used by Gall) took as its starting point the view that "the brain is composed of as many particular organs as there are propensities, sentiments and faculties which differ essentially from each other." Gall's project was to identify dissociable mental faculties on the basis of observation and to correlate them with specific cortical organs: "the important search always is for these independent powers, for, it is only for them that organs exist in the brain" (Gall 1835, p. 105). Gall's imaging tool was the shape and thickness of the skull, and thus organology was destined to fail. However, several of his twenty-seven "sentiments and propensities" hit the mark. The faculties of attending to words (faculty 14), spoken language (faculty 15), relations of tones (faculty 17), distinguishing colors (faculty 16), and relations of space (faculty 12) form the bedrock of current imaging research.

Flourens's position was one of unitary consciousness. He followed Descartes's thesis of the unity of the *moi*, arguing that understanding/intellect was a unitary faculty; hence its seat, the cerebrum, must itself be a unitary organ. He was dismissive of Gall's theory of multiple dissociable faculties: "Now here is the sum of and the substance of Gall's psychology. For the understanding, essentially a unitary faculty, he substitutes a multitude of little understandings

or faculties distinct and isolate" and "the consciousness tells me I am one, and Gall insists I am multiple" (see Robinson 1998, p. 167; 347).

Imaging Consciousness

An imaging study of consciousness that follows the tradition of Gall is very different from one that follows the tradition of Flourens. A Flourensian approach would be to compare the "conscious" and the "non-conscious" brain—consciousness being taken here in its unitary, holistic sense. The experiment seems a simple one, but in practice it is not. The problem is in finding an example of a "non-conscious" control state. An obvious candidate is sleep, but the difference between wakefulness and sleep is not simply the presence or absence of consciousness, as sensory input to the cortex is largely switched off during sleep. Thus, a simple comparison of the two states will identify many areas that may have nothing to do with consciousness.

Gall would argue that we have imaged consciousness from the very start. Every imaging study reveals the neural correlate of consciousness-for-some-attribute. The difference between seeing a colored object and seeing the same object in black-and-white is consciousness-for-color; hence the neural correlate of consciousness-for-color forms part of the differential brain activity revealed by fMRI or PET. The problem for the Gallian tradition is not how to activate the correlate of consciousness but how to dissect it from other neural activities. In contrast, a Flourensian interpretation of the same experiment would be that while color may be present in one experimental condition and absent in another, unitary "consciousness" is present throughout—a constant. In this interpretation any increases in activity are not the correlates of consciousness that we are interested in. Flourens labels as "unconscious" the same activity that Gall labels "conscious."

Which tradition is correct? The truth is that we do not know, and that imaging alone may not answer the question. This is not meant to imply that imaging studies of consciousness are uninformative. At the very least, these studies help define the minimal requirements of a neurobiological description of "seeing." Presented below are two recent fMRI experiments that provide new insights into this neurobiology.

Visual Hallucinations

From the modular perspective, a typical imaging experiment identifies a mixture of brain activities, some of which correlate with consciousness and some of which do not. The problem is how to differentiate one class of activity from the other. As pointed out above, one way is to study a visual system in which visual consciousness has become dissociated from sensory input. Such dissociation can follow a sudden deterioration in visual abilities in patients who are, in other respects, normal (Lepore 1990; Holroyd et al. 1992; Teunisse et al. 1996). The spontaneous visual percepts (visual hallucinations) experienced by such patients are identical in quality and intensity to the true percepts of normal "seeing", although patients often recognize the experiences as unreal on the basis of their bizarre and often amusing character and, given their impaired visual abilities, by the fact that they are usually "seen" in greater detail than real stimuli. Patients typically report hallucinations of vivid colors; textures described as grids, lattices, or fences; trees, shrubs, or hedges; disembodied, distorted faces; small figures, often in a costume or uniform and wearing distinctive hats; copies of the same object arranged in rows or columns; or complex landscapes and scenes (ffytche and Howard 1999).

Rob Howard, Mike Brammer, and I have had the opportunity to study several such patients at the Institute of Psychiatry in London. We set out to establish which brain regions were active

during different types of hallucination, using fMRI (ffytche et al. 1998). Patients were asked to report the beginning and end of a hallucination, and the timing of these perceptual events was correlated with the recorded brain activity. It is important to realize that apart from the appearance and disappearance of the hallucinations, nothing changed during the experiment (the patients signaled the onset and offset of each hallucination, but these motor responses were controlled for in the analysis). Two examples of the results are displayed in figure 14.2. In patients who hallucinated colors, the most significant correlations were found in the color area; hallucinations of faces were associated with activity in the face area; hallucinations of objects were associated with activity in the object area; and so forth. There was a simple cerebral logic to hallucination content: activity in color area + activity in object area = hallucination of colored object; activity in texture area without activity in color area = hallucination of achromatic texture. The most important finding was that hallucinations failed to correlate with activity outside specialized visual areas. Interestingly, the fMRI signal within each area increased before the hallucination was reported. Although the observed time scale was shorter, Logothetis reported the same inverted temporal relationship between cerebral activity and percept in his binocular rivalry studies (Leopold and Logothetis 1996).

What do these results tell us of conscious vision? One interpretation—a modular view—is that the activities identified are the neural correlates of consciousness-for-faces, consciousness-for-colors, and consciousness-for-objects. In other words, activity in specialized cortex is sufficient for us to see a face, color, or object. An equally valid unitary interpretation is that the early activities are as close as we can get to the neural correlate of consciousness but are not the correlates themselves. By Flourens's reasoning, our patients were "conscious" throughout

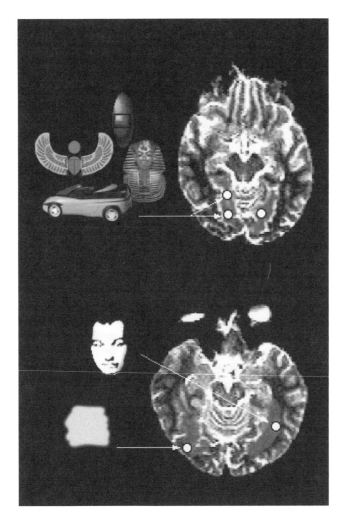

Figure 14.2
Visual hallucinations. Two transverse MRI slices through the ventral occipital lobe (the left of each slice is the left of the brain, the top of each slice is the front of the brain). Areas correlating with the timing of the hallucinations are shown as white disks. Illustrations of the hallucinations are shown on the left of each slice with an arrow to the visual area specialized for the particular visual attribute(s) illustrated. Both patients hallucinated in color.

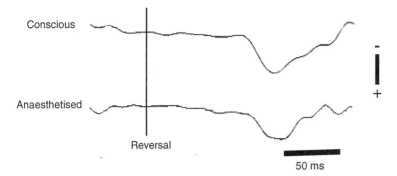

Conscious

Anaesthetised

Reversal

50 ms

Figure 14.3
Visual evoked responses. The response to a reversing checkerboard recorded from the scalp while the patient was conscious (top) and from the cortex while the patient was unconscious (bottom). The amplitude scale bar for each experiment is different (5 μV for scalp and 15 μV for cortical recordings).

the hallucination experiments, and hence our methodology will be blind to the neural activity underlying consciousness. In this conception, our experiments merely reveal those brain activities which feed into or emerge from the "seeing" module, not the "seeing" module itself.

Quantitative Consciousness

The simplicity of a modular consciousness is appealing—you see color when there is activity in the color area. However, there is a weight of evidence to suggest that there is no simple one-to-one mapping of activity and experience. For example, the early macaque recordings were carried out on anesthetized animals, and it is probable that one could substitute anesthetized for awake humans in the classical color, motion, and form PET and fMRI experiments without influencing the results. Figure 14.3 shows a visual evoked response monitoring occipital function before and during a neurosurgical procedure. The response evoked from the scalp while the patient was conscious seems identical to the response evoked directly from the cortex while the patient was unconscious.

Do these examples of the invariance of cerebral activity in different states of consciousness imply that functionally specialized cortex is nonconscious, and that the modular view of consciousness is wrong?

Experiments performed at the Wellcome Department of Cognitive Neurology by Semir Zeki and me reconcile the anesthetic evidence with a modular view. We have investigated a patient (GY) with a lesion of his left striate cortex and consequent blindness in his right visual field (Zeki and ffytche 1998). Previous studies have shown that this blindness is selective—with some stimuli, GY reports a crude conscious perceptual experience; with others, GY denies any percept (Barbur et al. 1980; Barbur et al. 1993; Weiskrantz et al. 1995). In general, if GY sees something, however crude that "seeing" might be, he is able to identify it from a small choice of alternatives; if he sees nothing, he cannot. However, it is the occasional variable dissociation of GY's perceptual and discriminatory responses that make him interesting from the consciousness point of view. Sometimes GY perceives the stimulus without being able to identify it, and on other occasions he identifies it without perceiving it (Zeki and ffytche 1998). We were able

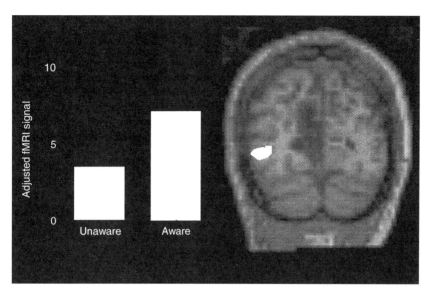

Figure 14.4
Quantitative consciousness. A coronal slice of GY's brain is shown on the right. The area of differential activation (fast or slow motion versus a blank gray screen) is shown in white (left of the slice is the left of the brain). The increases in signal intensity for unaware (slow-motion) and aware (fast-motion) stimuli are shown on the left of the image.

to characterize the respective neurobiologies of these two states by presenting GY with fast- and slow-moving stimuli and recording his cerebral activity with fMRI. GY identified the direction of both types of stimuli; however, his conscious experience of the two was quite different. He saw most of the fast-moving stimuli but almost none of the slow-moving stimuli. The results are presented in figure 14.4.

As was the case with color, object, and face hallucinations, GY's crude motion percepts did not correlate with activity outside the motion area. An important finding was that the degree of activation within motion cortex was significantly different for the two velocities, fast motion (aware) being associated with a greater increase in signal than slow motion (unaware). For GY, the difference between discriminating with "seeing" and discriminating without "seeing" is the amount of activity in the motion area. It is as if activity here allows him to identify the stimulus, but only a certain level of that activity is associated with a crude percept of motion. Exactly what the "seeing"-associated increase in fMRI signal means in neurobiological terms is not known. It may reflect the recruitment of additional subsets of neurons colocalized within the same specialized area—the motion area equivalent of color neurons in the color area (see Zeki 1980). Alternatively, the increase may result from more complex processing of the same neuronal population. Whichever explanation is chosen, the finding helps explain why the same spatial pattern of cerebral activity may be produced in the anesthetized or awake state. The point is that the difference between conscious and unconscious processing is not coded in the location of the activity but in the type of processing performed.

Conclusion

Visual consciousness correlates with some neural activities within areas specialized for the attribute perceived. Those who follow Flourens will interpret this activity as close to the neural correlate of consciousness but ultimately separate from it. Those who follow Gall will argue that the activity is the neural correlate of consciousness for the attribute under consideration. To date, imaging's contribution to our understanding of visual consciousness has been to limit the neurobiological requirements of both the modular and the unitary accounts—activity in specialized visual areas need not pass along an extended hierarchical pathway to be perceived— and to introduce quantitative considerations. Ironically, techniques developed to investigate the brain as a whole have led us back to its parts.

Acknowledgment

This work was supported by the Wellcome Trust.

References

Barbur, J. L., Ruddock, K. H., and Waterfield, V. A. (1980). Human visual responses in the absence of the geniculo-calcarine projection. *Brain* 103: 905–928.

Barbur, J. L., Watson, J. D. G., Frackowiak, R. S. J., and Zeki, S. (1993). Conscious visual perception without V1. *Brain* 116: 1293–1302.

Clarke, E., and Jacyna, L. S. (1987). *Ninteenth-Century Origins of Neuroscience Concepts*. Berkeley: University of California Press.

Crick, F., and Koch, C. (1998). Consciousness and neuroscience. *Cerebral Cortex* 8: 97–107.

ffytche, D. H., Howard, R. J., Brammer, M. J., David, A., Woodruff, P., and Williams, S. (1998). The anatomy of conscious vision: An fMRI study of visual hallucinations. *Nature Neuroscience* 1: 738–742.

ffytche, D. H., and Howard, R. J. (1999). The perceptual consequences of visual loss: Positive pathologies of vision. *Brain* 122: 1247–1260.

Gall, F. J. *On the Functions of the Brain*. (1835). Boston: Marsh, Capen and Lyon.

Holroyd, S., Rabins, P. V., Finkelstein, D., Nicholson, M. C., Chase, G. A., and Wisniewski, S. C. (1992). Visual hallucinations in patients with macular degeneration. *American Journal of Psychiatry* 149: 1701–1706.

Leopold, D. A., and Logothetis, N. K. (1996). Activity changes in early visual cortex reflect monkeys' percepts during binocular rivalry. *Nature* 379: 549–553.

Lepore, F. E. (1990). Spontaneous visual phenomena with visual loss. *Neurology* 40: 444–447.

Logothetis, N. K., and Schall, J. D. (1989). Neuronal correlates of subjective visual perception. *Science* 245: 761–763.

McKeefry, D. J., and Zeki, S. (1997). The position and topography of the human color centre as revealed by functional magnetic resonance imaging. *Brain* 120: 2229–2242.

Robinson, D. (1998). *The Mind*. Oxford: Oxford University Press.

Salzman, C. D., Murasugi, C. M., Britten, K. H., and Newsome, W. T. (1992). Microstimulation in visual area MT: Effects on direction discrimination performance. *Journal of Neuroscience* 12: 2331–2355.

Sereno, M. I., Dale, A. M., Reppas, J. B., Kwong, K. K., Belliveau, J. W., Brady, T. J., Rosen, B. R., and Tootell, R. B. H. (1995). Borders of multiple visual areas in humans revealed by functional magnetic resonance imaging. *Science* 268: 889–893.

Teunisse, R. J., Cruysberg, J. R., Hoefnagels, W. H., Verbeek, A. L., and Zitman, F. G. (1996). Visual hallucinations in psychological normal people: Charles Bonnet's syndrome. *Lancet* 347: 794–797.

Van Essen, D. C., Anderson, C. H., and Felleman, D. J. (1992). Information processing in the primate visual system: An integrated systems perspective. *Science* 255: 419–423.

Watson, J. D. G., Myers, R., Frackowiak, R. S. J., Hajnal, J. V., Woods, R. P., Mazziotta, J. C., Shipp,

S., and Zeki, S. (1993). Area V5 of the human brain: Evidence from a combined study using positron emission tomography and magnetic resonance imaging. *Cerebral Cortex* 3: 79–94.

Weiskrantz, L., Barbur, J. L., and Sahraie, A. (1995). Parameters affecting conscious versus unconscious visual discrimination with damage to the visual cortex (V1). *Proceedings of the National Academy of Sciences USA* 92: 6122–6126.

Young, R. M. (1970). Mind, Brain and Adaptation in the Ninteenth Century. Oxford: Clarendon Press.

Zeki, S. (1980). The representation of colors in the cerebral cortex. *Nature* 284: 412–418.

Zeki, S. (1990). A century of cerebral achromatopsia. *Brain* 113: 1721–1777.

Zeki, S. (1991). Cerebral akinetopsia (visual motion blindness)—A review. *Brain* 114: 811–824.

Zeki, S., and Bartels, A. (1998). The asynchrony of consciousness. *Proceedings of the Royal Society of London* B265: 1583–1585.

Zeki, S., and ffytche, D. H. (1998). The Riddoch syndrome: Insights into the neurobiology of conscious vision. *Brain* 121: 25–45.

Zeki, S., and Shipp, S. (1988). The functional logic of cortical connections. *Nature* 335: 311–317.

Zeki, S., Watson, J. D. G., Lueck, C. J., Friston, K. J., Kennard, C., and Frackowiak, R. S. J. (1991). A direct demonstration of functional specialization in human visual cortex. *Journal of Neuroscience* 11: 641–649.

15 Binocular Rivalry and Human Visual Awareness

Erik D. Lumer

What structures and processes in the human brain are associated with visual awareness? This question has long attracted the attention of scientists and philosophers interested in the neural basis of consciousness, but only recently have technical and methodological advances in neuroscience made its empirical study possible. In this chapter, I review recent research that may provide the beginnings of an answer to this question. This research uses functional magnetic resonance imaging (fMRI) in humans to examine the relationship between brain activity and visual awareness during binocular rivalry, an unstable viewing condition that dissociates subjective perception from sensory input. I will describe evidence that relates conscious visual experience during rivalry to covariation of activity in multiple cortical areas in both ventral and dorsal visual pathways, and in prefrontal cortex. The coordination of activity among these areas is not locked to external sensory or motor events; rather, it relates to internally generated changes in perception. Such evidence suggests that conscious vision reflects the interactions between widely distributed cortical centers, including regions lying outside the visual cortex, rather than the activity in specific visual areas or pathways. I will argue that these interactions contribute to phenomenal awareness by integrating distributed neural processes involved in object representation, in attentional selection, and in temporal integration.

Dissociating Subjective Perception from Retinal Input

Visual stimuli falling on the retina automatically evoke neuronal responses in the central nervous system, but not all such responses lead to phenomenal awareness (Maunsell 1995). How are we to differentiate brain activity specific to consciousness from unconscious neuronal responses to visual stimuli? Bistable percepts, in which a single pattern of retinal input gives rise to two alternating perceptual interpretations, provide a basis for such differentiation. Because changes in perception occur in the absence of any change in the stimulus itself, concomitant variation in brain activity can be related directly to subjective perception.

Necker cubes and ambiguous figures are classical examples of bistable perception. Perceptual instability also arises when dissimilar images are presented to the two eyes. Because the images cannot be fused by the cyclopean visual system, perception alternates spontaneously every few seconds between each monocular view. This phenomenon is called binocular rivalry. Since virtually any pair of dissimilar images can be made to rival when presented dichoptically, binocular rivalry provides a powerful paradigm to study the neural correlates of perceptual organization and visual awareness. This approach has been pioneered by Logothetis and his colleagues, working in the macaque visual system (Logothetis and Schall 1989). These researchers trained monkeys to report their percepts during rivalry. They then recorded spiking activity from single neurons located at several stages in the visual pathway (Leopold and Logothetis 1996). These experiments have demonstrated that whereas the firing of most neurons in primary visual cortex (V1) reflects the visual input and not the percept during rivalry, activity at higher levels in the ventral pathway show increasing correlation with the perceptual state of the animal. Thus, binocular rivalry appears to involve interactions between binocular neurons at several stages in the ventral visual pathway. Neural processing in this pathway culminates in the inferior temporal (IT) cortex, where most neurons modulate their firing in concert with perception during rivalry (Sheinberg and Logothetis 1997). At this stage of processing, activity therefore reflects the brain's internal view of a visual scene rather than the retinal stimulus.

These results lend strong support to a view held at the turn of the twentieth century by Helmholtz and others: that binocular rivalry reflects central selective processes which take effect subsequent to the analysis of both monocular stimuli (see review by Walker 1978). However, they also raise a number of questions. Does perceptual alternation during rivalry rely on functionally and anatomically distinct neural mechanisms, or are neuronal interactions within the ventral object vision pathway sufficient to select among competing stimulus representations? Does modulation of activity related to perception also occur in the occipito-temporal (ventral) pathway in humans? Is activity in the ventral pathway sufficient for the conscious perception of a visual stimulus, or does visual awareness require processing in other brain regions, particularly the parietal and frontal lobes?

Perceptual Representations in Human Occipito-Temporal and Prefrontal Cortex

To address these questions, we measured brain activity with fMRI in humans exposed to binocular rivalry, in which a drifting horizontal grating was presented to one eye, and a face was presented to the other eye (Lumer et al. 1998). To induce binocular rivalry, subjects wore stereoscopic glasses that brought the monocular images into superposition. They used key presses to report perceptual alternations from the grating to the face or vice versa. Brain activity was also monitored during a second viewing condition, in which subjects were exposed to a replay of their perceptual experience during rivalry. During the replay condition, the stimulus alter-

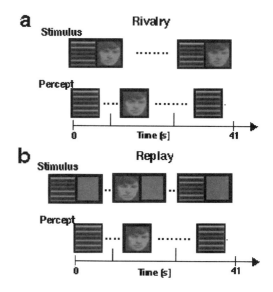

Figure 15.1
Schematic depiction of the viewing conditions used in the first fMRI experiment. (A) During binocular rivalry, subjects viewed pairs of monocular stimuli consisting of a red drifting grating shown to one eye and a green face shown to the other eye. This stimulation produced a bistable percept, alternating spontaneously between face and grating (vertical lines on the time axis mark the transition points). Subjects reported these perceptual alternations with keypresses. This viewing condition was presented in epochs lasting forty-one seconds. (B) During replay, the external stimulus alternated between presentations of the face alone and of the grating alone, in a sequence specified by the keypress reports during the previous rivalrous epoch.

nated between nonrivalrous monocular presentations of either face or grating alone, using the identical temporal sequence of alternations reported during the previous rivalry epoch. These viewing conditions are illustrated in figure 15.1.

Functional MRI scans were acquired over the whole brain and later analyzed in an event-related fashion time-locked to the subjects' reports of perceptual transitions. In the first instance, this analysis allowed us to identify brain areas where activity consistently correlated with the perceptual state of the subjects during rivalry. In particular, we tested for regions where activity was significantly higher during perceptual dominance of the face stimulus compared with phases during which the face was unseen (figure 15.2). Such modulation of activity was found bilaterally in occipito-temporal areas of the ventral visual pathway, including parts of the fusiform gyrus previously implicated in the processing of faces (Kanwisher et al. 1997). Using a paradigm similar to ours, Tong and colleagues further established that fMRI activity in these fusiform areas virtually returns to baseline levels during perceptual suppression of the face stimulus (Tong et al. 1998). Thus, responses in these areas do not depend solely on the visual features associated with a face but also are contingent on the visual awareness of the face stimulus.

Our analysis revealed multiple prefrontal areas where activity reflected the perceptual state. Three distinct prefrontal areas in both hemispheres were identified that all showed increased activity during perceptual dominance of the face stimulus compared with periods of perceptual suppression of the same stimulus: one in the posterior middle and inferior frontal gyri (Brodmann area [BA] 44), a second in the inferior frontal gyrus and insula (BA 45/47), and a third in the anterior middle frontal cortex, also known as dorsolateral prefrontal cortex (BA 46). These results extend findings from nonhuman primates by demonstrating that in human cortex, activity in multiple, functionally distinct, visual and prefrontal regions is correlated with conscious perception during binocular rivalry. The functional significance of such correlates in prefrontal cortex probably relates to its interconnectivity with extrastriate visual areas and to its involvement in the temporal organization of behavior. I shall return later to the possible role of prefrontal cortex in conscious vision.

How Does the Brain Resolve Perceptual Ambiguity?

A major question left unanswered by these observations concerns the neural mechanisms underlying the ongoing perceptual alternations during rivalry. Psychophysical observations suggest that these perceptual alternations result from the same neural operations underlying other multistable perceptual phenomena, such as depth reversal and ambiguous figures, which show temporal dynamics similar to those of binocular rivalry. Although less pronounced, similar perceptual alternations can also be experienced in normal vision (Andrews and Purves 1997). They may therefore reflect a basic perceptual strategy to resolve visual ambiguities and select the contents of visual awareness.

By comparing rivalry against a nonrivalrous replay of the perceptual experience during rivalry, we were able to test whether a specific neural machinery mediates the ongoing selection among conflicting neural representations. Because the rivalry and replay conditions yield similar perception and motor reports, we expected them to engage common neural pathways associated with the internal representation of visual scenes and with the generation of keypress reports. This was confirmed by the fMRI data: Statistically equivalent responses were observed in both conditions in visual areas of the occipito-temporal pathway and in cortical areas associated with movement. However, the rivalry and replay conditions differ in the way they achieve perceptual alternations. Whereas perceptual transitions during rivalry reflect an endogenous neural instability in the absence of any change in the retinal image, during replay they are due to an exogenous manipulation of the visual input. Thus, we reasoned that any differential modulation of activity at transition times between the two conditions would reflect this difference. In particular, it would expose

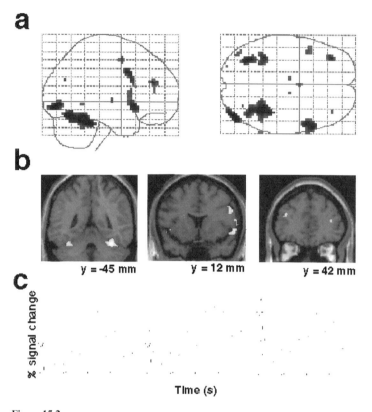

Figure 15.2
Neural correlates of perceptual state during rivalry. (A) Brain areas showing greater fMRI activity during perceptual dominance of the face compared with periods during which the face was unseen are shown as see-through
projections onto lateral (left) and horizontal (right) representations of standard stereotactic space. (B) Activation
maps during face perception in selected coronal sections, overlaid onto normalized anatomical MRIs.Activity is
shown in the fusiform gyri (left), middle and inferior frontal gyri (center), and dorsolateral prefrontal cortex (right).
Distance from the anterior commissure is indicated below each coronal section. (C) Peristimulus time histograms of
fMRI activity locked to the time of reported perceptual transitions from grating to face are shown for selected volumes in the fusiform gyrus (left), inferior frontal gyrus (center), and dorsolateral prefrontal cortex (right). A Siemens
Vision scanner, operating at 2 T, was used to acquire bold contrast functional images. The regional activations
represent averages over six subjects, thresholded at a level of statistical significance of P < 0.05, after correction for
multiple comparisons.

brain structures involved specifically in the on-going selection between conflicting visual representations during rivalry, a conflict that is not evoked by the replay condition.

To tease apart transient fMRI signals associated with perceptual alternation per se from other physiological effects of viewing conditions, we modeled the predicted hemodynamic response to each transition event and tested for the presence of such responses in the data. Differential transition-related activation during rivalry compared with replay was found in a distributed network of cortical areas that included a region in the middle occipital gyrus, at the junction of Brodmann areas 18 and 19, and regions of the inferior parietal cortex, superior parietal cortex, and middle and inferior frontal cortex (figure 15.3). This regional activation was strongly lateralized to the right hemisphere. These results suggest that a distributed right occipito-parietal and frontal network mediates the perceptual switches experienced during rivalry.

Similar cortical areas have been implicated in selective attention. Indeed, visuospatial neglect syndromes occur most frequently following lesions to the inferior parietal and frontal cortex (Mesulam 1981). Moreover, functional imaging studies by Corbetta and others have implicated the superior parietal and frontal regions delineated by our analysis in shifts of spatial attention (reviewed in Corbetta 1998). Finally, differential activation of right extrastriate areas has been reported in tasks directing attention to global aspects rather than local details of visual figures (Fink et al. 1996). But our results show that these areas are also involved in a phenomenon, rivalrous perceptual alternation, that, unlike shifts of attention, recurs in the absence of voluntary control. Why, then, should binocular rivalry and visual attention involve overlapping regions in right frontoparietal cortex? It is striking that both phenomena involve the selective suppression of information from conscious perception. Monocular stimuli become periodically invisible during rivalry; similarly, sensory events associated with unattended stimuli have a diminished impact on awareness. These effects occur in both cases in spite of a rather constant retinal input. Both phenomena may therefore rely on common neural mechanisms in fronto-parietal cortex, which is involved in the selection of neural events leading to visual awareness.

The dorsal visual pathway has traditionally been associated with spatial processing. However, the involvement of frontoparietal structures in resolving perceptual ambiguity during rivalry implies that this pathway plays a more general role in conscious perception than previously thought, biasing the content of visual awareness toward abstract internal representations of visual scenes rather than simply toward space. This view is consistent with recent observations that lesions of inferior parietal and frontal cortex cause disorders of nonspatial forms of perceptual selection, as well as spatial disorders (Husain et al. 1997), and that parietal neurons show selectivity for complex combinations of visual features, akin to the response specificity observed in the temporal lobe (Sereno and Maunsell 1998).

The Neural Integration of Conscious Perception

Our results indicate that conscious experience during rivalry depends on processing in multiple extrastriate ventral, parietal, and prefrontal cortical areas. How do these distributed neural processes interact to produce a unified perception of the visual world?

To determine the nature of the interactions between the cortical areas associated with conscious vision, we again measured brain activity with fMRI in humans exposed to dichoptic stimuli consisting of a drifting grating shown to one eye and a face shown to the other eye (Lumer and Rees 1999). However, in contrast with our earlier imaging study of rivalry, subjects were not instructed to make, nor did they make, any motor or verbal report to indicate perceptual transitions. This avoided any possible contami-

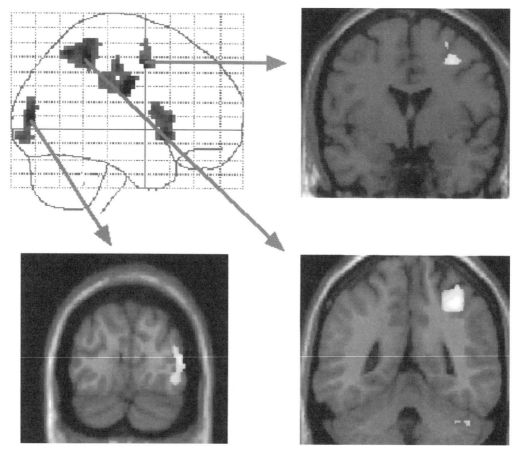

Figure 15.3
Differential transition-related activity during rivalry. Brain regions showing greater modulation of activity at times of perceptual alternations during rivalry compared with the nonrivalrous replay condition are shown as see-through projections onto a lateral representation of stereotactic space (upper left), and in selected coronal sections. These sections show such contrasts in the precentral sulcus (upper right), middle occipital gyrus (lower left), and intra-parietal sulcus (lower right).

nation of the data by motor processes. Correlation of activity between brain areas was used as an index of their functional interactions. To test for the presence of such correlation in the data, the temporal response in each brain area was analyzed by using multiple regression with regressors specified by the activity in selected cortical loci. We first chose as regressors the activity in two cortical loci. One locus was selected in early extrastriate cortex, at the junction of Brodmann areas 18 and 19 (BA 18/19), in a region shown to reflect reported perceptual alternations in our previous experiment. The second locus was chosen in the primary visual cortex, where activity shows little relation to changes in perception during rivalry.[1] This analysis allowed us to identify brain areas where activity was consistently correlated with that in BA 18/19, which served as a surrogate for perceptual reports, as well as brain areas where activity was correlated with that in V1, which served as an indicator of spatial correlation in the fMRI signals unrelated to perception.

All subjects showed significant modulation of activity in multiple visual cortical areas that was significantly correlated with the responses in the selected region of BA 18/19. This pattern of coactivation extended in both hemispheres, dorsally in middle and inferior segments of the occipital and temporal gyri, and ventrally in the fusiform gyrus. In particular, responses that correlated with activity in BA 18/19 were detected in fusiform areas previously associated with the processing of faces, and in the V5 motion-processing complex (figure 15.4). The presence of correlated modulation of activity in these areas is therefore consistent with their involvement in the alternating perception of a face and a moving stimulus experienced by the subjects. In addition to areas that respond specifically to visual stimuli, several regions lying outside the classical definition of visual cortex showed significant correlation with activity in BA 18/19. They were located in the superior and inferior parietal lobe, and in posterior superior, middle, and inferior

frontal cortices. In sharp contrast with the extended pattern of coactivation associated with BA 18/19, only a few, scattered sites in posterior cortices were correlated with the fMRI signals measured in V1. We repeated these covariation analyses, using regressors derived from activity in other cortical sites associated with reported perceptual transitions, in the fusiform gyrus and parietal cortex. The same pattern of coactivation associated with BA 18/19 was produced by these analyses. In addition, we found a more anterior region of dorsolateral prefrontal cortex, in Brodmann area 46, whose responses varied in concert with parietal and fusiform activity.

In our previous imaging study, we showed that activity in similar visual and nonvisual cortical areas was correlated with reported perceptual changes during rivalry. Taken together, these results demonstrate that covariation of activity in a distributed network of extrastriate visual, parietal, and prefrontal cortical areas is associated specifically with subjective perception, independent of motor reports. The coordination of activity between these areas probably reflects the massively parallel and reciprocal organization of cortico-cortical connections. Neuroanatomical and electrophysiological observations in monkeys indicate that parietal and prefrontal structures are reciprocally connected and act in concert with secondary visual areas in the temporal lobe (Fuster 1989; Chaffee and Goldman-Rakic 1998). Consistent with these earlier findings in monkeys, the present results imply a network organization that allows the human parietal and prefrontal cortex to operate with extrastriate visual areas as an integrated unit.

Representation, Selection, and Temporal Integration

The primate visual system is conventionally divided into two processing pathways originating in primary visual cortex (Ungerleider and Haxby 1994). One pathway extends dorsally, in the

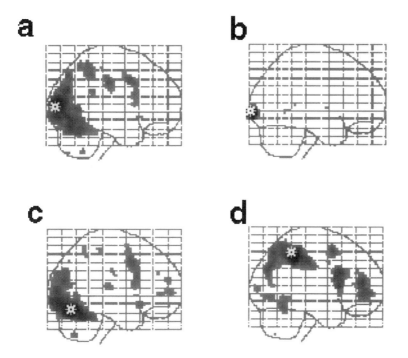

Figure 15.4
Covariation maps in the second fMRI experiment. Brain regions where activity significantly correlates with that in selected cortical loci (white markers) are shown as see-through projections onto lateral representations of stereotactic space. The activity used for such covariation analyses was taken from volumes in (a) the middle occipital gyrus, (b) the primary visual cortex, (c) the fusiform gyrus, and (d) the superior parietal lobe.

occipito-parietal lobe; the other pathway extends ventrally in the occipito-temporal lobe. Neurons in the parietal pathway appear to be specialized for the processing of spatial attributes of the visual scene, and are responsible for the coordinate transformations necessary to support visually guided behavior. The ventral visual pathway is involved in object representation and recognition. Several studies have emphasized the key role played by the ventral pathway in conscious visual perception (Logothetis 1998). Physiological evidence for this role comes from single-cell recordings in awake monkeys that demonstrate shape-selective responses in the temporal lobe which reflect the subjective perception of visual

objects and are modulated by attention (Desimone and Duncan 1995; Sheinberg and Logothetis 1997). Consistent with these observations, lesions in the temporal lobe lead to profound impairments in visual recognition and awareness (Farah 1990; Milner and Goodale 1995).

The picture that emerges from the imaging studies described in this chapter is that the ventral pathway is not sufficient to produce conscious visual perception; rather, these studies suggest that awareness of a visual stimulus is accomplished by the coactivation of neurons distributed over multiple brain regions, including cortical areas in both ventral and dorsal visual pathways, and in the prefrontal lobe. The functional properties of these areas further suggest that their coactivation combines three distinct capacities which appear crucial for the formation of conscious perceptual states: to extract higher-order features of the visual input, to select among countless alternative interpretations of how these features make up a visual scene, and to integrate the selected scene into the broader temporal and behavioral context in which it occurs. The neural substrates of the first two capacities have already been discussed: They encompass distributed networks in the temporal and parietal systems, respectively. The third capacity, temporal integration, is usually attributed to prefrontal structures involved in short-term memory and motor set.

Visual short-term, or working, memory refers to the ability to keep in mind a visual scene after its associated retinal image has disappeared, and while new sensory and motor events reach consciousness. In working-memory tasks, sustained activity is found in prefrontal cortex, and probably reflects reciprocal interactions between frontal and visual areas (Goldman-Rakic 1995). This sustained activity reflects both the maintained response to a past visual stimulus and the preparation of motor plans. It therefore appears to play a central role in resolving cross-temporal contingencies (Fuster 1989). That this capacity is brought to bear in conscious vision is suggested by the striking similarity between the distributed network of visual and prefrontal regions associated with the perceptual dominance of faces in our study and that recently implicated in the maintenance of facial representations in working memory (Courtney et al. 1997).

Conclusion

Although traditional views on visual awareness localize its neural basis to circumscribed visual areas or pathways, it has been suggested that conscious perception reflects the functional integration of widely distributed neural processes.

Yet, the evidence for either account of conscious experience has remained tenuous. In this chapter, I have discussed recent evidence in humans that argues in favor of the latter view. This evidence suggests that subjective visual perception is associated specifically with covariation of activity in multiple extrastriate ventral, parietal, and prefrontal cortical areas. Because this coactivation is internally generated, it implies a network organization that allows the human prefrontal and parietal cortex to operate with temporal areas as an integrated system. The integration of anatomically distinct and functionally specialized circuits involved in representation, selection and disambiguation, and temporal integration of the visual scene may provide the necessary ingredients for what William James described as the hallmarks of conscious experience: its unity, its extraordinary variety, and its continuity across time (James 1890).

Acknowledgment

This research was supported by the Wellcome Trust.

Note

1. These observations were based on recording techniques that are sensitive to mean levels of activity in neuronal populations. They do not exclude the possibility that changes in relative spike timing within V1 may contribute to interocular aspects of binocular rivalry. Such a possibility is suggested by electrophysiological observations in amblyopic cats (Fries et al. 1997) and predicted by computational models (Lumer 1998).

References

Andrews, T. J., and Purves, D. (1997). Similarities in normal and binocularly rivalrous viewing. *Proceedings of the National Academy of Sciences USA* 94: 9905–9908.

Chaffee, M. V., and Goldman-Rakic, P. S. (1998). Matching patterns of activity in primate prefrontal area 8a and parietal area 7ip neurons during a spatial working memory task. *Journal of Neurophysiology* 79: 2919–2940.

Corbetta, M. (1998). Frontoparietal cortical networks for directing attention and the eye to visual locations: Identical, independent, or overlapping neural systems? *Proceedings of the National Academy of Sciences USA* 95: 831–838.

Courtney, S. M., Ungerleider, L. G., Keil, K., and Haxby, J. V. (1997). Transient and sustained activity in a distributed neural system for human working memory. *Nature* 386: 608–611.

Desimone, R., and Duncan, J. (1995). Neural mechanisms of selective visual attention. *Annual Review of Neuroscience* 18: 193–222.

Farah, M. (1990). *Visual Agnosia*. Cambridge, MA: MIT Press.

Fink, G., Halligan, P. W., Marshall, J. C., Frith, C. D., Frackowiak, R. S. J., and Dolan, R. J. (1996). Where in the brain does visual attention select the forest and the trees? *Nature* 382: 626–628.

Fries, P., Roelfsema, P. R., Engel, A. K., Konig, P., and Singer, W. (1997). Synchronization of oscillatory responses in visual cortex correlates with perception in interocular rivalry. *Proceedings of the National Academy of Sciences USA* 94: 12699–12704.

Fuster, J. M. (1989). *The Prefrontal Cortex: Anatomy, Physiology, and Neuropsychology of the Frontal Lobe.* New York: Raven.

Goldman-Rakic, P. S. (1995). Cellular basis of working memory. *Neuron* 14: 477–485.

Husain, M., Shapiro, K., Martin, J., and Kennard, C. (1997). Abnormal temporal dynamics of visual attention in spatial neglect patients. *Nature* 385: 154–156.

James, W. (1890). *The Principles of Psychology*. New York: Holt.

Kanwisher, N., McDermott, J., and Chun, M. M. (1997). The fusiform face area: A module in human extrastriate cortex specialized for face perception. *Journal of Neuroscience* 17: 4302–4311.

Leopold, D., and Logothetis, N. K. (1996). Activity changes in early visual cortex reflect monkeys' percepts during binocular rivalry. *Nature* 379: 549–553.

Logothetis, N. K. (1998). Object vision and visual awareness. *Current Opinions in Neurobiology* 8: 536–544.

Logothetis, N. K., and Schall, J. D. (1989). Neural correlates of subjective visual perception. *Science* 245: 761–863.

Lumer, E. D. (1998). A neural model of binocular integration and rivalry based on the coordination of action-potential timing in primary visual cortex. *Cerebral Cortex* 8: 553–561.

Lumer, E. D., Friston, K. J., and Rees, G. (1998). Neural correlates of perceptual rivalry in the human brain. *Science* 280: 1930–1934.

Lumer, E. D., and Rees, G. (1999). Covariation of activity in visual and prefrontal cortex associated with subjective visual perception. *Proceedings of the National Academy of Sciences USA* 96: 1669–1673.

Maunsell, J. H. R. (1995). The brain's visual world: Representation of visual targets in cerebral cortex. *Science* 270: 764–869.

Mesulam, M.-M. (1981). A cortical network for directed attention and unilateral neglect. *Annual Review of Neurology* 10: 309–325.

Milner, D., and Goodale, M. A. (1995). *The Visual Brain in Action*. Oxford: Oxford University Press.

Sereno, A. B., and Maunsell, J. H. R. (1998). Shape selectivity in primate lateral intraparietal cortex. *Nature* 395: 500–503.

Sheinberg, D. L., and Logothetis, N. K. (1997). The role of temporal cortical areas in perceptual organization. *Proceedings of the National Academy of Sciences USA* 94: 3408–3413.

Tong, F., Nakayama, K., Vaughan, J. T., and Kanwisher, N. (1998). Binocular rivalry and visual awareness in human extrastriate cortex. *Neuron* 21: 753–859.

Ungerleider, L. G., and Haxby, J. V. (1994). What and where in the human brain. *Current Opinions in Neurobiology* 4: 157–165.

Walker, P. (1978). Binocular rivalry: Central or peripheral selective processes? *Psychological Bulletin* 85: 376–389.

IV CANDIDATES FOR THE NCC III: CONSCIOUSNESS, ANESTHESIA, AND THE NMDA RECEPTOR COMPLEX

One obvious, although long neglected, strategy in searching for the physical mechanisms enabling conscious experience consists in analyzing the conditions under which it *disappears*. Investigating the mechanisms of action of general anesthetics and looking for a common denominator might be one such strategy. This section relates recent research on the mechanisms of anesthesia to the question of consciousness. It is structured like a small symposium, with a target article written by Hans Flohr and three commentaries contributed by Valerie Hardcastle, Nick Franks and Bill Lieb, and Jackie Andrade.

Hans Flohr is the prototypical example of an active neuroscientist with a long-standing, deep, and serious interest in the philosophical issues related to mind–brain research. For a number of years he has been working on what he calls a "realization theory of consciousness," a theory that will render the relations between brain events and states of consciousness intelligible. Such a theory would order the diverse empirical correlations and define which causes are relevant or proximal, and which are trivial. His approach also contains a philosophical element: phenomenal content is the content of *higher-order representations*. Therefore, Flohr says, the search for the neural correlate of consciousness converges with the search for a computational mechanism generating the integrated, large-scale neural assemblies to which those higher-order representations will necessarily belong. Flohr's hypothesis states that in human cortex this function is implemented by the NMDA receptor complex. Important empirical observations on which his argument rests are (1) the normal functioning of the NMDA synapse is a necessary condition for consciousness, and (2) all other physiological or computational brain processes that remain intact after a selective blockade of the NMDA receptor, taken together, are not sufficient for the occurrence of conscious states. However, if the normal functions of the NMDA receptor are restored by removing the channel blockade, a physiological situation will arise that is a sufficient condition for consciousness. Any (almost) complete inhibition of the NMDA-dependent processes, either directly or indirectly induced, leads to a loss of consciousness, because it is the final common pathway of anesthetic action and of other causes of unconsciousness.

The cortical NMDA synapse mediates a specific class of computational processes, those which produce higher-order, self-reflexive representational structures. The NMDA synapse plays this crucial role because it implements the binding mechanism that the brain uses to produce large-scale neuronal cell assemblies. According to Hans Flohr, the formation of large-scale assemblies depends on the rate at which changes in synaptic strength take place, and this in turn depends on the depolarization of the postsynaptic membrane of cortical neurons. Large-scale assemblies will automatically emerge if the degree of depolarization of the postsynaptic membrane is kept near the activation threshold of the NMDA receptor. And the occurrence of higher-order self-reflexive representations in turn is necessary *and sufficient* for the occurrence of phenomenal states.

In the context of Flohr's proposal, the relevance of a number of methodological questions becomes particularly obvious: How do we pick out the neural correlate of consciousness from the enormous number of other spurious coincidences in the system? Valerie Gray Hardcastle points out that this is a nontrivial question, not exhausted by simply seeking an event both necessary and sufficient for the emergence of subjective experience. Focusing on this larger issue from the perspective of philosophy of science, she draws attention to the well-known concept of a "screening-off relation": One putative cause, A, screens off another, B, from the effect we are interested in if the probability of the effect occurring is the same regardless of whether we have A and B occurring or just A, but the probability is not the same if we have just B. Having B does not add anything to the system; A is actually doing the causal work. However, a screening-off analysis can be run either horizontally or vertically. That is, we can use it to determine which cause is "closest" to the explanans and thus is the most proximal cause (see also chapter 2, this volume). Or we can use it to determine which level of organization of matter is the appropriate one for describing the phenomena (see also chapter 4, this volume).

Hardcastle points out that isolating the neural correlates of consciousness currently is very much a vertical problem: What level of organization in the brain is appropriate for understanding consciousness? Even if we take a pragmatic approach to the horizontal aspect of the problem by adopting real-world constraints and simple relevance criteria, this issue remains: Are smaller units of explanation—for instance, computational properties of NMDA receptor sites versus the global dynamics of large cell assemblies (see chapters 8 and 9)—*really* always the right choice in the search for the NCC? In her contribution Hardcastle highlights these methodological aspects and shows that they also pertain to the route taken by Hans Flohr.

Nick Franks and Bill Lieb have assessed Flohr's theory of consciousness from a strictly pharmacological perspective. They contrast the mechanisms of action and the general properties exhibited by ketamine and by etomidate, then go on to criticize the "nonphilosophical" part of Flohr's argument: the claim that all general anesthetics ultimately inhibit NMDA receptor activity, and that this activity is a necessary condition for consciousness. This is a difficult hypothesis to test, since it depends on what assumptions are made about the unknown relative distributions of various ion channels. One prediction is that drugs like etomidate, which appear to act via direct binding to GABA(A) receptors, must *indirectly* inhibit NMDA receptor activity. Etomidate and ketamine both cause unconsciousness, but differ widely with respect to other pharmacological properties (for example, etomidate does not produce analgesia). The

questions remain not only of testability but also of whether or not the special additional assumptions needed to explain this divergence of effects would in principle leave intact Flohr's theory that the NMDA receptor complex is an essential type of necessary condition for the emergence of phenomenal experience.

Jackie Andrade investigates the utility of Flohr's proposal in trying to explain a number of contradictory findings that have emerged from the study of cognition during amnesia, presenting some of her own research in the field. One challenge she formulates for his theory is to explain how catecholamines interact with the NMDA-mediated cell assemblies that, according to his hypothesis, underlie consciousness and long-term memory. She proposes that we may be dealing with two learning mechanisms: one that is closely coupled to consciousness and is dependent on plasticity in NMDA synapses, and one that is independent of consciousness and dependent on or influenced by catecholamines. This second mechanism could then be the one responsible for the apparently preserved learning of simple stimuli and stimulus pairings during anesthesia. Andrade concludes by once more drawing readers' attention to the utility of anesthetics as a research tool in consciousness studies, especially in delineating the *cognitive* correlates of consciousness.

Further Reading

Andrade, J. (1995). Learning during anesthesia: A review. *British Journal of Psychology* 86: 479–506.

Andrade, J. (1997). Investigations of hypesthesia: Using anesthetics to explore relationships between consciousness, learning, and memory. *Consciousness and Cognition* 5: 562–580.

Andrade, J., and Jones, J. G. (1997). Awareness in anesthesia. In G. Hall and M. Morgan, eds., *Short Practice of Anesthesia*. London: Chapman and Hall.

Flohr, H. (1991). Brain processes and phenomenal consciousness: A new and specific hypothesis. *Theory and Psychology* 1: 245–262.

Flohr, H. (1995). An information processing theory of anaesthesia. *Neuropsychologia* 33: 1169–1180.

Flohr, H., Glade, U., and Motzko, D. (1998). The role of the NMDA synapse in general anesthesia. *Toxicology Letters* 100–101: 23–29.

Franks, N. P., and Lieb, W. R. (1994). Molecular and cellular mechanisms of general anaesthesia. *Nature* 367: 607–614.

Hardcastle, V. G. (1993). The naturalists versus the skeptics: The debate over a scientific understanding of consciousness. *Journal of Mind and Behavior* 14: 27–50.

Hardcastle, V. G. (1995). *Locating Consciousness.* Amsterdam: John Benjamins Press.

Hardcastle, V. G. (1996). Discovering the moment of consciousness I: Bridging techniques at work; II: An ERP analysis of priming using novel visual stimuli. *Philosophical Psychology* 9: 149–196.

Tomlin, S. L., Jenkins, A., Lieb, W. R., and Franks, N. P. (1998). Stereoselective effects of etomidate optical isomers on gamma-aminobutyric acid type A receptors and animals. *Anesthesiology* 88: 708–717.

16 NMDA Receptor–Mediated Computational Processes and Phenomenal Consciousness

Hans Flohr

Around 1966 Corssen and Domino described the anesthetic and psychotomimetic effects of two new drugs, phencyclidine and ketamine. When administered in high doses, these drugs cause a unique state of unconsciousness which is quite different from that produced by classic anesthetic agents such as halothane or barbiturates. This state is characterized by a rather selective loss of conscious functions. Patients are in a trancelike cataleptic state, profoundly analgesic and disconnected from the surroundings. Given in sub-hypnotic doses, these drugs induce altered states of consciousness. Patients experience abnormal perceptions, sensory illusions, visual and auditory hallucinations, and disorganized thought. In particular, they report bizarre ego disorders that resemble schizophrenic states.

The NMDA Receptor as the Ultimate Target of Anesthetic Action

It was discovered later that ketamine and phencyclidine act as noncompetitive antagonists of the *N*-methyl-D-aspartate (NMDA) receptor. This receptor (figure 16.1) is unique in several respects. The opening probability of the receptor-associated ion channel is both voltage- and transmitter-dependent. It opens under two conditions. First, the presynapse must release the transmitter glutamate and, second, the postsynaptic membrane must be depolarized to about -35 mV. When the membrane potential assumes a value nearly equivalent to the resting potential, the channel will be blocked by a magnesium ion that binds in a voltage-dependent manner to a site in the lumen of the channel. This blockade will be removed if the membrane is depolarized. The receptor-operated channel is permeable to Na^+, K^+, and Ca^{2+}. The permeation of Ca^{2+} through the open NMDA channel triggers a number of biochemical changes inside the postsynaptic terminal that modify the strength of the synapse. Ca^{2+} activates the enzyme nitric oxide synthase (NOS) that catalyzes the production of nitric oxide (NO). NO, a gas that rapidly diffuses through the cell membrane, acts as a retrograde messenger and induces rapid and transient changes in both presynaptic transmitter release and postsynaptic sensitivity to the released transmitter. In addition, Ca^{2+} triggers posttranslational changes of neuronal proteins and changes in protein synthesis that are responsible for persistent modifications of synaptic strength.

The NMDA receptor channel complex is a potential target for many different drugs:

1. The receptor-associated ion channel contains a binding site (PCP receptor) for noncompetitive antagonists, to which ketamine and phencyclidine belong. These antagonists block the influx of Na^+ and Ca^{2+} ions and thereby antagonize (1) the depolarization of the postsynaptic membrane induced by the agonist glutamate and (2) the induction of plastic changes by Ca^{2+}.

2. The recognition site for the endogenous agonist glutamate can be blocked by specific competitive NMDA antagonists.

3. A strychnine-insensitive glycine binding site, the coactivation of which is necessary for receptor activation, can be blocked by glycine antagonists.

4. A binding site for polyamines can be blocked by polyamine antagonists.

5. The enzyme NOS can be inactivated by various NOS inhibitors.

Ketamine and phencyclidine bind to the PCP receptor and block the influx of Ca^{2+} and Na^+. Like most noncompetitive NMDA antagonists, they are not fully selective but also interact with other components of the CNS. But these side effects are not able to fully account for the drugs' anesthetic and psychotomimetic properties. It

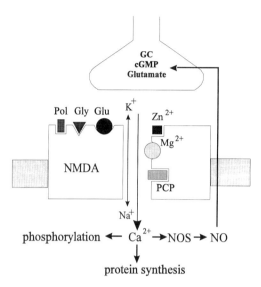

Figure 16.1
Schematic representation of the *N*-methyl-D-aspartate (NMDA) synapse. The receptor contains binding sites for the endogenous agonist glutamate (Glu), for glycine (Gly) and for polyamines (Pol). The receptor-associated channel is blocked by Mg^{2+} ions in a voltage-dependent manner. Noncompetitive antagonists bind to the PCP recognition site within the channel. Ca^{2+} activates the enzyme nitric oxide synthase (NOS), which synthesizes NO from L-arginine. NO acts as a retrograde messenger on the transmitter release of the presynaptic terminal.

seems safe to assume that both anesthetic and psychoactive effects are caused by their NMDA antagonism. First, all substances known so far to bind to the PCP receptor produce a similar anesthetic state. Among them is the selective high-affinity antagonist MK–801 (Koek et al. 1989; Scheller et al. 1989; Daniell 1990; Löscher et al. 1991; Irifune et al. 1992; Perkins and Morrow 1992a). Second, the anesthetic potency of these compounds is highly correlated with their relative affinity to the PCP receptor (Koek et al. 1989; Perkins and Morrow 1992b). Ketamine exists in two enantiomers, R(−) and S(+) ket-

amine, for which the PCP receptor displays stereoselectivity. S(+) ketamine has a three times higher affinity than R(−) ketamine. This corresponds to the anesthetic potency, S(+) ketamine being three times more potent (Marietta et al. 1977; Ryder et al. 1978; White et al. 1980; Lodge et al. 1982; Schüttler et al. 1987; Zeilhofer et al. 1992). The same is true for the subjective psychoactive effects of subanesthetic doses, as indicated by animal discrimination studies (Martin and Lodge 1988), and for the psychotomimetic effects in humans, including the characteristic ego disorders (Vollenweider 1998). Third, the anesthetic effects of the noncompetitive NMDA antagonists can be modified by changing their binding kinetics. Agonists of the glutamate and glycine receptors increase the open time of the NMDA receptor channel and thereby accelerate the dissociation rate of ligands bound within it. Both agonists antagonize the anesthetic effects of the noncompetitive antagonists (Irifune et al. 1992). This antianesthetic effect of glutamate and glycine can be reversed by selective glutamate and glycine antagonists.

From these observations one can draw the following conclusions:

1. The normal functioning of the NMDA synapse is a necessary condition for consciousness.

2. All other physiological or computational brain processes that remain intact after a selective blockade of the NMDA receptor are, taken together, not sufficient for the occurrence of conscious states.

3. If, however, the normal functions of the NMDA receptor are restored by removing the channel blockade, a physiological situation will arise that is a sufficient condition for consciousness.

A loss of consciousness, it appears, is not necessarily due to an unspecific, global depression of *all* neural activity, but to the disruption of a specific subset of processes that depend on the normal functioning of the NMDA receptor.

If these assumptions are correct, it will follow that not only noncompetitive antagonists, like ketamine, but all other drugs that interfere with this complex molecular entity, should have similar anesthetic and psychotomimetic effects. Figure 16.2 summarizes what is currently known in this respect. In fact, it appears that *any* of the possible direct interventions which inhibit the activation of the receptor or the subsequent processes triggered by Ca^{2+} inevitably produce anesthetic effects. This is true not only for a large number of noncompetitive antagonists that bind to the PCP receptor, but also for all competitive NMDA antagonists that block the glutamate receptor, such as AP5, CPP, CGS 19755 and D-CPP-ene (Koek et al. 1986; Boast and Pastor 1988; Woods 1989; France et al. 1990; Daniell 1991; Irifune et al. 1992; Perkins and Morrow 1992a; Kuroda et al. 1993); for glycine antagonists such as ACEA (McFarlane et al. 1995); and for polyamine antagonists such as spermidine and spermine (Daniell 1992). All these drugs have been shown to decrease the minimum alveolar concentration (MAC) for halothane and/or to increase the sleeping time in a standard barbiturate narcosis. Recently, it was found that nitrous oxide (laughing gas) inhibits the ionic currents mediated through the NMDA receptor, possibly by a mixed competitive/noncompetitive mechanism (Jevtovic-Todorovic et al. 1998). This interesting finding would explain the long-known specific psychopharmacological profile of laughing gas, which is very similar to that of ketamine.

A role for the NO-signaling pathway in general anesthesia is suggested by an increasing number of studies. The inhibition of NO synthesis with the unspecific NOS inhibitor nitro$_G$-L-arginine methyl ester (L-NAME) potentiates the effects of halothane, isoflurane, and alcohol (Johns et al. 1992; Adams et al. 1994; Ichinose et al. 1995). The brain selective NOS inhibitor 7-nitro-indazole (7-Ni) dose-dependently prolongs the duration of a barbiturate narcosis (Motzko et al. 1998) and also reduces the isoflurane MAC

(Pajewski et al. 1996). Moreover, the involvement of this pathway has been shown for a number of anesthetics, such as halothane, enflurane, and isoflurane (Zuo and Johns 1995; Zuo et al. 1996; Tonner et al. 1997), barbiturates (Morgan et al. 1991; Terasako et al. 1994) and alpha 2-adrenergic agonists (Vuilliemoz et al. 1996).

For a large number of anesthetics, however, it is known that they do *not* act *directly* upon the NMDA synapse. For example, it is assumed that the $GABA_A$ receptor is the primary site of action for intravenous anesthetics like barbiturates, benzodiazepines, steroids, etomidate, and propofol. $GABA_A$ receptors are typically located in the immediate vicinity of the NMDA receptor. Their activation causes hyperpolarization of the postsynaptic membrane. According to what has been said before, this will alter the working conditions of the NMDA receptor complex. It is therefore possible that the anesthetic action of $GABA_A$ agonists is due to an *indirect* inhibition of NMDA receptor activity. In fact, there is some experimental evidence that supports this assumption. Figures 16.3 and 16.4 show an attempt to visualize the activation state of the cortical NMDA synapses directly, under in vivo conditions, by means of an autoradiographic technique (Flohr et al. 1998). A radioactively labeled noncompetitive NMDA antagonist ($[^3H]$-MK-801) that is able to associate with the open, but not with the closed, NMDA channel was used to label activated channels. The rate at which the indicator is bound to its recognition site under nonequilibrium conditions depends on the number of activated channels and on the mean opening times of the individual channels.

Figure 16.3 shows the in vivo uptake in the brain of the awake rat. The binding sites are distributed unevenly, with highest densities occurring in the cortex and the hippocampal formation. The picture obtained under awake conditions resembles conventional in vitro receptor autoradiographs that depict the regional concentration of NMDA receptors. This means

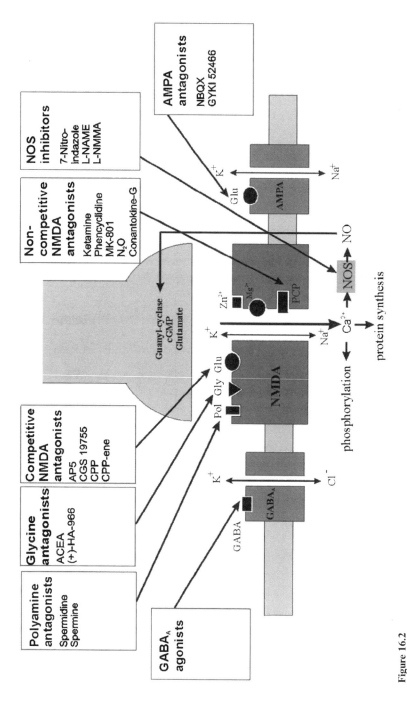

Figure 16.2

The NMDA synapse as a target for anesthetics. Schematic representation of the NMDA receptor channel complex with its regulatory sites and of neighboring AMPA and GABA receptors by which the working conditions of the NMDA receptor can be influenced. All agents mentioned possess anesthetic properties; arrows indicate the interaction sites.

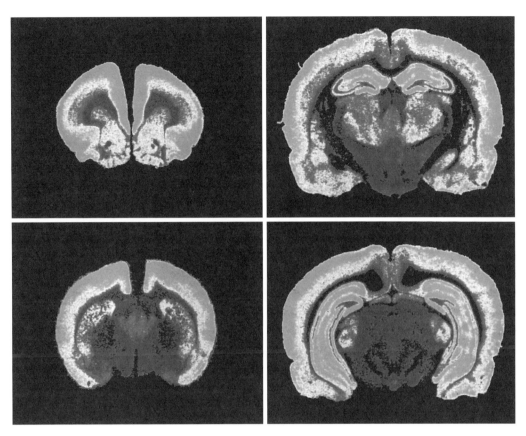

Figure 16.3
In vivo uptake of [^{3}H]-MK-801 in the rat brain under awake conditions. [^{3}H]-MK-801 was dissolved in saline and injected through a vene catheter at a dose of 600 μCi/kg. The animals were sacrificed by swift decapitation 1 min after the administration of the tracer. The brain was rapidly removed and frozen. Frozen sections were washed with TRIS maleate buffer to minimize nonreceptor-associated bindings, and subsequently air-dried. The sections were juxtaposed to [^{3}H] Hyperfilm (Amersham, Buchler) for 60 days. See color insert.

that under awake conditions, most of the NMDA synapses present have been activated during the time period when the indicator was present in the extracelluar space. In ketamine narcosis (figure 16.4b), the indicator uptake is considerably reduced, which is not surprising because ketamine acts as a channel blocker. A very similar uptake pattern, however, is obtained in barbiturate (figure 16.4c) and propofol (figure 16.4f) narcosis, indicating that the cortical NMDA synapse is suppressed by GABAergic inhibition. A similar inhibitory effect can be observed with other anesthetics, such as halothane (figure 16.4d) and alcohol (figure 16.4e).

Antagonists of excitatory synapses in the vicinity of the NMDA receptor, such as the glutamatergic (AMPA) receptor, in theory should have similar indirect effects. In fact, it has been shown that 2,3 dihydroxy–6-nitro–7-sulfamoylbenzo(F)quinoxaline (NBQX), a selective AMPA antagonist, possesses anesthetic properties (McFarlane et al. 1992).

Taken together, one can conclude (1) that an anesthetic potency has been shown for all kinds of agents that directly interfere with the function of the NMDA receptor channel complex or the subsequent plastic processes; and (2) that the action of anesthetics which primarily interact with other targets, such as the GABA synapse, can eventually be explained as an indirect effect on the NMDA synapse. These data support the hypothesis that NMDA receptor-dependent processes are the ultimate target of anesthetic action (Flohr 1995b).

The Role of the Ascending Reticular Activating System

The NMDA receptor may also be the ultimate target of other causes of unconsciousness. Since the pioneering studies of Moruzzi and Magoun it has been known that awareness critically depends on the ascending reticular activating system (ARAS), which originates in the upper brain stem reticular formatio and projects through synaptic relays in the thalamus to the cortex, where it diffusely increases excitability. Bilateral lesions of the reticular formatio lead to coma, a global loss of consciousness. Discrete unilateral lesions of the ascending pathways lead to focal disturbances of consciousness, such as attentional neglect.

This role of the ARAS in the generation of consciousness has been known for a long time. But it has not been convincingly explained. It remained unclear what an arousal state of the cortex really is, what effect it has on cortical information processing, and why the diffuse activation of the cortex is necessary for consciousness.

According to the hypothesis outlined here, the nature of the arousal state can be defined more precisely: It corresponds to the membrane potential of the postsynaptic membranes in which the NMDA receptor is embedded. Only if this potential is kept near the threshold of the activation of this receptor will these synapses participate in cortical information processing. The unspecific activation of the cortical neurons determines the rate at which NMDA-dependent processes take place. A minimum activation of the cortical NMDA system is a necessary condition for the mechanisms underlying consciousness.

A Binding Mechanism for Large-Scale Neuronal Assemblies

The fact that the NMDA receptor is voltage-dependent *and* ligand-gated qualifies this synapse as a Hebbian coincidence detector that detects coincident pre- and postsynaptic activity. The occurrence of coincident pre- and postsynaptic activity induces diverse changes in synaptic strength. First, if the activation threshold is reached, this synapse will be switched on in addition to already active excitatory connections converging at the postsynaptic membrane. This

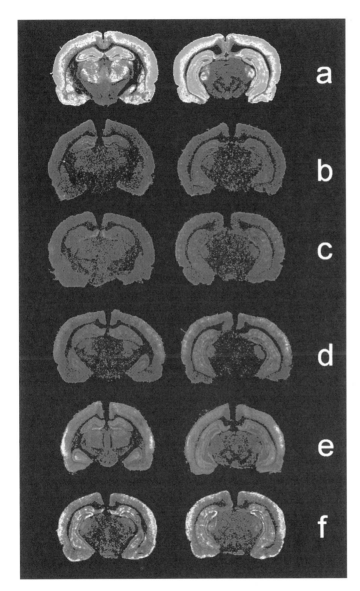

Figure 16.4
In vivo uptake of [^{3}H]-MK-801 under (b) ketamine (175 mg/kg), (c) Na-pentobarbital (110 mg/kg), (d) halothane, (e) ethanol (4 g/kg), and (f) propofol (180 mg/kg) anesthesia. Compared with the awake condition (a), the cortical indicator uptake is reduced in all forms of anesthesia. See color insert.

means that non-NMDA receptor-mediated depolarizations which exceed a certain critical voltage or frequency are amplified. This leads to a rapid change in the connection strength between simultaneously active neurons. The activity of these neurons is enhanced and coordinated via positive feedback loops. They form a Hebbian cell assembly. Second, Ca^{2+} that permeates through the activated channel acts as a second messenger which induces several reactions in the postsynaptic terminal. It activates the NO synthase, and thereby NO production. As mentioned above, this is a second mechanism that leads to rapid and reversible modifications in synaptic strength. In addition, Ca^{2+} presumably is also responsible for slow and long-lasting alterations of synaptic efficacy. Thus, the NMDA synapse realizes the Hebb principle in multiple ways. It possesses a repertoire of mechanisms to bring about changes in synaptic strength. It controls rapid and reversible synaptic modifications as well as long-term changes.

Following the activation by glutamate, the NMDA receptor channel complex remains in an activated state for several hundred milliseconds. This endows the postsynaptic membrane with a relatively long memory for the detection of correlated activity. The receptor, therefore, plays a role not only in the initiation of long-term memory but also in working memory, the ability to store and manipulate information over periods of time ranging from seconds to minutes. A large time window is also necessary for detecting widely distributed correlated activity, and consequently for establishing Hebbian assemblies that connect very distant neurons. The concept of the cell assembly is one of the most commonly used in brain theory. Hebb's (1959) central idea was that the spatiotemporal activity of a cell assembly is identical with the physiological instantiation of a mental representation. In his words, "[T]he assembly activity is the simplest case of an image or an idea: a representative process."

The NMDA synapse appears to be ideally suited to tie together and integrate widely distributed activities and to organize large-scale neuronal assemblies. Such assemblies detect coincident lower-level neuronal events in segregated specialized cortical areas, and bind them into a coherent percept that represents a higher level of correlation between *internal* events. It instantiates self-reflexive representations of the system itself and of its current state. The activation state of the NMDA receptor determines the probability with which plastic changes occur. Thus, it determines the size and the complexitiy of large-scale representational structures that can be built up in a given period of time. Large and complex assemblies will automatically develop if the plastic changes are accomplished at a critical rate. If the cortical NMDA system is inhibited, large-scale representational structures will not occur.

If these assumptions are correct, the empirical findings described above will support a representational theory of consciousness. The occurrence of states of consciousness depends on the presence of specific global representational structures and specific binding mechanisms that lead to their formation.

The Instantiation of Higher-Order Representations

Representational theories of consciousness come in different versions. One important position in the current debate is that consciousness is a kind of metarepresentation—either a higher-order perception or a higher-order thought. Such ideas have a long history in the philosophy of mind that dates back to John Locke, Gottfried Wilhelm Leibniz, Immanuel Kant, William James, and Franz Brentano. Important modern versions have been worked out by Armstrong (1980), Churchland (1985), Rosenthal (1986, 1990, 1993a, 1993b), and Metzinger (1993). Roughly speaking, to be conscious, in this view, is to be in a specific cognitive state, that of having a mental representation by which the system represents its own actual state as its own state. Being conscious of something means that a mental representation is accompanied by, or embedded in, a second, higher-order representation to the effect that the system itself is in a certain state. The attractive feature of such concepts is that they could be a point of departure for the development of concrete hypotheses on the *realization* of such states in brains and possibly in other systems as well.

The higher-order representation (HOR) concept implies that phenomenal states cannot be understood in isolation. It resembles the concept that Kant introduced in the context of rejecting Hume's associationism. Phenomenal experience is not merely a succession or a "heap" of different cognitive states, but an integrated experience of a world of objects and of ourselves as subjects within it (Strawson 1966; van Gulick 1993). Phenomenal states are cognitive events that presuppose a model of the world and of the self, to which first-order representations can be bound. Information from different modalities and memory stores must be joined to one coherent representational structure.

If such representational structures are instantiated in a neural net, it will necessarily require the binding of segregated, widely distributed data into one Hebbian assembly. Thus, one consequence of the HOR concept would be to postulate the existence of large-scale neuronal assemblies and also a specific binding mechanism that makes such assemblies possible. The core of my hypothesis is that the NMDA synapse implements the binding mechanism that the brain uses to produce these large-scale representations to which HORs belong (Flohr 1991).

Baars (1988) proposed that one of the computational functions of consciousness is to broadcast information throughout the central nervous system. According to the present hypothesis, a rich set of activated associative links and widely available information is both the *precondition* for the occurrence of conscious states and the reason for the specific computational role they have. For

inner states Kant assumed a similar necessary interdependence between their connectedness, consciousness, and functional role. According to Kant's concept of synthesis, inner states must at least be capable of being connected with all other cognitive states in one consciousness to acquire the functional status of a mental representation (Kant 1781, A116; Strawson 1966; Kitcher 1990).

Psychedelic States

Having HORs—and that is a frequently heard objection against such theories—would require the ability to refer to oneself. And this, in turn, seems to entail the possession of some notion of the self, the representation of oneself to which other representational states can be bound. As mentioned above, it is typical for noncompetitive NMDA antagonists like ketamine and phencyclidine to cause bizarre ego disorders. Patients report what has been called an ego dissolution, a loosening of the ego boundaries that may end up in a feeling of merging with the cosmos, and an ego disintegration, i.e., a loss of control over thought processes. Like the anesthetic effects, these psychotomimetic effects of the noncompetitive NMDA antagonists are highly correlated with their relative affinity for the NMDA receptor. S(+) ketamine, which has a high affinity, is much more potent than the R(−) enantiomer (Vollenweider 1998). It follows that NMDA-dependent processes not only are essential for the occurrence of conscious states as such, but also determine the phenomenal content of these states. In particular, they are responsible for the HOR content that says I am in this very mental state. This is in accordance with the HOR hypothesis, which assumes that first-order representations must be connected with the representation of the self in order to produce the subjective character of conscious states. If this binding operation is disturbed, it will result in HORs whose phenomenal content seems different.

Psychedelic states can be caused by a variety of drugs. Most of these compounds are analogues of transmitter molecules and act preferentially upon specific synapses. Apart from the noncompetitive NMDA antagonists, four major groups of psychedelics are known that interact with cholinergic, noradrenergic, dopaminergic, or serotonergic synapses. Surprisingly, the psychological effects of these different drugs are very similar. All of them produce a psychosis-like syndrome that shares a number of symptoms with schizophrenia. In particular, all of these compounds produce ego disorders (Vollenweider 1998).

There have been attempts to explain the similarity of symptoms. Vollenweider (1998) has proposed that the disturbances arise from defects of sensory information processing in several cortico-striato-thalamo-cortical feedback loops. He assumes that in these loops cholinergic, noradrenergic, dopaminergic, serotonergic, and glutamatergic synapses are arranged in series so that pharmacological blockades at different links of the chain have the same outcome.

On the basis of the present hypothesis, however, an alternative explanation for the similarity of psychedelic states can be proposed that joins the pharmacology of psychedelic drugs with a realization theory for altered states of consciousness. The ascending reticular activating system consists—as we now know—of several discrete subsystems, each using a single neurotransmitter. *Cholinergic* projections arise in the nucleus basalis of Meynert; *dopaminergic*, in the ventral tegmental area; *noradrenergic*, in the locus coeruleus; and *serotonergic*, in the brain stem raphe nuclei. The cortical projections of all four subsystems are widely distributed, reaching into all cortical areas. It is therefore possible that the similar effects of pharmacological interventions into these different projection systems result from their convergence on a common cortical target, the cortical NMDA receptor.

Thus, the cortical NMDA receptors could be the final common target not only of anesthetics but also of psychedelic drugs. A similar mechanism has been suggested for the psychotic symptoms in schizophrenia (Flohr 1992). According to the present hypothesis, the primary cause of schizophrenic symptoms could be either a malfunction of the cortical NMDA synapses themselves (as stated by the NMDA hypothesis of schizophrenia), or, which is also possible in the account of the present hypothesis, a defect of subcortical systems (as is stated, for instance, by the dopamine hypothesis). In any case, the ultimate common cause of the altered states of consciousness would have to be located at the level of cortical information processing.

A Short Comment on Neural Correlates and Theories of Consciousness

Spotting a physiological state that is correlated with a conscious state or is a necessary condition for it does not *automatically* lead to an understanding of the relationship between brain processes and states of consciousness. Phenomenal states have numerous necessary conditions and countless physiological correlates. Most of them, it appears, are theoretically irrelevant. The problem consists in identifying the causally relevant factors that are close to the explanans.

How can this be done? The only possibility to decide upon the relevance or irrelevance of an empirical finding is within the framework of a theory. Brute correlations will not suffice. Beyond doubt, what is needed is a realization theory that will render the relations between brain events and states of consciousness intelligible. Such a theory would order the diverse empirical correlations and define which causes are relevant or proximal, and which are trivial.

Higher-order representation theories of consciousness attempt to reduce phenomenal states to specific cognitive events, the occurrence of higher-order, self-reflexive representations. They maintain that having such states is not only necessary but also sufficient for having phenomenal

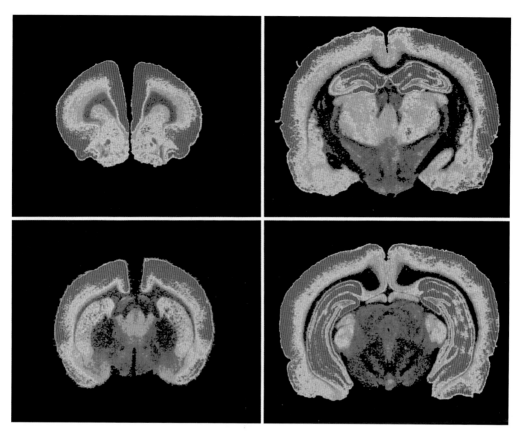

Plate 1

In vivo uptake of [³H]-MK-801 in the rat brain under awake conditions. [³H]-MK-801 was dissolved in saline and injected through a vene catheter at a dose of 600 mCi/kg. The animals were sacrificed by swift decapitation 1 min after the administration of the tracer. The brain was rapidly removed and frozen. Frozen sections were washed with TRIS maleate buffer to minimize nonreceptor-associated bindings, and subsequently air-dried. The sections were juxtaposed to [³H] Hyperfilm (Amersham, Buchler) for 60 days.

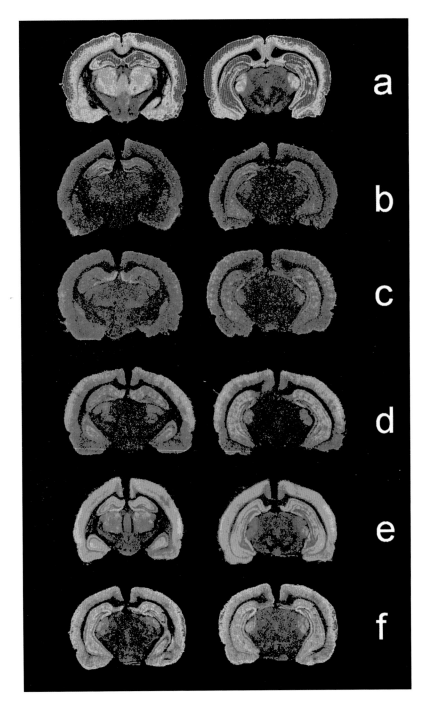

Plate 2

In vivo uptake of [^{3}H]-MK-801 under (b) ketamine (175 mg/kg), (c) Na-pentobarbital (110 mg/kg), (d) halothane, (e) ethanol (4 g/kg), and (f) propofol (180 mg/kg) anesthesia. Compared with the awake condition (a), the cortical indicator uptake is reduced in all forms of anesthesia.

experiences. This is an important step toward demystifying the notion of phenomenal states and, therefore, toward a realization theory. I do not share objections that this line of argumentation merely leads to a brute fact explanation or misses the explanandum, which is the phenomenal, subjective, experiential character of conscious states (Flohr 1994, 1995a). The explanatory value of the higher-order representation concepts, however, crucially depends on whether or not they can be made concrete and experimentally testable. What is needed is to transpose philosophical propositions into neurophysiological terms. The basic problem here is to develop hypotheses on how self-referential, higher-order representational states could be realized and generated in the brain. The attractive feature of the higher-order representation concept is that this is not impossible.

Summary

In this short review I have described a number of empirical facts demonstrating that the cortical NMDA synapse plays a key role in such physiological processes that instantiate consciousness, and I have tried to relate them to contemporary higher-order representation theories of consciousness. I have proposed six hypotheses:

1. The occurrence of brain states instantiating states of consciousness critically depends on a specific class of computational processes, those which produce higher-order, self-reflexive representational structures. These processes are mediated by the cortical NMDA synapse.

2. The NMDA synapse plays this crucial role because it implements the binding mechanism that the brain uses to produce large-scale neuronal cell assemblies. The spatiotemporal activity pattern of such assemblies instantiates higher-order mental representations.

3. The formation of large-scale assemblies depends on the rate at which changes in synaptic strength take place, and this in turn depends on the depolarization of the postsynaptic membrane of the cortical neurons. The state of the postsynaptic membrane determines the rate at which complex representational structures are actually developed. Large-scale assemblies will automatically emerge, if the degree of depolarization of the postsynaptic membrane is kept near the activation threshold of the NMDA receptor.

4. The occurrence of higher-order self-reflexive representations is necessary *and sufficient* for the occurrence of phenomenal states.

5. An (almost) complete inhibition of the NMDA-dependent processes, either directly or indirectly induced, leads to a loss of consciousness. It is the final common pathway of anesthetic action and of other causes of unconsciousness.

6. Partial inhibition of these processes leads to altered states of consciousness. It is the final common cause for drug-induced and naturally occurring psychotic states.

References

Adams, M. L., Meyer, E. R., Sewing, B. N., and Cicero, T. J. (1994). Effects of nitric oxide-related agents on alcohol narcosis. *Alcoholism, Clinical and Experimental Research* 18: 969–975.

Armstrong, D. (1980). *The Nature of Mind and Other Essays.* Ithaca, NY: Cornell University Press.

Baars, B. J. (1988). *A Cognitive Theory of Consciousness.* Cambridge: Cambridge University Press.

Boast, C. H., and Pastor, G. (1988). Characterization of motor activity patterns induced by N-methyl-D-aspartate antagonists in gerbils. *Journal of Pharmacology and Experimental Therapeutics* 247: 556–561.

Churchland, P. (1985). Reduction qualia and the direct introspection of brain states. *Journal of Philosophy* 82, no. 1: 2–28.

Corssen, G., and Domino, E. F. (1966). Dissociative anesthesia: Further pharmacologic studies and first clinical experience with the phencyclidine derivative CI–581. *Anesthesia and Analgesia* 45: 29–40.

Daniell, L. C. (1990). The non-competitive NMDA antagonists MK–801, phencyclidine and ketamine increase the potency of general anesthetics. *Pharmacology, Biochemistry and Behavior* 36: 111–115.

Daniell, L. C. (1991). Effects of CGS 19755, a competitive *N*-methyl-D-aspartate antagonist, on general anesthetic potency. *Pharmacology, Biochemistry and Behavior* 40: 767–869.

Daniell, L. C. (1992). Alteration of general anesthetic potency by agonists and antagonists of the polyamine binding site of the *N*-methyl-D-aspartate receptor. *Journal of Pharmacology and Experimental Therapeutics* 261: 304–310.

Flohr, H. (1991). Brain processes and phenomenal consciousness: A new and specific hypothesis. *Theory and Psychology* 1: 245–262.

Flohr, H. (1992). Qualia and brain processes. In A. Beckermann, H. Flohr, and J. Kim, eds., *Emergence or Reduction*, 220–238. Berlin and New York: De Gruyter.

Flohr, H. (1994). Die physiologischen Bedingungen des Bewußtseins. In H. Lenk and H. Poser, eds., *Neue Realitäten—Herausforderung der Philosophie*, 222–235. Berlin: Akademie Verlag.

Flohr, H. (1995a). Sensations and brain processes. *Behavioral Brain Research* 71: 157–161.

Flohr, H. (1995b). An information processing theory of anaesthesia. *Neuropsychologia* 33: 1169–1180.

Flohr, H., Glade, U., and Motzko, D. (1998). The role of the NMDA synapse in general anesthesia. *Toxicology Letters* 100–101: 23–29.

France, C. P., Winger, G. D., and Woods, J. H. (1990). Analgesic, anesthetic and respiratory effects of the competitive *N*-methyl-D-aspartate (NMDA) antagonist CGS 19755 in rhesus monkeys. *Brain Research* 526: 355–358.

Hebb, D. O. (1959). A neuropsychological theory. In S. Koch, ed., *Psychology: A Study of Science*, vol. 1, 622–643. New York: McGraw-Hill.

Ichinose, F., Huang, P. L., and Zapol, W. D. (1995). Effects of targeted neuronal nitric oxide synthase gene disruption and nitroG-L-arginine methylester on the threshold for isoflurane anesthesia. *Anesthesiology* 83: 101–108.

Irifune, M., Shimizu, T., Nomoto, M., and Fukuda, T. (1992). Ketamine-induced anesthesia involves the *N*-methyl-D-aspartate receptor-channel complex in mice. *Brain Research* 596: 1–9.

Jevtovic-Todorovic, V., Todorovic, S. M., Mennerick, S., Powell, S., Dikranian, K., Benshoff, N., Zorumski, C. F., and Olney, J. W. (1998). Nitrous oxide (laughing gas) is an NMDA antagonist, neuroprotectant and neurotoxin. *Nature Medicine* 4: 460–463.

Johns, R. A., Moscicki, J. C., and DiFazio, C. A. (1992). Nitric oxide synthase inhibitor dose-dependently and reversibly reduces the threshold for halothane anesthesia. *Anesthesiology* 77: 779–884.

Kant, I. (1781). *Kritik der reinen Vernunft*, 1 Aufl. Riga: Hartknoch.

Kitcher, P. W. (1990). *Kant's Transcendental Psychology*. New York: Oxford University Press.

Koek, W., Woods, J. H., and Ornstein, P. (1986). Phencyclidine-like behavioral effects in pigeons induced by systemic administration of the excitatory amino acid antagonist, 2-amino–5-phosphono-valerate. *Life Sciences* 39: 973–978.

Koek, W., Colpaert, F. C., Woods, J. H., and Kamenka, J. M. (1989). The phencyclidine (PCP) analog *N*-[1-(2-benzo (B)thiophenyl) cyclohexyl] piperidine shares cocaine-like but not other characteristic behavioral effects with PCP, ketamine and MK 801. *Journal of Pharmacology and Experimental Therapeutics* 250: 1019–1027.

Kuroda, Y., Strebel, S., Rafferty, C., and Bullock, R. (1993). Neuroprotective doses of *N*-methyl-D-aspartate receptor antagonists profoundly reduce the minimum alveolar anaesthetic concentration (MAC) for isoflurane in rats. *Anesthesia and Analgesia* 77: 795–800.

Lodge, D., Anis, N. A., and Burton, N. R. (1982). Effects of optical isomers of ketamine on excitation of cat and rat spinal neurons by amino acids and acetylcholine. *Neuroscience Letters* 29: 281–286.

Löscher, W., Fredow, G., and Ganter, M. (1991). Comparison of pharmacodynamic effects of the non-competitive NMDA receptor antagonists MK 801 and ketamine in pigs. *European Journal of Pharmacology* 192: 377–382.

Marietta, M. P., Way, W. L., Castagnoli, N., and Trevor, A. J. (1977). On the pharmacology of the ketamine enantiomorphs in the rat. *Journal of Pharmacology and Experimental Therapeutics* 202: 157–165.

Martin, D., and Lodge, D. (1988). Phencyclidine receptors and *N*-methyl-D-aspartate antagonism: Electrophysiologic data correlate with known behaviors. *Pharmacology, Biochemistry, and Behavior* 31: 279–286.

McFarlane, C., Warner, D. S., Nader, A., and Dexter, F. (1995). Glycine receptor antagonism. Effects of ACEA 1021 on the minimum alveolar concentration for halothane in the rat. *Anesthesiology* 82: 961–968.

McFarlane, C., Warner, D. S., Todd, M. M., and Nordholm, L. (1992). AMPA receptor competitive antagonism reduces halothane MAC in rats. *Anesthesiology* 77: 1165–1170.

Metzinger, T. (1999). *Subjekt und Selbstmodell.* Paderborn: Mentis.

Morgan, W. W., Bermudez, J., and Chang, X. (1991). The relative potency of pentobarbital in suppressing the kainic acid- or the *N*-methyl-D-aspartate acid-induced enhancement of cGMP in cerebellar cells. *European Journal of Pharmacology* 204: 335–338.

Motzko, D., Glade, U., Tober, C., and Flohr, H. (1998). 7-nitro indazole enhances methohexital anesthesia. *Brain Research* 788: 353–355.

Pajewski, T. N., DiFazio, C. A., Moscicki, J. C., and Johns, R. A. (1996). Nitric oxide synthase inhibitors, 7-nitro indazole and nitroG-L-arginine methyl ester, dose dependently reduce the threshold for isoflurane anesthesia. *Anesthesiology* 85: 1111–1119.

Perkins, W. J., and Morrow, D. R. (1992a). A dose-dependent reduction in halothane MAC in rats with a competitive *N*-methyl-D-aspartate (NMDA) receptor antagonist. *Anesthesia and Analgesia* 74: 233.

Perkins, W. J., and Morrow, D. R. (1992b). Correlation between anesthetic potency and receptor binding constant for non-competitive *N*-methyl-D-aspartate receptor antagonists. *Anesthesiology* 77: A742.

Rosenthal, D. (1986). Two concepts of consciousness. *Philosophical Studies* 49: 329–359.

Rosenthal, D. (1990). *A Theory of Consciousness.* Report no. 40/1990 on Mind and Brain, Perspectives in Theoretical Psychology and the Philosophy of Mind. ZiF, University of Bielefeld.

Rosenthal, D. (1993a). Thinking that one thinks. In M. Davies and G. Humphreys, eds., *Consciousness,* 197–223. Cambridge, MA: Blackwell.

Rosenthal, D. (1993b). Higher-order thoughts and the appendage theory of consciousness. *Philosophical Psychology* 6: 155–166.

Ryder, S., Way, W. L., and Trevor, A. J. (1978). Comparative pharmacology of the optical isomers of ketamine in mice. *European Journal of Pharmacology* 49: 15–23.

Scheller, M. S., Zornow, M. H., Fleischer, J. E., Shearman, G. T., and Greber, J. F. (1989). The noncompetitive NMDA receptor antagonist, MK 801, profoundly reduces volatile anesthetic requirements in rabbits. *Neuropharmacology* 28: 677–681.

Schüttler, J., Stanski, D. R., White, P. F., Trevor, A. J., Horai, Y., Verotta, D., and Sheiner, L. B. (1987). Pharmacodynamic modeling of the EEG effects of ketamine and its enantiomers in man. *Journal of Pharmacokinetics and Biopharmacy* 15: 241–253.

Strawson, P. F. (1966). *The Bounds of Sense: An Essay on Kant's Critique of Pure Reason.* London: Methuen.

Terasako, K., Nakamura, K., Miyawaki, I., Toda, H., Kakuyuma, M., and Kenjiro, M. (1994). Inhibitory effects of anesthetics on cyclic guanosine monophosphate (cGMP) accumulation in rat cerebellar slices. *Anesthesia and Analgesia* 78: 823–830.

Tonner, P. H., Scholz, J., Lamberz, L., Schlamp, N., and Schulte am Esch, J. (1997). Inhibition of nitric oxide synthase decreases anesthetic requirements of intravenous anesthetics in Xenopus laevis. *Anesthesiology* 87: 1479–1485.

van Gulick, R. (1993). Understanding the phenomenal mind: Are we all just armadillos? In M. Davies and G. Humphreys, eds., *Consciousness,* pp. 137–154. Cambridge, MA: Blackwell.

Vollenweider, F. X. (1998). Advances and pathophysiological models of hallucinogenic drug action in humans: A preamble to schizophrenia research. *Pharmacopsychiatry* 31: 92–103.

Vuilliemoz, Y., Shen, H., and Virag, L. (1996). Alpha-2-adrenoreceptor agonists decrease cyclic guanosine 3′,5′-monophosphate in the mouse brain. *Anesthesiology* 85: 544–550.

White, P. F., Ham, J., Way, W. L., and Trevor, A. J. (1980). Pharmacology of ketamine isomers in surgical patients. *Anesthesiology* 52: 231–239.

Woods, J. M. (1989). Consciousness. *Pharmacology, Biochemistry and Behavior* 32: 1081.

Zeilhofer, H. U., Swandulla, D., Geisslinger, G., and Brune, K. (1992). Differential effects of ketamine enantiomers on NMDA receptor currents in cultured neurons. *European Journal of Pharmacology* 213: 155–158.

Zuo, Z., De Vente, J., and Johns, R. A. (1996). Halothane and isoflurane dose-dependently inhibit the cyclic GMP increase caused by *N*-methyl-D-aspartate in rat cerebellum: Novel localization and quantitation by in vitro autoradiography. *Neuroscience* 74: 1069–1075.

Zuo, Z., and Johns, R. A. (1995). Halothane, enflurane, and isoflurane do not affect the basal or agonist-stimulated activity of partially isolated soluble and particulate guanyl cyclases of rat brain. *Anesthesiology* 83: 395–404.

Valerie Gray Hardcastle

Consciousness studies, like most areas of study, is replete with cottage industries and fads. Last year it was the "Hard Problem" (see Chalmers 1996), the follow-up to the "Explanatory Gap" (see Levine 1983). This year, perhaps in response to the difficulties in convincing skeptics that the Hard Problem is really an Easy Problem or No Problem at All, finding the neural correlates of consciousness (the NCC) is in vogue. At first blush this might seem a more reasonable puzzle to tackle than something like the Hard Problem, since being a "correlate" is ontologically neutral. All we are doing is looking for the physiological differences between someone who is conscious and someone who is not. Seeking the NCC is feasible even if one has not solved—or dissolved—the Hard Problem.

Still, uncovering the NCC is not as straightforward as it may seem, for which correlates should count as *the* NCC is a nontrivial question. It is not an empirical difficulty I am alluding to here, though obviously it is that, too. I am concerned with a deeper and prior methodological or philosophical question: How do we pick out the correlate from boundless other spurious coincidences, given that we have to draw our conclusion from spotty and indirect evidence? This is a question about the appropriate level of analysis in the brain for understanding and explaining cognitive events, and a question about how to make convincing cases for inductive inferences using less than stellar data.

I focus here on this larger issue. I take as my stalking horse Flohr's identification of the NCC with the NMDA receptors in cortex, for this is a particularly rich and well-developed proposal. I note that there are others, including Baars and Newman's reticular formation, Crick and Koch's (and others') 40 Hz oscillations, my own activation in parietal cortex, and Hameroff's microtubules (Baars and Newman 1994; Crick and Koch 1990; Hardcastle 1995; Hameroff

1994). The worries I raise here are equally applicable to any and all of these.

Flohr's Hypothesis

Flohr claims Hebb is right (see Hebb 1949. The present section draws on Flohr 1992, 1995a, 1995b; Flohr et al. 1998). Brains are plastic. Any activity between synapses strengthens the connections, so postsynaptic neurons fire more readily the next time around. Inactivity weakens synaptic connections, so postsynaptic cells are more difficult to provoke into firing later. The brain's mantra is "use it or lose it." This so-called Hebbian learning rule means that brains will develop complexes of neurons which prefer to fire together when a subset of them is stimulated. These assemblies, say Flohr and Hebb, are the building blocks for mental representations.

Unlike Hebb, though, Flohr, along with von der Malsburg (1981), holds that there are two ways to create cell assemblies. Permanent change occurs slowly, over a period of considerable time and repeated activations. Transient assemblies are also possible, and these occur quite rapidly, on the order of 100 msecs. Flohr's research has indicated that the NMDA receptors are responsible for both types of changes.

Some of the rapid, transient cell assemblies, some representations, are conscious. Conscious representations are the self-reflexive cell assemblies, the cell assemblies that refer to the current state of the brain as well as to something external to the brain, those which refer to the brain itself referring to something else. According to Flohr, being a system that has second-order representations is a necessary condition for having phenomenal experiences. Whether it is also sufficient is still unclear.

A second neurophysiological item important for consciousness is the ascending reticular activating system. Bilateral lesions of the reticular formation lead to deep coma and, Flohr presumes, unconsciousness. Somehow the reticular formation, an unspecific activating system, interacts with specific transient cell assemblies to produce, enhance, or modify consciousness. Flohr hypothesizes that this system determines how likely it is that a cell assembly forms as well as aids in binding together several simple assemblies into more complex representational states. If cell assemblies are created quickly enough, then the system is conscious: "An unconscious state is present if the rate at which plastic changes take place falls below a critical threshold" (Flohr 1995b: 160).

In his theory, Flohr outlines many of different events in the brain that covary with consciousness: self-reflexive representations, rapidly changing cell assemblies, activation in the reticular formation, NMDA receptor-driven synaptic change. It strikes me that all are possible candidates for *the* NCC. Flohr, however, has no difficulty in choosing the one item he believes is crucially responsible for consciousness: "The occurrence of states of consciousness critically depends on a specific class of computational processes that are mediated by the NMDA synapse." Because "the direct or indirect disruption of NMDA-dependent processes is the common operative mechanism of anesthetic action," he concludes that "the essential difference between anesthetized brains and conscious brains consists in the presence or absence of NMDA-dependent computational processes" (Flohr et al. 1998: 28). According to Flohr, NMDA-sponsored computations are the NCC we have been looking for.

Let us leave aside some of the potential difficulties of this view—for example, why Flohr wants to claim that NMDA synapses are crucial for consciousness, even though their activity is just as essential for nonconscious cell assemblies (the nonreflexive ones, or the ones that do not fluctuate rapidly enough). Let us just assume that Flohr's theory is correct in its entirety: A

phenomenological experience boils down to a reflexive cognitive thought, which, neurophysiologically speaking, is a complex and transient cell assembly in cortex, underwritten by activity from the reticular formation and made possible by the NMDA receptors and their computational properties.

So which *is* the NCC? The cell assembly itself, as I have argued? The reticular formation, as Baars and Newman claim? The NMDA receptors with their computational properties, as Flohr believes? Or perhaps their internal quantum effects, as Hammeroff holds? And how do we know that *this* is the NCC? All are correlated with the qualia, after all.

Screening Off

The trivial answer to this concern is to seek the event that is both necessary and sufficient for consciousness. Can creatures with cell assemblies but no reticular activating systems be conscious? How about those with a reticular activating formation but no NMDA receptors? Or NMDA receptors with different computational effects? Or the same computational effects but with different underlying quantum interactions? If we just run the right sort of experiment, we should be able to separate the genuine effect from mere experimental artifact or interesting coincidence.

The investigative strategy that philosophers of science advocate for determining the actual cause of an event is to determine which putative cause "screens off" the others (see Cartwright 1970; Eells 1988; Hardcastle 1991, 1998; Salmon 1971; Wimsatt 1984). In general, we say that one putative cause, A, screens off another, B, from the effect we are interested in if the probability of the effect occurring is the same regardless of whether we have A and B occurring or just A, but the probability is not the same if we have just B. In other words, having B does not add anything to the system; A is actually doing the causal work.

To see how the screening-off relation functions, consider an example unrelated to consciousness: the units of selection controversy in evolutionary biology (see Brandon 1982). We would say that the phenotype A screens off the genotype B—and hence is the causally relevant factor—with respect to reproductive success if (1) we can affect reproductive success by changing the phenotype, (2) we can change the phenotype without altering the genotype, and (3) changing the genotype does not affect reproductive success.

A screening-off analysis can be run either horizontally or vertically. That is, we can use it to determine which cause is "closest" to the event to be explained and thus is the most proximal cause. Or we can use it to determine which level of organization of matter is appropriate for describing the phenomena. The units of selection debate can be understood as an example of the former case. Phenotypes emerge through the interaction of genes, the various kinds of RNA, and the environment. DNA comes first; the phenotype later. Since phenotypes screen off genotypes, we know that phenotypic traits are the most proximate relevant causal factor in reproductive success.

The conflict between psychiatric and neurobiological explanations in relation to something like depression illustrates the vertical dimension of a causal analysis. On the one hand, we might want to claim Fred is depressed because he learned that he has cancer. The cognitive event of understanding that one has a potentially fatal disease is the causally relevant factor in explaining Fred's change in mood. On the other hand, we might also want to claim that Fred is depressed because the amount of norepinephrine in his brain has dropped. The amount of a particular neurotransmitter is the causally relevant factor in explaining Fred's change in mood. Which explanation is the correct one? Which one picks out *the* cause of Fred's depression?

To answer these questions, we need to know whether cognitive events screen off neuro-physiological ones, or vice versa. Is the probability greater that Fred will get depressed if he learns he has cancer or if he learns he has cancer and his norepinephrine level drops? Or is the probability greater that Fred will get depressed if his norepinephrine level drops, but he hasn't learned anything new? Research indicates that neurotransmitter levels are better indicators of depression—Fred is more likely to get depressed if his norepinephrine level drops than if he receives some bad news—hence, we should look to neurophysiology and biochemistry to understand large-scale mood swings. In this case, changes in our brain chemistry screen off psychological events.

Discerning the neural correlates of consciousness is also a vertical problem. We want to know which level of organization in the brain is the appropriate one for understanding consciousness. Which events in the brain—the assemblies themselves, NMDA computations, or microtubule activity—are most closely associated with conscious experiences? Which predict its appearance best?

At the moment, it is too early to tell. Nevertheless, the sorts of experiments we have to run in order to determine whether NMDA computations screen off the other possibilities are clear.

Experiments in Consciousness Studies

Naturally, running the right sorts of experiments is easier said than done. In fact, it is probably impossible to do. The first (and very obvious) point is that we have only indirect access to conscious experience. In general, we take verbal reports (or related behaviors) to be by-and-large veridical descriptions of phenomenological experiences. And we take lack of verbal report as evidence for not being conscious. These facts mean that whatever we believe about the presence or absence of consciousness is going to be skewed by our beliefs about language and mnemonic processing, on the one hand, and subjects' capacities for self-report and memory, on the other. While we all recognize that saying something doesn't make it so, in practice it is much more difficult to devise experimental tasks that do not explicitly assume this.

Our reliance on verbal reports of either previous or current experiences, and reporting's dependence on linguistic and mnemonic capacities, means that we cannot be entirely sure when someone or something is conscious. Most researchers hold that anesthesia, stage 4 sleep, and deep coma render organisms unconscious. These are dubious assumptions at best. Why would they think this? It is true that one can only rarely, and then only with difficulty, report any phenomenological experiences when roused from one of those states. However, it is not at all clear that this isn't a problem with memory—we cannot remember what we experience when we are in those states. Or perhaps it is a problem with linguistic access to these memories—we can remember these states, but we cannot put these memories into words. Since both memory and language mediate our access to others' conscious mental states, we cannot devise experiments that compare test subjects with phenomenological experiences against nonexperiencing controls in a reasonably pure form. Though we may have paradigm instances of conscious experiences, we certainly do not have pure and uncontroversial cases of unconsciousness (except perhaps in the case of death, but then there are too many other confounding features for good experimental practice).

This latter fact is important because most consciousness theorists rely on juxtaposing paradigm cases of conscious experience with presumed cases of nonconsciousness to support their pet hypotheses. But if we cannot be certain that someone is unconscious, we cannot use the differences between that person and our conscious subject to support any ideas concerning what in the brain is associated with phenomenological processing. Consequently, we lose all contrastive data used in the NCC discussions,

and this accounts for most of the data in consciousness studies.

Bilateral lesions in the reticular formation cause deep coma from which patients cannot be roused. It is reasonable to conclude that the reticular formation is somehow tied to alertness. But what does this fact have to say about conscious experience? Next to nothing, I should think, since people in a deep coma cannot report what their experiences are like, or if they had any. If we already knew that the reticular formation is the NCC, then we could predict that patients with damaged reticular formations have diminished consciousness; but we don't know that yet.

Certainly, the differences between alert and anesthetized patients drive Flohr's theory. Patients under anesthesia cannot be roused. It is reasonable to conclude that anesthesia is also tied to level of alertness. But, again, what does this fact have to say about conscious experience? Still next to nothing, since patients under anesthesia cannot report what their experiences are like, or if they had any. If we already knew that anesthesia blocks consciousness, then we could predict that patients under anesthesia are unconscious; but we don't know that yet. In short, most evidence touted as relevant to consciousness is still nonevidence. Designing the appropriate experiments for uncovering the neurophysiological event that screens off the others vertically is a nontrivial task.

The Pragmatics of Consciousness Research

What should we do? Given the constraints on gathering data, how are we supposed to determine the NCC? Even if we suppose that Flohr's theory is correct, how can we prove that NMDA computations screen off everything else?

The short answer is that we should turn to the pragmatic aspects of explanation and the various explanatory heuristics that science has adopted (for better or ill) over time. Wimsatt (1984) argues that we should relax our notion of screening off. In actual science, with real-world constraints, we perform a cost-benefit analysis so that we would say A "effectively" screens off B if adding B to our explanation increases our understanding of the effect by only a small amount and B is difficult or expensive to procure. Determining whether some variable screens off another is partially a pragmatic decision. In all explanations, some otherwise relevant events are set aside as not being significant enough to warrant including. Not all causal influences are created equal, and we need worry about only the most obvious in our explanations and research.

Which NCC we choose will be at least partially determined by which gives us the most bang for the buck, as it were. This concession to the social pressures on science goes a bit of the way toward solving our problem. We need not worry about the conscious experiences of creatures with brains very different from our own, since we have little to no access to their mental lives—what is it like to be a bat—and such data would be very difficult to get.

But it does not solve our central concern, the vertical question of which event, at which level of organization, in the human brain is most closely associated with consciousness. Data that separate NMDA receptor computations from their quantum effects or the formation of cell assemblies are, at least for the moment, impossible to get for intact brains. Is determining the NCC an insurmountable problem, too?

We have one explanatory move left to us, and that is to turn to previously accepted explanatory heuristics in science: Simpler is better; consilience and parsimony are preferred; and so forth. These set the standards for ideal explanations. The best explanation of some phenomenon is one that is very simple to model mathematically, contains few variables, and dovetails nicely with previously accepted theories. These sorts of explanatory goals inform scientists' hypothesizing. No one is going to propose, much less have accepted, a complicated theory if there is a simpler one available.

In biology and neuroscience, there has been a distinct bias toward reductionism: the assumption is that the smaller the unit of analysis, the better, for the more fundamental processes occur at the lower levels of organization. With this bias in place, we should say that the NCC is most likely the smallest unit we can discern which covaries with consciousness. In this case, someone like Flohr or Hammeroff would be right: The neural correlate of consciousness is probably something like receptor computations or quantum effects.

Recently, however, this propensity toward "smallism" has come under fire. (I take the term "smallism" from Wilson 1999.) With the increasing popularity of large-scale dynamical systems explanations of brain phenomena, we are losing our unspoken agreement that the real stuff occurs down below and the surface appearances are mere reflections of the underlying causal interactions. We are finding champions of "largism" at every turn. They disdain the small as irrelevant data, and seek true understanding in the large-scale patterns that emerge out of the mess of tiny interactions, each of which is insignificant when considered alone. A largist would claim that the complex cell assemblies are the true NCC, whereas the microtubules and NMDA receptors merely support the assemblies.

Which way should we jump? Which explanatory bias should we adopt in consciousness studies? Unfortunately, the answer is not forthcoming at the moment. We are caught in an odd time; a war over explanatory biases in the biological sciences is being fought in journals and laboratory hallways around the world. Some neurobiological explanations are reductionistic; others are not. And neither type has the upper hand at the moment with respect to explanatory power, funding decisions, centrality in the profession, and the like (see Hardcastle 1999).

Hence, we cannot say with any certainty how we should understand the NCC. We are simply going to have to wait and see which side wins. Whether we should be smallists or largists in our biological explanations of mental events is currently undetermined. For now, we have only educated guesses, personal declarations of faith, and a plethora of individual research programs. But much basic research remains to be done and, more important for our concerns, our fundamental theoretical scaffolding remains to be constructed. For now, the NCC remains a truly Hard Problem with no solution in sight.

References

Baars, B., and Newman, J. (1994). A neurobiological interpretation of global workspace theory. In A. Revonsuo and M. Kampinen, eds., *Consciousness in Philosophy and Cognitive Neuroscience*, 211–226. Hillsdale, NJ: Lawrence Erlbaum.

Brandon, R. N. (1982). The levels of selection. In *PSA 1982*, vol. 1, 315–323. East Lansing, MI: Philosophy of Science Association.

Cartwright, N. (1979). Causal laws and effective strategies. *Nous* 13: 419–437.

Chalmers, D. (1996). *The Conscious Mind: In Search of a Fundamental Theory*. New York: Oxford University Press.

Crick, F. H. C., and Koch, C. (1990). Towards a neurobiological theory of consciousness. *Seminars in Neuroscience* 2: 263–275.

Eells, E. (1988). Probabilistic causal laws. In B. Skyrms and W. I. Harper, eds., *Causation, Chance, and Credence*, vol. 1, 109–133. New York: Reidel.

Flohr, H. (1992). Qualia and brain processes. In A. Beckerman, H. Flohr, and J. Kim, eds., *Emergence or Reduction? Essays on the Prospects of Nonreductive Physicalism*, 220–238. New York: Walter de Gruyter.

Flohr, H. (1995a). An information processing theory of anesthesia. *Neuropsychologia* 33: 1169–1180.

Flohr, H. (1995b). Sensations and brain processes. *Behavioral Brain Research* 71: 157–161.

Flohr, H., Glade, U., and Motzko, D. (1998). The role of the NMDA synapse in general anesthesia. *Toxicology Letters* 100–101: 23–29.

Hameroff, S. (1994). Quantum coherence in microtubules: A neural basis for emergent consciousness. *Journal of Consciousness Studies* 1: 91–118.

Hardcastle, V. G. (1991). Partitions, probabilistic laws, and Simpson's paradox. *Synthese* 86: 209–228.

Hardcastle, V. G. (1995). *Locating Consciousness*. Amsterdam: John Benjamins Press.

Hardcastle, V. G. (1998). On the matter of mental causation. *Philosophy and Phenomenological Research*, IVIII: 1–25.

Hardcastle, V. G. (1999). What we do not know about the brain. *Journal of the History and Philosophy of the Biological and Medical Sciences* 30: 69–89.

Hebb, D. O. (1949). *The Organization of Behavior*. New York: Wiley.

Levine, J. (1983). Materialism and qualia: The explanatory gap. *Pacific Philosophical Quarterly* 64: 354–361.

Salmon, W. (1971). *Statistical Explanation and Statistical Relevance*. Pittsburgh: University of Pittsburgh Press.

von der Malsburg, C. (1981). The correlation theory of brain functioning. Internal Report 81–2. Göttingen: Max-Planck Institut. for Biophysical Chemistry. Reprinted in Schulten, K., and von Hemmen, J. (1994) *Models of Neural Networks*, Band 2. Berlin.

Wilson, R. A. (1999). The individual in biology and psychology. In V. G. Hardcastle, ed., *Biology Meets Psychology: Conjectures, Connections, Constraints*. Cambridge, MA: MIT Press.

Wimsatt, W. C. (1984). Reductive explanation: A functional account. In E. Sober, ed., *Conceptual Issues and Their Biases in the Units of Selection Controversy*, 142–183. Cambridge, MA: MIT Press.

18 The Role of NMDA Receptors in Consciousness: What Can We Learn from Anesthetic Mechanisms?

Nicholas P. Franks and William R. Lieb

How general anesthetics are able to render a patient unconscious and insensible to pain has sometimes been thought to be almost as mysterious as consciousness itself. General anesthetics obey none of the conventional pharmacological rules: No specific chemical groups are necessary for their activity, there are no known antagonists (except, bizarrely, high pressure), and anesthetic agents vary from complex molecules such as steroids and barbiturates to "inert" gases such as xenon (Franks and Lieb 1982, 1987, 1994). It seems reasonable to suppose that an understanding of how anesthetics exert their effects in the brain might cast some light on the neuronal basis of consciousness. This chapter addresses this issue, with particular reference to the hypothesis that NMDA receptors at glutamatergic synapses play a central role both in the conscious state and as the ultimate targets for anesthetic action (Flohr 1995a, 1995b).

What Is General Anesthesia?

The first thing to appreciate about general anesthetics is that they are capable of doing far more than simply rendering a patient unconscious. As the anesthetic concentration increases, a whole spectrum of neurological and physiological effects occur, and these can be rather different for different anesthetics (although obviously the ability to cause loss of consciousness is shared by all agents). Table 18.1 outlines four "stages" of anesthesia, first described for diethyl ether.

Given this complex spectrum of effects, general anesthesia usually is operationally defined as the loss of a well-defined and easily measured end point. Although several have been used over the years, there are two of particular importance. First is the failure of a patient to respond purposefully to a verbal command. Roughly speaking, one can consider this as corresponding to a loss of consciousness. Second, at higher concentrations, a patient will not respond purposefully to a painful stimulus (such as a surgical incision). This "depth" of anesthesia would be appropriate for a surgical procedure.

For any given general anesthetic, therefore, concentrations can be determined that achieve either of these end points in 50 percent of a population of subjects. Such EC_{50} concentrations for the intravenous general anesthetic thiopental are given in table 18.2. As can be seen, the concentration of thiopental needed to render a patient unconscious is considerably less than that needed to prevent the response to a painful stimulus. A similar picture emerges with other anesthetics. For comparison, concentrations are also given in table 2 for two end points used with rats (failure to respond to a painful stimulus,

Table 18.1
Four stages of progressively deepening general anaesthesia

Stage	Description
Stage I	Analgesia. The patient is conscious but drowsy. The degree of analgesia depends greatly on the anesthetic.
Stage II	Excitement. The patient loses consciousness and will not respond to a nonpainful stimulus. The subject may move and talk incoherently, and may exhibit respiratory and cardiovascular irregularities.
Stage III	Surgical anesthesia. Spontaneous movement ceases and respiration becomes regular. As anesthesia deepens, various reflexes are lost and the muscles relax.
Stage IV	Medullary depression. Respiration and vasomotor control cease, leading to death.

Source: Rang et al. 1995.

Table 18.2
Anesthetic endpoints and free aqueous concentrations for thiopental

Human		Rat	
End point	Thiopental (μM)	End point	Thiopental (μM)
Response to verbal command	9	Righting reflex	9
Response to painful stimulus (surgical incision)	23	Response to painful stimulus (tail clamp)	22

Sources: Becker 1978; Hung et al. 1992; Gustafson et al. 1996.

such as a tail clamp, and the loss of the righting reflex). It is worth noting that, for many anesthetics, the concentrations required to prevent the response to a verbal command in humans are comparable with the concentrations required to cause a loss of righting reflex in other animals.

Most emphasis in general anesthesia research has, understandably, been directed toward identifying those targets which are relevant to the state of surgical anesthesia rather than loss of consciousness. For those interested in consciousness, therefore, this should be borne in mind when reading the anesthesia literature.

Which Molecular Targets Are Relevant to General Anesthesia?

During the 1990s, great progress was made toward understanding how general anesthetics act at the molecular level. The traditional view was that anesthetics are very "nonselective" and act by dissolving in the lipid bilayer portions of nerve membranes and changing their properties in such a way as to disrupt the functioning of some crucial membrane proteins (such as ion channels). This idea dates back to the turn of the twentieth century, when Meyer and Overton independently showed that anesthetic potency was well correlated with fat solubility. However, it has since been shown that not only are lipid bilayers very little affected by clinically relevant concentrations of general anesthetics (Franks and Lieb 1982, 1978), but the Meyer-Overton correlation can be more plausibly interpreted in terms of the anesthetics binding directly to protein molecules (Franks and Lieb 1984). Moreover, this explanation readily accounts for certain exceptions to the Meyer-Overton correlation (e.g., anesthetic optical isomers often have different anesthetic potencies) (Franks and Lieb 1994). The idea that anesthetics act by binding directly to proteins rather than lipids has led to an appreciation that anesthetics can be quite selective at the molecular level, with some targets being much more sensitive than others. But which ones are important for general anesthesia?

Certain criteria need to be addressed when considering whether a particular molecular target is relevant or not. The first is whether its function is significantly perturbed at pharmacologically relevant concentrations of anesthetics. This may seem obvious, but it has not always been easy to establish, because researchers have often been uncritical about which anesthetic concentrations to use experimentally. A common error is to use free aqueous anesthetic concentrations far higher than needed to produce general anesthesia. Also, even when relevant concentrations are used, it can be difficult to know whether or not an effect observed at the molecular level is physiologically significant.

Work with voltage-gated calcium channels provides an excellent example. These ubiquitous channels are responsible, among other things, for triggering the release of neurotransmitter at a chemical synapse when the presynaptic nerve terminal is depolarized by an action potential. It is probably fair to say that the majority of papers which have concluded that anesthetic effects on these channels are substantial used concentrations considerably in excess of those which are pharmacologically relevant. In fact, these channels are, like most voltage-gated channels, relatively insensitive to general anesthetics, although small inhibitions are observed at appropriate concentrations (Franks and Lieb 1993, 1994; Hall et al. 1994). The question then remains: Given the importance of voltage-gated calcium channels, are these small inhibitions nonetheless pharmacologically relevant? Conversely, some ion channels are "too sensitive" to anesthetics. For example, volatile agents can inhibit neuronal nicotinic acetylcholine receptors at extremely low concentrations (Violet et al. 1997), but their relevance to anesthesia is difficult to assess because their importance in CNS function is unclear. Clearly, additional criteria (other than sensitivity) are needed.

One useful criterion exploits the fact that general anesthesia often displays stereoselectivity (Franks and Lieb 1994). In other words, for optically active anesthetics, the optical isomers (enantiomers) often display different anesthetic potencies. The strategy here is to use these animal potencies as a guide to which molecular targets are most relevant. One important result that has emerged from these studies is the possibility that some agents may act predominantly on a small number of molecular targets. This conclusion has been drawn from the fact that the stereoselectivities observed in vitro for a given anesthetic are never much greater than those found in animals. This implies there cannot be a large number of genetically unrelated targets. For some anesthetics a single target can account for many of the central actions of the drug, and it is useful to consider two such agents, etomidate and ketamine, when considering the validity of the NMDA receptor hypothesis.

Etomidate and Ketamine

Etomidate is a potent intravenous general anesthetic that has minimal effects on the cardiovascular and respiratory systems. It is a carboxylated imidazole compound that contains a single asymmetric carbon atom and thus exists in two mirror-image enantiomeric forms, with R(+)-etomidate being approximately 15 times more potent as an anesthetic than S(−)-etomidate (Tomlin et al. 1998). It turns out that there are relatively few molecular targets that show any significant sensitivity to R(+)-etomidate, with one notable exception: the GABA$_A$ receptor. This important inhibitory neurotransmitter-gated receptor channel is markedly potentiated by etomidate at clinically relevant concentrations and, importantly, it displays a stereoselectivity toward etomidate comparable with that found for anesthetic potencies in animals (Tomlin et al. 1998). (Incidentally, according to Tomlin et al. [1998], etomidate shows no stereoselectivity when interacting with lipid bilayers.) It has recently been found that GABA$_A$ receptors which contain either the β_2 or β_3 subunits show a particularly high sensitivity to etomidate (Belelli et al. 1997). It is highly likely that etomidate acts very selectively and exerts its major effects by potentiating the activities of GABA$_A$ receptor channels, with little involvement of other CNS targets.

Ketamine is another intravenous anaesthetic that may exert its effects largely at a single molecular target, although not the GABA$_A$ receptor. (In fact, ketamine is one of the very few anesthetics that do not potentiate the GABA$_A$ receptor [Franks and Lieb 1994; Brockmeyer et al. 1995]. It appears to act by blocking the aqueous pore of the NMDA receptor channel [MacDonald et al. 1987]). This conclusion has been drawn not only on grounds of sensitivity (Anis et al. 1983) but also because the NMDA receptor displays a stereoselectivity for ketamine very similar to that found for general anesthesia in animals, with the S(+) enantiomer being approximately three times more potent than the R(−) enantiomer (Lodge 1982; Zeilhofer et al. 1992; White et al. 1985; Ryder et al. 1978).

Although it is certainly possible that other molecular targets will be found which are important in the anesthetic states induced by these agents (particularly ketamine), it seems safe to conclude that, at the very least, these anesthetics cause loss of consciousness by directly binding to and affecting very different molecular targets: Etomidate potentiates the inhibitory $GABA_A$ receptor channel, while ketamine inhibits the excitatory NMDA receptor channel. How does this bear on the NMDA hypothesis?

Critique of the NMDA Hypothesis

Hans Flohr has developed two distinct lines of argument (Flohr 1995a, 1995b) to support his hypothesis: (1) a philosophical argument, based on the idea that NMDA receptor activity is capable of forming "representational states" in the brain, and (2) an argument which claims that all general anesthetics ultimately inhibit NMDA receptor activity, and hence NMDA receptor activity must be essential for consciousness. We will leave the philosophical argument to the philosophers, although we are bound to say that we find the arguments for and against far from compelling. The argument based on experimental evidence, however, is tantalizing.

There is no doubt that ketamine causes loss of consciousness at high enough doses. There is also good evidence that it acts predominantly on NMDA receptors (although there remains some doubt that this is its only important target) (Hirota and Lambert 1996). Thus one probably can safely conclude that the normal functioning of NMDA receptors is *necessary* for consciousness. But of course the normal functioning of all sorts of molecular and cellular systems must be necessary for consciousness. Flohr's hypothesis is far more specific, and interesting, because it states that the normal functioning of NMDA receptors is directly responsible for consciousness. It therefore follows that drugs like etomidate, which, as discussed above, almost certainly act via $GABA_A$ receptors, must indirectly inhibit NMDA receptor activity. This is certainly easy

to imagine, and there is some experimental evidence that supports this view (as discussed in chapter 16). If we suppose, as seems reasonable, that the normal firing of a certain subset of neurons in the brain is necessary for consciousness, and these neurons contain NMDA receptors, then obviously anesthetics that act by blocking NMDA receptors would act directly on these neurons, among others. Anesthetics that acted via $GABA_A$ receptors, on the other hand, could do so either because these receptors were present on the same neurons, or because they inhibited another set of neurons which then inhibited the critical "consciousness neurons."

There is, however, the difficult question of whether the state of unconsciousness induced by ketamine is the same as that induced by etomidate. Both drugs certainly cause unconsciousness (using the simplest of criteria), but the pharmacological profiles of ketamine and etomidate differ in a number of important ways. For example, ketamine induces powerful psychotomimetic effects (Bowdle et al. 1998) and is a potent analgesic (Marshall et al. 1996). Indeed, these properties seem characteristic of several NMDA antagonists. Etomidate, however, does not have these properties (Marshall et al. 1996). If etomidate acts by ultimately inhibiting NMDA receptors, why does it not produce analgesia? The answer could lie in the different distributions of NMDA and $GABA_A$ receptors in the brain and spinal cord, or on neuronal connectivity.

Unfortunately, these sorts of explanations open up a slippery slope of special pleading arguments that make the hypothesis less and less appealing because, we feel, they could be used to explain away almost any experimental result that challenged the theory. Overall, then, our view is that one of the apparent strengths of this interesting idea is also one of its weaknesses— namely, that it is capable of explaining almost everything. Nonetheless, Flohr's ideas are certainly of sufficient interest to justify serious attempts to design experiments that may provide definitive tests of his NMDA hypothesis.

References

Anis, N. A., Berry, S. C., Burton, N. R., and Lodge, D. (1983). The dissociative anaesthetics, ketamine and phencyclidine, selectively reduce excitation of central mammalian neurones by N-methyl-aspartate. *British Journal of Pharmacology* 79: 565–575.

Becker, K. E., Jr. (1978). Plasma levels of thiopental necessary for anesthesia. *Anesthesiology* 49: 192–196.

Belelli, D., Lambert, J. J., Peters, J. A., Wafford, K., and Whiting, P. J. (1997). The interaction of the general anesthetic etomidate with the γ-aminobutyric acid type A receptor is influenced by a single amino acid. *Proceedings of the National Academy of Sciences USA* 94: 11031–11036.

Bowdle, T. A., et al. (1998). Psychedelic effects of ketamine in healthy volunteers: Relationship to steady-state plasma concentrations. *Anesthesiology* 88: 82–88.

Brockmeyer, D. M., and Kendig, J. J. (1995). Selective effects of ketamine on amino acid-mediated pathways in neonatal rat spinal cord. *British Journal of Anaesthesia* 74: 79–84.

Flohr, H. (1995a). An information processing theory of anaesthesia. *Neuropsychologia* 33: 1169–1180.

Flohr, H. (1995b). Sensations and brain processes. *Behavioural Brain Research* 71: 157–161.

Franks, N. P., and Lieb, W. R. (1978). Where do general anaesthetics act? *Nature* 274: 339–342.

Franks, N. P., and Lieb, W. R. (1982). Molecular mechanisms of general anaesthesia. *Nature* 300: 487–493.

Franks, N. P., and Lieb, W. R. (1984). Do general anaesthetics act by competitive binding to specific receptors? *Nature* 310: 599–601.

Franks, N. P., and Lieb, W. R. (1987). What is the molecular nature of general anaesthetic target sites? *Trends Pharmacological Sciences* 8: 169–174.

Franks, N. P., and Lieb, W. R. (1993). Selective actions of volatile general anaesthetics at molecular and cellular levels. *British Journal of Anaesthesia* 71: 65–86.

Franks, N. P., and Lieb, W. R. (1994). Molecular and cellular mechanisms of general anaesthesia. *Nature* 367: 607–614.

Gustafsson, L. L., Ebling, W. F., Osaki, E., and Stanski, D. R. (1996). Quantitation of depth of thiopental anesthesia in the rat. *Anesthesiology* 84: 415–427.

Hall, A. C., Lieb, W. R., and Franks, N. P. (1994). Insensitivity of P-type calcium channels to inhalational and intravenous general anesthetics. *Anesthesiology* 81: 117–123.

Hirota, K., and Lambert, D. G. (1996). Ketamine: Its mechanism(s) of action and unusual clinical uses. *British Journal of Anaesthesia* 77: 441–444.

Hung, O. R., Varvel, J. R., Shafer, S. L., and Stanski, D. R. (1992). Thiopental pharmacodynamics. II. Quantitation of clinical and electroencephalographic depth of anesthesia. *Anesthesiology* 77: 237–244.

Lodge, D., Anis, N. A., and Burton, N. R. (1982). Effects of optical isomers of ketamine on excitation of cat and rat spinal neurones by amino acids and acetylcholine. *Neuroscience Letters* 29: 281–286.

MacDonald, J. F., Miljkovic, Z., and Pennefather, P. (1987). Use-dependent block of excitatory amino acid currents in cultured neurons by ketamine. *Journal of Neurophysiology* 58: 251–266.

Marshall, B. E., and Longnecker, D. E. (1996). General Anesthetics. In J. G. Hardman et al., eds., *Goodman and Gilman's The Pharmacological Basis of Therapeutics*, 9th ed., 307–330. New York: McGraw-Hill.

Rang, H. P., Dale, M. M., and Ritter, J. M. (1995). *Pharmacology*, 3rd ed. Edinburgh: Churchill Livingstone.

Ryder, S., Way, W. L., and Trevor, A. J. (1978). Comparative pharmacology of the optical isomers of ketamine in mice. *European Journal of Pharmacology* 49: 15–23.

Tomlin, S. L., Jenkins, A., Lieb, W. R., and Franks, N. P. (1998). Stereoselective effects of etomidate optical isomers on gamma-aminobutyric acid type A receptors and animals. *Anesthesiology* 88: 708–817.

Violet, J. M., Downie, D. L., Nakisa, R. C., Lieb, W. R., and Franks, N. P. (1997). Differential sensitivities of mammalian neuronal and muscle nicotinic acetylcholine receptors to general anesthetics. *Anesthesiology* 86: 866–874.

White, P. F., et al. (1985). Comparative pharmacology of the ketamine isomers. Studies in volunteers. *British Journal of Anaesthesia* 57: 197–203.

Zeilhofer, H. U., Swandulla, D., Geisslinger, G., and Brune, K. (1992). Differential effects of ketamine enantiomers on NMDA receptor currents in cultured neurons. *European Journal of Pharmacology* 213: 155–158.

19 NMDA Receptor–Mediated Consciousness: A Theoretical Framework for Understanding the Effects of Anesthesia on Cognition?

Jackie Andrade

Anesthetics are a diverse class of drugs that cause loss of consciousness and, to various extents, analgesia and muscle relaxation. In smaller doses they have more diverse effects. General anesthetics such as isoflurane and propofol cause sedation, whereas dissociative anesthetics such as ketamine and phencyclidine cause visual disturbances, hallucinations, dysphoria, and thought disorder. Flohr hypothesizes that all anesthetics act, directly or indirectly, as antagonists of the NMDA receptor channel complex. He argues that modulation of the NMDA synapse is central to their effects on consciousness, because NMDA synapse activity underlies normal conscious experience. From a cognitive viewpoint, Flohr's theory contains some intriguing ideas. He proposes that the hallucinations and thought disorder caused by dissociative anesthetics are evidence that they target consciousness more directly than general anesthetics. Conversely, the sedation caused by general anesthetics is a side effect, not a necessary feature of impaired consciousness. He predicts that loss of long-term memory will occur before loss of consciousness (Flohr 1992; see also chapter 16). If his theory is correct, then loss of long-term memory should occur before loss of short-term memory and attention. This paper assesses the utility of Flohr's theory for explaining the rather contradictory findings that have emerged from studies of cognition during anesthesia.

When viewed as research into consciousness, much of the research into the cognitive effects of general anesthetics looks rather haphazard. A reason for this is that many studies were inspired by practical rather than theoretical concerns. Researchers tested the cognitive effects of small doses of anesthetic to discover whether the performance of operating theater staff was impaired by gases leaking from the anesthetic equipment. Many studies in the 1990s explored the extent to which information processing and learning continued despite clinically adequate anesthesia; studies of "therapeutic suggestions" (e.g., "The operation is going very well, you will make a rapid recovery") asked whether this continued learning could aid recovery.

Meanwhile, in mainstream cognitive psychology, there was an explosion of interest in unconscious processing. Numerous studies showed that unconscious, or implicit, memory was preserved under conditions of divided attention or organic amnesia that impaired conscious, or explicit, memory (Schacter 1987). Lack of attention or awareness at study affected conscious memory considerably more than unconscious memory (e.g., Merikle and Joordens 1997). Such studies led to the expectation that patients would have unconscious but not conscious memory for stimuli presented during general anesthesia. However, there was little theorizing about what types of stimuli would be remembered, or what the underlying mechanisms of the preserved learning might be.

Learning During General Anesthesia

Studies of learning during general anesthesia have employed a range of auditory stimuli from single familiar words to sentences and novel stimuli such as melodies, nonsense words, or fictitious names. Typically, these stimuli are played to patients during surgery and learning is assessed on recovery by an indirect memory test. Indirect tests measure people's tendency to select presented stimuli from filler items, or to respond with presented stimuli when asked to say the first thing that comes to mind in response to a cue. No mention is made of the study phase and there is little incentive to retrieve studied items to complete the test. For example, Jelicic showed that patients who were played the words "yellow banana green pear" during surgery were more likely than a control group to respond with those words when asked to give examples of fruits and colors (Jelicic et al. 1992a). Patients who were played fictitious, nonfamous names during anesthesia tended on recovery to identify those names as famous (the false fame effect). Those who were played statements such as "Queen Beatrix came to the throne in 1980" during anesthesia answered more general knowledge questions correctly on recovery (Jelicic et al. 1992b).

These observations suggest that patients had learned the information presented during anesthesia. However, since approximately half the studies of learning during anesthesia obtained null results, the conclusion that learning persists during general anesthesia is controversial. Learning may occur only in moments of consciousness during surgery. The problem is that the level of unconsciousness, or depth of anesthesia, fluctuates and is hard to measure if, as is often the case, patients are given a muscle relaxant to facilitate surgery. Research using the isolated forearm technique, which keeps one hand free of the muscle relaxant and thereby lets patients move if they wake up, suggests that many patients are conscious for moments during surgery though they recollect nothing about the surgery when they recover from the anesthetic (Russell 1986, 1993). Although patients sometimes learn information presented during surgery, it is not clear whether this learning is conscious or unconscious (for further discussion, see Andrade 1995; Bonebakker et al. 1997; Ghoneim and Block 1997).

Without a theory of the processes underlying consciousness and their role in learning and memory, or of the effects of different anesthetics on those processes, it is hard to predict the circumstances under which learning will persist despite anesthesia. Neuropsychological studies show that the frontal lobes play a role in aspects of conscious cognition such as selective attention and planning (Shallice 1988). Drawing on neuropsychological evidence, Caseley-Rondi (1996) hypothesized that the effects of anesthetics on

learning were a consequence of selective disruption of frontal lobe function. Priming of single words would persist during anesthesia, but learning of complex information would not, because it required frontal functions such as integration of information into a single representation. Positron emission tomography shows that anesthetics cause global depression of cerebral metabolism (Alkire et al. 1995), but single-cell electrophysiological recordings (Angel 1993) suggest that they block information flow via the thalamus, starving the frontal cortex of information. This is consistent with the idea that the frontal cortex is the locus of the functional effects of anesthetics.

People with frontal lobe lesions tend to be distractable, but also to perseverate and confabulate. The affected cognitive processes of selective attention, task switching, and retrieval from long-term memory are functions of the hypothetical central executive of working memory (Baddeley 1996). If anesthetics selectively impair frontal functions, then performance on executive tasks should be particularly sensitive to the effects of small doses of anesthetics. Some support for this prediction is provided by research into the cognitive effects of anesthetics in the small amounts that might leak from operating theater equipment. Small doses of enflurane impaired short-term memory (Adam and Collins 1979) and caused people to make riskier decisions (Bentin et al. 1978a); they also impaired learning (Bentin et al. 1978b). Trace concentrations of halothane, enflurane, and nitrous oxide impaired attention (Bruce and Bach 1975, 1976). These studies suggest that working-memory function is sensitive to small doses of anesthetic, but no one has yet shown that it is more sensitive than other aspects of cognition.

Learning and Short-Term Memory During Conscious Sedation with Propofol

We conducted a study that bears on this issue, although it did not originally aim to do so. We wanted to compare the effects of light anesthesia on conscious and unconscious memory, so we played lists of fictitious names to volunteers who were awake, lightly sedated with a small dose of propofol (a general anesthetic agent), or more deeply sedated with propofol. Participants remained conscious. With the smaller dose, they were drowsy but able to talk and respond to commands to open their eyes or raise their hand. With the larger dose, they were less responsive but still raised their hand to command. When the effects of propofol had worn off, participants listened to names and were asked to select those which were famous or those which they remembered hearing during the experiment. In laboratory studies, the tendency to mistake previously heard fictitious names for famous names—the false fame effect—occurs despite divided attention at study (Jacoby et al. 1989). Conscious, recognition memory is more sensitive to manipulations of attention at study. Therefore we predicted that memory for the names presented during sedation would show up on the fame judgment task but not on the recognition test.

Another aim of the study was to assess the coherent frequency, an EEG measure of auditory evoked responding, as an index of depth of anesthesia (Andrade et al. 1996). To do this, we compared coherent frequency with an objective measure of cognitive function, performance on a within-list recognition test. Participants listened to a list of unrelated words and responded to repeated words by raising their right thumb. Repeats occurred after varying numbers of intervening words, therefore good performance required attention and rehearsal of recently heard words, i.e., working memory.

The recognition and fame judgment tasks revealed memory only for names presented before propofol was administered. Neither task showed any evidence for learning during propofol infusion. With the smaller dose of propofol, performance on the within-list recognition test was impaired compared with performance when awake, but it was still reasonably good; participants identified approximately half the repeated

words. Thus participants had preserved working-memory function but no long-term learning during light propofol sedation. Following Caseley-Rondi (1996), we explained these data by suggesting that executive or frontal functions are needed to integrate or bind complex stimuli—in this case the fictitious names—before they can be encoded in memory (Andrade 1996).

Flohr's theory explains our data without recourse to assumptions about frontally mediated integration of stimuli. He proposes that NMDA cell assemblies function as Hebbian synapses, becoming more reactive with use through postsynaptic changes known as long-term potentiation, the cellular mechanism underlying fear conditioning and other types of learning (e.g., McKernan and Shinnick-Gallagher 1997). Flohr suggests that NMDA synapses also form transient assemblies which organize themselves into the higher-order representations underlying normal conscious cognition and working memory. Calcium ions are a secondary messenger in both types of plasticity. They promote transient changes by increasing transmitter release from the presynaptic membrane (by increasing synthesis of nitric oxide, which is released into the synaptic cleft) and more permanent changes by altering protein synthesis in the postsynaptic membrane. The more Ca^{2+} that passes through the ion channel of the NMDA receptor, the longer the duration of the synaptic change. Therefore long-term memory formation requires more Ca^{2+}, and generally more activity in the NMDA receptor complex, than awareness and attention. This explains the coincident loss of awareness and loss of memory for particular stimuli in conditions such as agnosia, and the amnesic effects of dissociative anesthetics (see Flohr 1992).

A stronger prediction can also be made: For any anesthetic, there will be a dose that preserves awareness and working-memory function but prevents long-term learning. The data from our volunteer study support this prediction, as does Harborne et al.'s (1996) finding that a subanesthetic dose of ketamine impaired verbal learning and memory but had little effect on attention and measures of frontal function. The various demonstrations of learning during clinical anesthesia contradict it, unless one assumes that all patients with implicit memory for intraoperative events were at least momentarily conscious during surgery. An alternative, ad hoc explanation of the clinical data is that when words are presented during anesthesia, stored representations of those words are temporarily activated in a way that alters performance on the memory tests but is not dependent on formation of NMDA-mediated cell assemblies.

The Role of Surgery in Learning During Sedation and Anesthesia

Two further studies suggest that the situation is in any case more complex (see Andrade et al. 1999). In one study (Andrade et al. in preparation), we hypothesized that clinical studies tend to reveal memory for stimuli played during anesthesia, whereas volunteer studies tend not to, because the patients in the clinical studies are anxious about their operation and their anxiety promotes learning. Surgical stimulation may also promote learning. To test these hypotheses, we played words to patients shortly before they went into the operating theater and tested memory for those words on recovery from the anesthetic after surgery. During word presentation, one group of patients was lightly sedated with propofol, another group was anesthetized with propofol, and a third group was anesthetized with propofol and the words were played during intubation. This design allowed us to compare learning during anesthesia that was light because only a small dose of anesthetic was given, with learning during anesthesia that was light because the stimulating effects of intubation counteracted the sedative effects of the anesthetic.

We presented two types of word: the "yellow banana green pear" phrase for comparison with Jelicic et al.'s (1992a) clinical study, and Finnish words that patients did not comprehend. We tested memory directly, by asking participants to judge whether they recognized presented and new Finnish words, and indirectly by asking them to generate examples of fruits and colors and to rate how much they liked different Finnish words. This preference rating task measures the mere exposure effect, an increase in liking of previously encountered stimuli compared with new stimuli. Zajonc (e.g., Murphy and Zajonc 1993) has argued that this change in emotional response is more resistant to lack of consciousness than are cognitive changes picked up by tasks such as category generation. Our pilot study confirmed that recognition of the Finnish words was impaired by dividing attention at study, whereas the mere exposure effect was the same with full or divided attention.

Patients recognized and preferred the Finnish words presented before propofol infusion, compared with distracter words that had not been presented. However, none of the three groups showed statistically significant memory for category examples or Finnish words presented during propofol infusion. This study provides another example of consciousness without subsequent memory, and leaves unsolved the puzzle of why some studies seem to have demonstrated memory for words presented during clinical anesthesia. There was a hint of memory for words presented during intubation, suggesting that potentially painful stimulation promotes learning in some way.

Our third study therefore investigated memory for words played during minor surgery with propofol sedation or propofol anesthesia. Patients either were sedated with a relatively small dose of propofol supplemented with alfentanil, or were lightly anesthetized with a larger dose of propofol and somewhat less alfentanil (details will be reported in Stapleton and Andrade in press). The sedated patients remained responsive to command during surgery. All patients were played a list of common English words before propofol infusion and another list when surgery began. On recovery, memory was tested by playing word stems and asking patients to complete them. Traditionally, this word stem completion task is considered a measure of unconscious memory, because participants are asked to complete the stems with the first word that comes to mind. However, if no word comes to mind, participants may search conscious memory of the studied words for a suitable completion, so the test is not process-pure—it may pick up conscious as well as unconscious memory.

A solution is to encourage conscious retrieval of studied words but, for half the test items, to forbid participants to use the consciously retrieved words to complete the word stems. On this half of the test, the exclusion condition, unconscious memory increases the tendency to complete stems with presented words but conscious memory impedes it. On the other half of the test, the inclusion condition, both types of memory increase the number of completions with studied words. This so-called method of opposition, or process dissociation procedure, is widely used in cognitive psychology to estimate the contributions of conscious and unconscious memory to performance on a memory test (Jacoby et al. 1993). There is debate about the validity of the underlying assumption that the conscious and unconscious memory contributions are independent (e.g., Curran and Hintzman 1995, 1997; Jacoby et al. 1997; Russo and Andrade 1995), but the advantage of the technique is that it assesses conscious and unconscious memory using a single memory test.

In our study, patients used conscious and unconscious memory to complete word stems belonging to words presented before propofol infusion. For the words presented during surgery, their completions appeared to be driven by conscious memory. This finding may be artifactual, because in the exclusion condition patients may have rejected any words that seemed familiar rather than only those words they consciously recalled. A tendency to exclude all common

words would show up as a difference in responses to distracter items in the exclusion and inclusion conditions. This difference was not observed, baseline performance being comparable in the two conditions. However, if unconscious memory for presented words led to those words being excluded because they seemed familiar, this would lead to an overestimate of conscious memory, because those words would be treated in the calculations as though they were consciously recalled, and there would be a corresponding underestimate of unconscious memory.[1] Nonetheless, the interesting finding is that the patients in this study learned words presented during propofol infusion, even though the lightly sedated participants in our earlier studies had failed to do so. The amount of learning was comparable in the sedated and anesthetized patients.

Together, our three studies suggest that learning during anesthesia occurs only when surgery is present. We found no evidence of learning during sedation or light anesthesia when words were presented to patients before surgery, or to volunteers. By contrast, we observed learning during deeper anesthesia when words were presented during surgery. In our studies, surgery appears to be more critical for learning than is consciousness. Surgery is promoting learning in some way that is independent of its effect on depth of anesthesia.

A study by Lubke et al. (1999) indicates that level of consciousness influences learning during surgery. Lubke et al. played words to patients during surgery and tested their memory on recovery, using a word stem completion task with inclusion and exclusion instructions, as we did in our third experiment. They used a new EEG measure called the bispectral index to measure the depth of anesthesia at which each word was presented. This is the first study to assess the importance of depth of anesthesia for memory of individual stimuli. The outcome was a statistically significant but weak correlation between the bispectral index when words were presented and memory for the words on recovery. Lubke et al. tested trauma patients undergoing emergency surgery because their condition makes it difficult to maintain a stable depth of anesthesia during the operation. This meant that they could study the effects on learning of a wider range of depths of anesthesia than would be possible to obtain ethically in other patient groups. It is conceivable that the degree of surgical stimulation also varies widely in trauma surgery, compared with the minor surgery undergone by the patients in our studies. It would be interesting to know to what extent the variation in surgical stimulation explained the remaining variance in learning in Lubke et al.'s study.

Animal studies suggest that the effect of surgery on learning is due to increases in catecholamine release in response to tissue damage. Catecholamine levels would have been high in Lubke et al.'s trauma patients. Catecholamines enhance memory retention (McGaugh 1989) and may promote learning during anesthesia. Weinberger et al. (1984) and Dariola et al. (1993) have shown that anesthetized rats cannot learn pairings between fear-provoking and neutral stimuli. This is not surprising if anesthetics antagonize the long-term potentiation of NMDA synapses that underlies learning. However, Weinberger et al. and Dariola et al. showed that injections of adrenaline enabled fear conditioning despite anesthesia (but see El-Zahaby et al. 1994, for a failure to replicate). A challenge for Flohr is to explain how catecholamines interact with the NMDA-mediated cell assemblies that he hypothesizes underlie consciousness and long-term memory. Perhaps we are dealing with two learning mechanisms here: one that is closely coupled to consciousness and is dependent on plasticity in NMDA synapses, and another that is independent of consciousness and dependent on or influenced by catecholamines. This second mechanism may be the one responsible for the apparently preserved learning of simple stimuli and stimulus pairings during anesthesia.

Some Implications of Flohr's Theory

An important aspect of Flohr's argument is that dissociative anesthetics target conscious processes more directly and selectively than do general anesthetics, which inhibit nonconscious processes as well as antagonizing conscious processes. EEG recordings of primary auditory cortex activity during ketamine and general anesthesia are consistent with this view. Mid-latency evoked potentials are almost unchanged by ketamine anesthesia (Schwender et al. 1993), but truncated or absent with general anesthesia (e.g., Schwender et al. 1994). General sedation is probably a useful feature of clinically used anesthetics. The reduction in sensory input may "starve" higher-level conscious processes, facilitating loss of consciousness and helping to maintain unconsciousness even if the blockade of NMDA synapse activity is imperfect. However, Flohr suggests that dissociative anesthetics are better research tools for manipulating consciousness. If he is correct, drugs like ketamine may help to answer some of the questions posed by recent research into the cognitive effects of general anesthetics.

The outcome of this research with general anesthetics suggests that learning is impaired by smaller doses of anesthetic than is working memory, yet some learning persists even with large doses if stimuli are presented during surgery. We used a single anesthetic agent, propofol, so we could compare findings across experiments. However, Veselis et al. (1997) found that different general anesthetic agents differentially impair learning when administered in doses that cause equal sedation. To discover why this might be, one needs to know the how different anesthetics affect the neural mechanisms of consciousness and learning. Flohr's theory offers some suggestions for research into this issue. If the effect of an anesthetic on learning correlates with its impact on NMDA synapse activity, then dissociative anesthetics should impair learning more than general anesthetics. If, on the other hand, the degree of learning impairment correlates with the general sedative action of an anesthetic, then general anesthetics should impair learning more than dissociative anesthetics.

The appropriate studies have not been carried out, but it is probable that the outcome would depend on the type of learning assessed. If there is a type of learning that persists despite ketamine anesthesia, perhaps because it depends only on preserved processing in primary auditory cortex and not on the formation of NMDA-mediated cell assemblies, then an interesting question is what the neural mechanisms of that learning might be. Research into issues like this would help identify which types of learning are tightly bound to consciousness and which are truly unconscious.

Research into learning during anesthesia has been dogged by conflicting results, and it is unclear whether one should attribute different findings to differences in the stimuli, memory tests, or anesthetic agents used, or to different types of surgery or differences in depth of anesthesia. It now seems clear that whether learning occurs is not simply a question of whether patients are inadequately anesthetized, because surgery enables learning under anesthetic conditions that would otherwise prevent it. For the same reason, learning during anesthesia cannot depend solely on residual activity in NMDA synapses. Something more complex and more interesting is going on. A theory of the molecular mechanisms of anesthetics and of surgery, and of their combined effects on cognition, is needed to explain why patients can learn words presented during surgery but volunteers fail to learn words presented during lighter sedation with the same anesthetic.

Given the conflicting results in the literature on learning during anesthesia, it is hardly surprising that there have been relatively few studies of the effects of anesthetics on other aspects of human cognition. In principle, such studies could reveal which cognitive processes are most affected by loss of consciousness—in other words, the cognitive correlates of consciousness. In practice, though, many anesthetic effects could be attributed to sedation or to other actions unrelated to the impairment of consciousness. It is difficult to make principled decisions about which anesthetics and which cognitive tasks to study without a theory of how anesthetics cause loss of consciousness, at a molecular and cognitive level of explanation. By integrating pharmacology, neuroscience, and information processing, Flohr provides a much-needed theoretical basis for research into the cognitive effects of anesthetics, and increases the utility of anesthetics as a tool for researching consciousness.

Note

1. Thanks to Phil Merikle for this suggestion.

References

Adam, N., and Collins, G. I. (1979). Alteration by enflurane of electrophysiologic correlates of search in short-term memory. *Anesthesiology* 50: 93–97.

Alkire, M. T., Haier, R. J., Barker, S. J., Shah, N. K., Wu, J. C., and Kao, J. (1995). Cerebral metabolism during propofol anesthesia in humans studied with positron emission tomography. *Anesthesiology* 82: 393–403.

Andrade, J. (1995). Learning during anaesthesia: A review. *British Journal of Psychology* 86, no. 4: 479–506.

Andrade, J. (1996). Investigations of hypesthesia: Using anesthetics to explore relationships between consciousness, learning and memory. *Consciousness and Cognition* 5: 562–580.

Andrade, J., Englert, L., Harper, C., and Edwards, N. (manuscript in preparation). The effects of anaesthetic dose and stimulation on learning during propofol infusion.

Andrade, J., Sapsford, D., Jeevaratnum, R. D., Pickworth, A. J., and Jones, J. G. (1996). The coherent frequency in the EEG as an objective measure of cognitive function during propofol sedation. *Anesthesia and Analgesia*, 83: 1279–1284.

Andrade, J., Stapleton, C., Englert, L., Harper, C., Englert, L., and Edwards, N. (1999). The contribution of surgery to learning and memory in anaesthesia. In C. Jordan, D. J. A. Vaughn, and D. Newton, eds., *Memory and Awareness in Anaesthesia IV*, pp. 141–163. London: Imperial College Press.

Angel, A. (1993). Central neuronal pathways and the process of anaesthesia. *British Journal of Anaesthesia* 71: 148–163.

Baddeley, A. D. (1996). Exploring the central executive. *Quarterly Journal of Experimental Psychology* 49A: 5–28.

Bentin, S., Collins, G. I., and Adam, N. (1978a). Decision-making behaviour during inhalation of subanaesthetic concentrations of enflurane. *British Journal of Anaesthesia* 50: 1173–1177.

Bentin, S., Collins, G. I., and Adam, N. (1978b). Effects of low concentrations of enflurane on probability learning. *British Journal of Anaesthesia* 50: 1179–1183.

Bonebakker, A. E., Jelicic, M., Passchier, J., and Bonke, B. (1996). Memory during general anesthesia: Practical and methodological aspects. *Consciousness and Cognition* 5: 542–561.

Bruce, D. L., and Bach, M. J. (1975). Psychologic studies of human performance as affected by traces of enflurane and nitrous oxide. *Anesthesiology* 42: 194.

Bruce, D. L., and Bach, M. J. (1976). Effects of trace anaesthetic gases on behavioural performance of volunteers. *British Journal of Anaesthesia* 48: 871.

Caseley-Rondi, G. (1996). Perceptual processing during general anaesthesia reconsidered within a neuropsychological framework. In B. Bonke, J. G. Bovill, and N. Moerman, eds., *Memory and Awareness in Anaesthesia III*, 102–107. Assen: Van Gorcum.

Curran, T., and Hintzman, D. L. (1995). Violations of the independence assumption in process dissociation. *Journal of Experimental Psychology: Learning, Memory and Cognition* 21: 531–547.

Curran, T., and Hintzman, D. L. (1997). Consequences and causes of correlations in process dissociation. *Journal of Experimental Psychology: Learning, Memory and Cognition* 23: 496–504.

Dariola, M. K., Yadava, A., and Malhotra, S. (1993). Effect of epinephrine on learning under anaesthesia. *Journal of the Indian Academy of Applied Psychology* 19: 47–51.

El-Zahaby, M., Ghoneim, M. M., Johnson, G. M., and Gormezano, I. (1994). Effects of subanesthetic concentrations of isoflurane and their interactions with epinephrine on acquisition and retention of the rabbit nictitating membrane response. *Anesthesiology* 81: 229–237.

Flohr, H. (1992). Qualia and brain processes. In A. Beckermann, H. Flohr, and J. Kim, eds., *Emergence or Reduction? Essays on the Prospects of Nonreductive Physicalism*. Berlin: Walter de Gruyter.

Ghoneim, M. M., and Block, R. I. (1997). Learning and memory during general anesthesia: An update. *Anesthesiology* 87: 387–410.

Harborne, G. C., Watson, F. L., Healy, D. T., and Groves, L. (1996). The effects of sub-anaesthetic doses of ketamine on memory, cognitive performance and subjective experience in healthy volunteers. *Journal of Psychopharmacology* 10: 134–140.

Jacoby, L. L., Begg, I. M., and Toth, J. P. (1997). In defense of functional independence: Violations of assumptions underlying the process-dissociation procedure? *Journal of Experimental Psychology: Learning, Memory and Cognition* 23: 484–495.

Jacoby, L. L., Toth, J. P., and Yonelinas, A. P. (1993). Separating conscious and unconscious influences in memory: Measuring recollection. *Journal of Experimental Psychology: General* 122: 139–154.

Jacoby, L. L., Woloshyn, V., and Kelley, C. (1989). Becoming famous without being recognised: Unconscious influences of memory produced by divided attention. *Journal of Experimental Psychology: General* 118: 115–125.

Jelicic, M., Bonke, B., Wolters, G., and Phaf, R. H. (1992a). Implicit memory for words presented during general anaesthesia. *European Journal of Cognitive Psychology* 4: 71–80.

Jelicic, M., De Roode, A., Bovill, J. G., and Bonke, B. (1992b). Unconscious learning during anaesthesia. *Anaesthesia* 47: 835–837.

Lubke, G. H., Kerssens, C., Phaf, H., and Sebel, P. S. (1999). Dependence of explicit and implicit memory on hypnotic state in trauma patients. *Anesthesiology* 90: 470–480.

McGaugh, J. L. (1989). Dissociating learning and performance: Drug and hormone enhancement of memory storage. *Brain Research Bulletin* 23: 339–345.

McKernan, M. G., and Shinnick-Gallagher, P. (1997). Fear conditioning induces a lasting potentiation of synaptic currents in vivo. *Nature* 390: 607–611.

Merikle, P. M., and Joordens, S. (1997). Parallels between perception without attention and perception without awareness. *Consciousness and Cognition* 6: 219–236.

Murphy, S. T., and Zajonc, R. B. (1993). Affect, cognition, and awareness: Affective priming with optimal and suboptimal stimulus exposures. *Journal of Personality and Social Psychology* 64: 723–839.

Russell, I. F. (1986). Comparison of wakefulness with two anaesthetic regimens. *British Journal of Anaesthesia* 58: 965–968.

Russell, I. F. (1993). Midazolam-alfentanil: An anaesthetic? An investigation using the isolated forearm technique. *British Journal of Anaesthesia* 70: 42–46.

Russo, R., and Andrade, J. (1995). The directed forgetting effect in word fragment completion: An application of the process dissociation procedure. *Quarterly Journal of Experimental Psychology* 48A: 405–423.

Schacter, D. L. (1987). Implicit memory: History and current status. *Journal of Experimental Psychology: Learning, Memory, and Cognition* 13: 501–518.

Schwender, D., Klasing, S., Madler, C., Pöppel, E., and Peter, K. (1993). Mid-latency auditory evoked potentials during ketamine anaesthesia in humans. *British Journal of Anaesthesia* 71: 629–632.

Schwender, D., Madler, C., Klasing, S., Peter, K., and Pöppel, E. (1994). Anesthetic control of 40-Hz brain activity and implicit memory. *Consciousness and Cognition* 3: 129–147.

Shallice, T. (1988). *From Neuropsychology to Mental Structure*. Cambridge: Cambridge University Press.

Stapleton, C., and Andrade, J. (in press). An investigation of learning during propofol sedation and anaesthesia using the process dissociation procedure. *Anesthesiology*.

Veselis, R., Reinsel, R. A., Feshchenko, V. A., and Wronski, M. (1997). The comparative amnestic effects of midazolam, propofol, thiopental, and fentanyl at equisedative concentrations. *Anesthesiology* 87: 49–64.

Weinberger, N. M., Gold, P. E., and Sternberg, D. B. (1984). Epinephrine enables Pavlovian fear conditioning under anesthesia. *Science* 233: 605–607.

V TOWARD THE NEURAL CORRELATES OF SELFHOOD, AGENCY, AND SOCIAL COGNITION

Consciousness may have been a key factor in the transition from biological to cultural evolution. Social cognition seems to require an integrated self-representation, which makes self-related information globally available. The capacity to become the object of one's own attention,[1] to engage in self-reflexive cognition, and to voluntarily initiate self-directed actions are important steps through which the representational architecture of human beings unfolds, ontogenetically as well as from the point of view of evolutionary history. On the one hand, it seems obvious that mental capacities like these are necessary preconditions for the emergence of a phenomenal self as well as for genuinely cooperative forms of social activities. On the other hand, however, it appears very likely that there are higher-order, complex forms of phenomenal content which possess not only neural correlates but also *social* correlates: Some forms of consciousness seem to require a social context in order to be "booted." Certain types of phenomenal self-awareness—like tracking another human being's attention or mentally grasping his or her intention—seem to require that the organism in which they occur is *socially situated*, grounded in a network of social relationships, as it were. To develop a successful social strategy, one has to internally model those properties of other beings in the environment, which are not available "on-line," through sensory perception, and attribute this activity to oneself. In short, one's own phenomenal states can sometimes be driven by the intentional as well as the phenomenal states of other individuals.

After one has discovered this highly interesting point, a whole new class of questions immediately springs to mind: What is the causal relationship between neural and social correlates of consciousness? Are there sets of minimally sufficient conditions (see chapter 2 in this volume), describable on the functional level as well as on the level of phenomenal self-representation, that will lead to "social awareness" (i.e., to those forms of conscious experience which represent and are mediated by social interactions)? Can we

specify the *necessary* conditions that have to be met in order for any cultural dynamics to evolve from groups of conscious agents? And finally, in terms of methodology, what type of interdisciplinary cooperation would be required to tackle these questions in a rigorous manner?

Searching for the neural correlates of phenomenal selfhood, agency, and social cognition does not imply neglecting other relevant factors to be analyzed on other levels of description. The aim, of course, is not to arrive at a primitive reductionist stance of the "X is *nothing but* a set of neural events" type. Quite the contrary: The aim will have to be to investigate the logical relationships between neuroscientific, sociological, and cultural levels of description, relative to certain theoretical interests and in the light of current evidence. Empirical work investigating the necessary and sufficient neurobiological conditions for the conscious experience of self and other, for phenomenal subjectivity and intersubjectivity, is an important contribution to this project. It will soon make research programs in the humanities more successful—not only by adding precision and testable empirical content, but also by coupling them to the forceful dynamics of an explosive growth of scientific knowledge by which the field of consciousness research is characterized at the beginning of the twenty-first century.

However, first things first. Before one can even start to approach this newly emerging theoretical landscape, one needs a theory about what a *first-person perspective* really is. This theory has to be conceptually convincing, empirically plausible, and, most of all, open to new developments. The chosen conceptual framework must be able to accommodate progress. Its basic assumptions have to be plastic, as it were, so that new details and empirical data can continuously be fed into the theoretical model as it grows and becomes more refined.

Thomas Metzinger in his contribution makes an attempt at sketching the outlines of such a theory, offering a representationalist analysis of the phenomenal first-person perspective. Three phenomenal target properties are centrally relevant: "mineness" (I consciously experience *my* leg as subjectively having always belonged to me), "selfhood" (before initiating, and independently of, any intellectual operations, I am already "directly" acquainted with the contents of my self-consciousness) and "perspectivalness" (phenomenal space as a whole is organized around a center, a supramodal point of view). Metzinger analyzes these properties on a representational as well as on a functional level of description. In doing so, he introduces new conceptual tools plus two theoretical entities needed in order to understand what a first-person perspective is: "the phenomenal self-model" and "the phenomenal model of the intentionality relation." A phenomenal self-model is a multimodal representational structure, the contents of which form the contents of the consciously experienced self. It has two important features. First, it is the only representational structure that is anchored in the brain by a persistent functional link, namely, by a continuous source of internally generated input (see also chapter 7 in this volume). Second, large parts of the self-model are *transparent*: they cannot be recognized *as* representations by the system itself. It is therefore caught in what might be called a "naive-realistic self-misunderstanding."

If we now—this is the last step in Metzinger's argument—apply the transparency criterion to the internal representation of the dynamical relations between subject and object (e.g., to the representation of the system as being affected by certain perceptual objects), we arrive at complex forms of representational content. They can only be truthfully described by the system itself as (e.g.) "I *myself* [= the content of a transparent self-model] am now seeing *this object* [= the content of a transparent object representation], and I am seeing it *with my own eyes*" [= the simple story about immediate sensory perception, which sufficed for the brain's evolutionary purposes]. This deep representational structure,

Metzinger claims, is the essence of what makes phenomenal experience a *subjective* phenomenon, which is bound to the internal perspective of an individual agent.

The *perspectivalness* of phenomenal experience has two aspects: the subject-centeredness of perception/cognition and the subject-centeredness of action. *Agency* is certainly one of the most fascinating forms of phenomenal content. It is interesting to note that in schizophrenia, as well as in other psychiatric syndromes like depersonalization or the Cotard delusion, we find the subjective experience of agency deprivation (i.e., this specific form of mental content is missing from phenomenal space).

Joëlle Proust compares two current approaches to schizophrenia (associated with Chris Frith and Marc Jeannerod) from a philosophical perspective. In doing so, she introduces three new concepts: agency awareness, goal awareness, and sensorimotor awareness. Each concept denotes a special kind of phenomenal content. *Agency awareness* is typically a conscious realization that I—or someone else—did or did not perform an action. It is the state in which an organism finds itself when detecting its being active or passive in a particular situation. In particular, it is a state that is activated when interpreting input signals (afferences or reafferences) that in turn allow achieving a veridical perception of the environment. *Goal awareness* is the type of awareness that individuates the action through its intentional content. This dimension of action awareness allows categorizing actions according to their adaptive meaning. It focuses on the motive that drives the execution of the corresponding action. *Sensorimotor awareness* is related to the motor content of an action. It is the form of awareness that identifies an action through its dynamics (i.e., via the spatial and temporal properties of the bodily movement involved in the action). In utilizing these conceptual distinctions for an analysis of impoverished forms of phenomenal agency, Proust comes to a number of interesting conclusions. One of them is that schizophrenic subjects' failures in agency attribution may arise from a difficulty in comparing egocentric representations of an action with the allocentric cues provided by feedback reafferences; such a difficulty would be particularly prominent in contexts requiring an explicit, controlled type of processing.

In the concluding chapter of this book, Vittorio Gallese investigates how a certain type of representation in the human motor system could open a door from the world of subjective experience into the universe of social cognition. He begins by pointing out that many of the brain's properties can be understood only by analyzing the dynamic interplay between the biological agent, who possesses the brain, and the external world. The external world consists not only of objects but also of other agents and their intentions. However, intentions of fellow human beings and other animals are not something we can access on the level of sensory experience. How, then, can brains construct the bridge from conscious, subjective experience to conscious, *intersubjective* experience? Gallese proceeds by describing a certain class of neurons in area F5 of the ventral premotor area of the monkey, which code movements in a rather abstract way, namely, as relations between an agent and the object of his action.

An interesting new concept, originally introduced by Giacomo Rizzolatti and coworkers, is "motor vocabulary": What is coded are not control commands for individual movements, but whole action representations and their temporal and teleological aspects (e.g., grasp, precision grip, or aperture phase). "Canonical neurons" are a class of neurons that respond to classes of visually perceived 3D objects by coding them according to the "affordance" (e.g., of a specific grasping movement), that is, in *relation* to the effect of the interaction with an agent. A second class of premotor neurons, which was discovered some time ago, has been called "mirror neurons." Mirror neurons, localized in the same brain region and motorically similar to

canonical neurons, are visually activated only when another *agent* is observed as acting in a purposeful way with his hand or mouth upon objects. Mirror neurons seem to constitute the neural correlate of an observation/execution matching system: In many of them we find a strict congruence between the observed action and the executed action effective in driving exactly the same motor response that has been observed. The link that is shared by both classes of representations is an allocentric goal representation: This goal is recognized by the observer through mapping it onto a shared motor representation. Understanding the intentions of other perceived agents in the environment could therefore consist in discovering an abstract kind of "motor equivalence."

This line of thought opens a completely new interpretation of the function of the human mirror system, namely as an "intentionality detector," which recognizes stimuli as volitional by detecting their goal. The elementary units of *inter*subjectivity and social awareness would then be of a preconceptual, prerational, and pretheoretical nature, a special kind of representational content fully embodied in the nonegocentric aspects of the human motor vocabulary. The importance of the work presented by Gallese lies in the fact that it makes conceivable future rigorous research programs that take the step from the phenomenal first-person perspective to all the other forms of conscious experience from which our rich social reality eventually emerges: The phenomenal experience of the "you," the "he-she-it," the phenomenal awareness of "us," "you," and "them." It gives us a first vision of how consciousness could actually have been the decisive step from biological to cultural evolution.

Note

1. This was the original, pragmatic definition of self-consciousness used by primatologists like Gordon Gallup. See Gallup 1970, 1991.

Further Reading

Frith, C. D. (1992). *The Cognitive Neuropsychology of Schizophrenia*. Hillsdale, NJ: Lawrence Erlbaum Associates.

Frith, C. D. (1994). Theory of mind in schizophrenia. In A. David, ed., *The Neuropsychology of Schizophrenia*. Hillsdale, NJ: Lawrence Erlbaum Associates.

Gallese, V., Fadiga, L., Fogassi, L., and Rizzolatti, G. (1996). Action recognition in the premotor cortex. *Brain* 119: 593–609.

Gallese, V., and Goldman, A. (1998). Mirror neurons and the simulation theory of mindreading. *Trends in Cognitive Sciences* 12: 493–501.

Gallup, G. (1970). Chimpanzees: Self-recognition. *Science* 167: 86–87.

Gallup, G. (1991). Toward a comparative psychology of self-awareness: Species limitations and cognitive consequences. In J. Strauss and G. R. Goethals, eds., *The Self: Interdisciplinary Approaches.* New York: Springer-Verlag.

Georgieff, N., and Jeannerod, M. (1998). Beyond consciousness of external reality: A "who" system for consciousness and action and self-consciousness. *Consciousness and Cognition* 7: 465–477.

Grivois, H., and Proust, J., eds. (1998). *Subjectivité et conscience d'agir: Approches clinique et cognitive de la psychose.* Paris: Presses Universitaires de France.

Jahanshahi, M., and Frith, C. D. (1998). Willed action and its impairments. *Cognitive Neuropsychology* 15: 483–533.

Jeannerod, M. (1994). The representing brain, neural correlates of motor intention and imagery. *Behavioral and Brain Sciences* 17: 187–245.

Jeannerod, M. (1997). *The Cognitive Neuroscience of Action.* Oxford: Basil Blackwell.

Metzinger, T. (1993; 2nd ed. 1999). *Subjekt und Selbstmodell. Die Perspektivität phänomenalen Bewußtseins vor dem Hintergrund einer naturalistischen Theorie mentaler Repräsentation.* Paderborn: mentis.

Metzinger, T., ed. (1995). *Conscious Experience.* Thorverton: Imprint Academic; Paderborn: mentis.

Metzinger, T. (2002). *Being No One: The Self-Model Theory of Subjectivity*. Cambridge, MA: MIT Press.

Proust, J. (1999a). Indexes for action. *Revue internationale de philosophie* 3: 321–345.

Proust, J. (1999b). Self-Model and Schizophrenia. *Journal of Consciousness Studies*.

Rizzolatti, G., Fogassi, L., and Gallese, V. (2000). Cortical mechanisms subserving object grasping and action recognition: A new view on the cortical motor functions. In M. Gazzaniga, ed., *Handbook of Cognitive Neurosciences*, 2nd ed. Cambridge, MA: MIT Press.

20

The *Subjectivity* of Subjective Experience: A Representationalist Analysis of the First-Person Perspective

Thomas Metzinger

Introduction: Finding the Neural Correlates of Consciousness Through a Representationalist Analysis

Why Is a Representationalist Analysis Useful?

In this chapter I will briefly sketch the outline of a representationalist theory of subjective experience. (See also Metzinger 1993, 2002). A representationalist theory is one that chooses to analyze its target properties—those aspects of the domain which eventually are to be explained—on a certain level of description: by describing conscious systems as *representational* systems and conscious states as *representational* states, one hopes to achieve progress with regard to the relevant properties. This first background assumption is shared by many philosophers today (see, e.g., Dretske 1995; Lycan 1996; Metzinger 1993; Tye 1995), and one may interpret it as a weak version of Brentano's intentionalism. William Lycan (e.g., 1996: 11) has called it the "hegemony of representation": The explanatory base for *all* mental properties is formed by a definite, exhaustive set of functional and representational properties of the class of systems under investigation. However, if in this way one also aims at achieving genuine scientific progress by naturalizing classical theoretical problems, these have to be transformed into an empirically tractable form. It is therefore vital that the underlying theory of representational content is itself empirically plausible, open to data-driven conceptual changes, and limited to a specific domain (Churchland 1989; Clark 1989). One such domain is biological nervous systems; a more specific domain would be human brains in waking or dream states. What, then, are the target properties of our domain and how are they to be treated?

Table 20.1 shows the seven most important theoretical problems connected with conscious experience, in terms of phenomenological constraints imposed on any representationalist theory of consciousness. According to this model, the typical way of generating an empirical research program in interdisciplinary cooperation would consist in moving through one of the rows in the table from left to right. When confronted with a conceptual interpretation of a certain element of subjective experience, the job would first consist in analyzing this element as a form of representational content, generated and utilized by the system in interaction with its environment. The second step would be an attempt to give a functional description of the relevant content-bearing states in the system, by individuating them through their causal role. This opens the functional level of analysis, on which the "functional correlates" of phenomenal experience have to be specified. As soon as the intended class of systems (e.g., humans, macaques, or certain artificial systems) has been delimited, experimental approaches can proceed to isolate the minimal set of basic physical properties (e.g., the *neural* correlates) that the system needs in order to exhibit the target properties by nomological necessity. In this way domain-specific reductive explanations become possible.

Of course, real-world cooperation between disciplines is much more complex. For instance, the rows shown above can also be read from right to left: Differentiated research into the physical correlates of phenomenal states can draw our attention to fine-grained differences in the actual functional role of these correlates. This may eventually lead us to being able to describe our conscious experience in a more fine-grained manner, thereby increasing the amount of information conveyed when speaking about our own introspective experience. In other

Table 20.1

What makes a neural representation a phenomenal representation?

The seven most important phenomenological constraints for any representationalist analysis of conscious experience

Phenomenological Constraint →	Representational Content →	Causal Role ("Functional Correlate") →	Neural Correlate
"Ultra-smoothness": homogeneity of sensory primitives ("qualia"; "grain problem")	*Presentational* content (see Metzinger 1997) • First-order properties; i.e. "elementary" features • representational atomicity; i.e. structureless "density" • indicator function • non-conceptual content	Stimulus-correlated information which is • attentionally/volitionally available, but: • *not* cognitively available • "memory constraint" (Raffman 1995); i.e. discrimination without categorization	? Synchronicity of feature detectors contributing to perceptual object, read out by higher-order mechanism?
Transparency	• Immediacy of epistemic contact • Introspective access exhausted by content properties • *Naive realism*	Internal causal history and temporal microstructure of phenomenal states is globally unavailable	? "Glossing over" by temporal coherence of neural responses?
Presence	Temporal internality: *de nunc* character of phenomenal content	Activation within a virtual "window of presence"	? Recurrent activity underlying formation of short-term memory?
Embeddedness into world model	Dynamic integration into highest-order situational context	*Global* availability of information: • attentional availability • volitional availability • cognitive availability	? Global coherence? "Dynamical core"? (see chapter 9, this volume) "Highest-order binding"? (Metzinger 1995)
Convolved holism	Multi-layered, flexible part-whole relationships	"Liquid architecture": Dynamic linkages on different time-scales	? Synchronous activity with multiple time-constants?
Dynamicity	Temporal macrostructure of causal interaction-domain	Unknown aspects of network dynamics	? Which anatomical subset?
Perspectivalness	*Access from "first-person perspective"; "Subjectivity"* (see text)	*Centeredness of world model* (see text)	? (research program needed)

Intended class of systems: *Homo sapiens* in nonpathological waking states.

words, one way of making progress can consist in increasing the *number* of rows in the left column.[1] There may also be oscillations between neighboring columns, as when philosophers discuss the adequacy of a representationalist conceptualization of experiential content, or when neuroscientists have doubts about a specific functional analysis offered by researchers in classical AI or cognitive science. And real-life science progresses through multiple loops: There are many trajectories through the problem landscape and across levels of description, and one and the same line of inquiry may return to the same vicinity again and again, at a slightly different angle.

For a philosopher, attempting to contribute to a reductive explanation of consciousness is never an ideology or an emotional substitute for religion. If it turns out that there are principled reasons why important features of subjective experience can never be epistemically grasped through a system of interdisciplinary cooperation like the one sketched above, she will be quite happy with this result, because the philosopher will then have achieved what she has always aimed at in the first place: epistemic progress, a growth of knowledge. All she will insist on is that those elements of consciousness purportedly resistant to any reductive approach are described with a maximum of conceptual clarity. So even antireductionists should, if only as a heuristic strategy, follow a reductionist methodology (Walter 1998).

In this essay I will select only one aspect of phenomenal experience, its *perspectivalness*. This very last aspect mentioned in the table above is crucial for interdisciplinary research programs, because it poses the greatest methodological and epistemological problems. Any serious scientific approach to consciousness will have to rely entirely on objective, third-person criteria for the ascription of phenomenal states to a given system. How, then, could it ever do justice to the essentially subjective, first-person character of the phenomenon? (See Metzinger 1993, 1996; Nagel 1974, 1986). Can the subjectivity of the target phenomenon itself ever be turned into an explanandum for the hard sciences?

Analysanda and Explananda: What Does the *Subjectivity* of Subjective Experience Consist in?

This could work only if, first of all, the concept of a "first-person perspective" is clarified in a way that makes the corresponding phenomenon empirically tractable. Our starting point therefore is an *analysandum*, a certain allegedly self-evident manner of speaking about ourselves and the structure of our conscious experiences. In order for this analysandum to be transformed into a set of experimentally tractable *explananda*, we have to choose a suitable level of description. My first claim would be that whenever we have in the past been speaking about the subjectivity of phenomenal experience in terms of having an experiential "first-person perspective," we have merely been employing a very soft "visuogrammatical" metaphor. Our visual space, as a matter of contingent, trivial fact, possesses a perspectival, geometrical structure:[2] This is the spatial part of the metaphor, which originates in the folk phenomenology of visual experience.

Then there is another, more abstract element of our metaphor: Self-ascriptions—for instance, of psychological properties—follow a certain logic; they take place from a grammatical "first-person" perspective. This is the grammatical aspect of the analogy, and prominent philosophers have in the past analyzed the underlying logic a lot (e.g., Castañeda 1966; Chisholm 1981; Lewis 1979; Perry 1993; Shoemaker 1996). However, if you want to understand how this logic of conceptual self-reference could ever come about, what our soft visuogrammatical metaphor actually refers to, you have to go much deeper: We have to understand what the deep representational structure is that enables beings like ourselves to pose philosophical questions of this type in the first place. Why do human beings employ visual metaphors in picking out global properties of their experiential space and in trying to understand the underlying logic of their linguistic abilities, like the self-ascription of psychological properties? What are the necessary and sufficient conditions for *any* representational system, when trying to understand its own mental properties, to run into the problem of the "immunity to error of misidentification," to eventually start wondering about "essential indexicals," "*de-se*-attitudes," or "objective selves"? Which class of representational architectures will inevitably lead all systems, that realize this architecture, into the theoretical landscape sketched at the beginning of this introduction? In order to answer this more fundamental question, one needs to produce an informative account of the neural and functional correlates of three very special phenomenal properties. To understand subjectivity on the logical, the epistemic or metaphysical level, one has to investigate what the *phenomenal* first-person perspective is.

A Representationalist Analysis of the Phenomenal First-Person Perspective

Three Phenomenal Target Properties

The "phenomenal first-person perspective" is one of the most fascinating natural phenomena we know, and in a certain sense we *are* this phenomenon ourselves: The essence of being a person seems to consist in the potential for being a conscious subject. It consists of three phenomenological target properties that in their conceptual interpretation constitute three different aspects of one and the same problem:

(1) *Mineness:* a higher-order property of *particular* forms of phenomenal content. Here are some typical examples of how we refer to these properties in folk psychological contexts: I experience *my* leg subjectively as always having belonged to *me*; I always experience *my* thoughts, *my* focal attention, and *my* emotions as part of my *own* consciousness; voluntary acts are initiated by *myself*.

(2) *Selfhood* ("prereflexive self-intimacy"): the phenomenal *target* property. Again, let us look at some examples of how we usually attempt to linguistically describe the phenomenal content of the representational states underlying these properties: I am *someone*; I experience myself as being *identical* through time; the contents of my phenomenal self-consciousness form a coherent *whole*; before initiating any intellectual operations, and independent of them, I am already "directly" acquainted with the contents of my self-consciousness.

What we frequently just call "the self" in a folk-psychological context is the *phenomenal* self: the content of self-consciousness, as given in subjective experience. We are therefore confronted with a higher-order phenomenal property that is constituted by different and constantly changing types of phenomenal content. Let us call this property "selfhood" or, to use a more technical term, "prereflexive self-intimacy" (e.g., Frank 1991). The phenomenal self arguably is the theoretically most interesting form of phenomenal content because, among other reasons, it endows our mental space with two highly interesting structural characteristics: centeredness and perspectivalness. As long as there is a phenomenal self, our conscious model of the world is a functionally centered model and is tied to what in philosophy of mind is called the "first-person perspective."

(3) *Perspectivalness:* a global, *structural* property of phenomenal space as a whole. It possesses an immovable center. According to subjective experience, the overall dynamics within this space is organized around a supramodal point of view. The phenomenal self is this center. And at this stage the conflict between first-person and third-person descriptions of our target properties becomes very obvious. This is what constitutes the philosophical puzzle: I am this center *myself*; to be phenomenally aware means to possess an inward perspective and to take this perspective on in the subjective experience of the world and of one's own mental states.

So phenomenal subjectivity—as opposed to subjectivity in an epistemological or ontological sense—simply amounts to the fact that under standard conditions, the dynamics of conscious experience unfolds in a space that is centered on a singular, temporally extended experiential self. What now has to be achieved is a representational and a functional analysis of these properties. The pivotal question is What is the minimal set of functional and representational properties that an information-processing system must possess in order to exemplify the *phenomenal* properties under investigation? Which of these low-level properties are necessary, and which are sufficient? What, precisely, does it mean for such a system to take a phenomenal first-person perspective on the world and on its own mental states?

Step 1:   What Is a Self-Model?

The first step of my analysis consists in introducing a new theoretical entity: the phenomenal *self-model*. It forms the representational instantiation basis of the phenomenal properties to be explained. The content of the phenomenal self-model, again, is what we often call "the self" in folk-psychological contexts; its content is the content of self-consciousness, bodily, emotional, and cognitive. My claim is that—ontologically speaking—no such things as selves exist in the world. What actually exists is a special kind of self-models and their contents, and this content makes us believe that we actually do have, or are identical to, a self.

The following can be said of the self-model:

• The self-model is an episodically active representational entity, the content of which is formed solely by properties of the system itself.

• A self-model can be described on multiple, subpersonal levels. For instance, we might describe it as an activation vector or as a trajectory through some suitable state-space. A trivial but important background assumption is that, in our own case, it also possesses a true *neurobiological*

description, for instance, as a complex neural activation pattern with a certain temporal fine structure. On a more abstract level the same pattern of physiological activity can also be described as a complex functional state.

• The *phenomenal* self-model is that partition of the presently active mental self-model which is currently embedded in the highest-order integrated structure, the global model of the world (see, e.g., Yates 1975; Baars 1988; see also row 4 of table 20.1). In other words, nonconscious but causally active self-models (or nonconscious subregions of such models) may exist (see also chapter 6 in this volume).

• In our own case the phenomenal self-model is a plastic, multimodal structure that is plausibly based on an innate and "hardwired" model of the spatial properties of the system (e.g., a "long-term body image"; see section "The Central Theoretical Problem on the Functional Level of Description," below, and O'Shaughnessy 1995; Bermúdez 1998; Damasio 1994; Kinsbourne 1995; Metzinger 1993, 2002), while being functionally rooted in elementary bioregulatory processes; e.g., those systems in the upper brain stem and hypothalamus achieving homeostasis and the stability of the internal chemical milieu (see chapter 7 and Damasio 1999). The content of this underlying form of primitive self-awareness is nonconceptual and subdoxastic.[3]

In order to better understand what a self-model actually is, you can develop a parallel description on the functional level of analysis. An active self-model is the physical realization of a subpersonal functional state. It plays a certain causal role; that is, under an analytical perspective it represents a discrete set of causal relations. It is likely that the neural microevents constituting the relevant causal matrix within the system have to be individuated on a very fine-grained, subsymbolic level including the temporal structure of these events (see Singer 1993, 1994; and especially chapter 8 in this volume). However, just to illustrate the core idea, you could also take a classical cognitivist perspective. Then the self-model could be described as a transient computational module, episodically activated by the system in order to regulate its interaction with the environment.[4]

The next step in defining the working concept of a self-model consists in integrating the biological history of our target phenomenon into the explanatory base. One may plausibly assume that it was, very obviously, *adaptive* to have something like a partly veridical, functionally active self-representation. Philosophers call this theoretical move a "teleofunctionalist assumption": The development and the activation of this neurocomputational module plays a role *for* the system. The functional properties of the self-model possess a true evolutionary description; that is, it is a weapon that was invented and optimized in the course of a "cognitive arms race" (a very apt and unromantic metaphor coined by Andy Clark; see Dennett 1987; Lycan 1996; Clark 1989, p. 62). The functional instantiation basis for a phenomenal first-person perspective, then, is a specific cognitive achievement: the capacity to open and employ centered representational spaces, to operate under egocentric world models. This amounts to the central necessary[5] (but not sufficient[6]) condition in ascribing subjective experience to a given system: weak subjectivity$_1$—phenomenal subjectivity (a subsymbolic, nonconceptual, first-person perspective) is a property that is instantiated only if the system in question activates a coherent self-model and embeds this into its global model of the world.

Before going on, let us take a short break and look at two examples. They will serve to illustrate the concept of a phenomenal self-model by some anecdotal evidence. Astronauts, after some time in space, tend to lose their phenomenal body axis, the subjective feeling of where the top and where the bottom of their body is. When trying to eat, for instance, this can be uncomfortable. Every astronaut knows how to help his buddy: He briefly touches the sole of his part-ner's foot, and instantly his phenomenal body image will lock into a subjective "top-bottom axis" again. Every astronaut also knows how to tease his partner: by tapping his head, thereby reversing the spatial frame of reference. This shows that the self-model of human beings is a *virtual* model which, if underdetermined by internally generated input (i.e., from gravitational acceleration affecting the *maculae utriculi* and *sacculi* in the vestibular organ), is highly context-dependent: Its content is a possibility and not a reality. Just as the phenomenal properties of external experience are properties of virtual objects, so the properties exemplified in inner experience are those of a virtual subject. Its content is simply the best hypothesis about the current state of the system, given all constraints and information resources currently available. Interestingly—and this seems to be one of the core characteristics of phenomenal experience—this possibility is depicted *as* a reality, as an untranscendable presence (see section "Step 3: Transparency and Naive Realism," below). The actuality of situated self-awareness is a *virtual* form of actuality.[7]

A second, even more vivid example of what is meant by the concept of a phenomenal self-model is demonstrated in Vilayanur Ramachandran's intriguing experiments on mirror-induced synesthesia and illusory movements in phantom limbs (see Ramachandran and Rogers-Ramachandran 1996; see also Ramachandran and Blakeslee 1998: 46pp). Phantom limbs are subjectively experienced limbs that typically remain after the loss of an arm or a hand as the result of an accident or surgical amputation (we will return to phantom limbs in the section "The Central Problem on the Functional Level of Description," below). In some situations, such as following a nontraumatic surgical amputation, patients are subjectively able to volitionally control and move their phantom limbs. The neurofunctional correlate of this phenomenal configuration could be that—since there is no contradictory feedback from the amputated limb—motor commands originating in motor cortex are still continuously monitored by the parietal lobes and thereby integrated into that part of the self-model which serves as an internal motor *emulator* (see Grush 1997, 1998: 174; Ramachandran and Rogers-Ramachandran 1996: 378; Metzinger 2002, chap. 7; for a recent review see Ramachandran and Hirstein 1998). In other situations, however, subjective motility and control over the phantom limb can be lost. Such a configuration may arise because of a pre-amputational paralysis due to peripheral nerve lesions or to a prolonged absence of confirming proprioceptive and kinesthetic feedback. The result on the phenomenal level of representation is a paralyzed phantom limb.

Ramachandran and colleagues constructed a "virtual reality box" by placing a vertical mirror inside a cardboard box with the top of the box removed. Two holes in the front of the box enabled the patient to insert his real and his phantom arm. A patient suffering from a paralyzed phantom limb for many years was then asked to view the reflection of his normal hand in the mirror, thus—on the level of visual input— creating the illusion of observing two hands, when in fact he was seeing only the mirror reflection of the intact hand. What would happen to the content of the phenomenal self-model when the subject was asked to try to make bilateral, mirror-symmetric movements? Ramachandran describes one typical outcome of the experiment:

I asked Philip to place his right hand on the right side of the mirror in the box and imagine that his left hand (the phantom) was on the left side. "I want you to move your right and left arms simultaneously," I instructed.

"Oh, I can't do that," said Philip. "I can move my right arm but my left arm is frozen. Every morning, when I get up, I try to move my phantom because it's in this funny position and I feel that moving it might help relieve the pain. But," he said, looking down at his invisible arm, "I never have been able to generate a flicker of movement in it."

"Okay, Philip, try anyway."

Philip rotated his body, shifting his shoulder, to "insert" his lifeless phantom into the box. Then he put his right hand on the other side of the mirror and attempted to make synchronous movements. As he gazed into the mirror, he gasped and then cried out, "Oh, my God! Oh, my God, doctor! This is unbelievable. It's mind-boggling!" He was jumping up and down like a kid. "My left arm is plugged in again. It's as if I'm in the past. All these memories from so many years ago are flooding back into my mind. I can move my arm again. I can feel my elbow moving, my wrist moving. It's all moving again."

After he calmed down a little I said, "Okay, Philip, now close your eyes."

"Oh, my," he said, clearly disappointed. "It's frozen again. I feel my right hand moving, but there's no movement in the phantom."

"Open your eyes."

"Oh, yes, now it's moving again."[8]

By now it should have become clear how these data serve to illustrate the new concept I have introduced: What is moving in this experiment is the phenomenal self-model. The sudden occurrence of kinesthetic qualia in the degraded subspace of the self-model was made possible by installing a second and perfectly superimposed source of "virtual information," restoring, as it were, the visual mode of self-representation and thereby making this information volitionally available. Once again, this experiment nicely demonstrates how phenomenal properties are determined "from below," by functional and representational properties.

Step 2: Representationalist Analysis of the Target Properties

The Phenomenal Property of "Mineness"   Now that the basic explanatory concept has been introduced, one can start developing an analysis of the target properties. Let us turn to the first target property, the phenomenal quality of "mineness." On a functional level of description, it is clear that it must be intimately associated with what is very likely the most fundamental partitioning of the neurocomputational state-space underlying conscious experience: the emergence of a self-world border. On the representational level of description there will be a simple and straightforward assumption that generates a large number of testable and more differentiated hypotheses. All representational states, which are being embedded into the currently active phenomenal self-model, gain the additional higher-order property of phenomenal mineness. Mineness therefore is a prereflexive, nonconceptual sense of ownership (e.g., Martin 1995; Bermúdez 1998). If the underlying integration process is being disturbed, different neuropsychological syndromes or altered states of consciousness result. Here are some examples:

• Consciously experienced thoughts are not *my* thoughts anymore: schizophrenia.

• My leg is not *my* leg anymore: unilateral hemineglect.

• My arm acts without *my* control: alien hand syndrome.

• I am a robot; I am transformed into a puppet; volitional acts are not *my own* volitional acts anymore: depersonalization.[9]

• I *am* the whole world, all events in the world are being initiated and controlled by my own volitional acts: mania.

What could be a more complex phenomenon than conscious experience? An empirically founded philosophical theory will eventually have to do full justice to the depth and complex topology of our phenomenal state-space. Historical experience in science has shown that one of the most promising general research heuristics in understanding a complex phenomenon consists in analyzing borderline cases and impoverished variations of it. Nonstandard situations in complex domains help us in pointing out implicit assumptions and deficits in existing theories, as well as intuitive fallacies. Let us therefore briefly take a closer look at these examples. (I discuss

more of such examples in Metzinger 1993, 1996, 2002).

• Schizophrenia is, on the level of phenomenal content, usually characterized by phenomena such as thought insertion, verbal-auditory hallucinations, or delusions of control. Thought insertion can be representationally analyzed as a situation where the content of currently active cognitive states and processes can not be integrated into the self-model, and therefore must be represented as external. Nevertheless, such nonsubjective thoughts are encoded as an element of objective reality, and their phenomenal presence (see table 20.1, rows 3 and 4) cannot be transcended by the experiential subject. If, as in hearing voices, internal speech production cannot be representationally integrated into the conscious self, a global phenomenal model of reality will emerge in which external voices are heard. The interesting phenomenon here seems to be the additional "pseudosensory" character of such hallucinations. Possibly they depend on an internal emulator for the generation of coherent speech acts, which, in the schizophrenic, transforms an efference copy of motor speech commands, used as input for an internal model of the ongoing process of speech production, into auditory format (Frith 1996; see also Grush 1997, 1998).

In regard to the third type of deficit classically associated with schizophrenia, according to the model here proposed, delusions of external control arise if the volitional acts preceding external motor behavior of the patient are no longer integrated into a phenomenal self-model. The attribution of such disconnected intentions to an external *person*, visible or invisible, may be a confabulatory reaction of the brain, still desperately trying to maximize the overall coherence of its model of reality. In those cases, where another person is experienced as the cause of one's own bodily actions, this may simply be the most economical way to still represent such actions as caused by *mental* events (i.e., to preserve a personal-level representation of such events). If a circumscribed neural module for "theory-of-mind" ascriptions should exist, it is well conceivable that such a module suffers from functional dedifferentiation (see Daprati et al. 1997; Frith 1996; for a more detailed philosophical interpretation of empirical data, see chapter 21 in this volume).[10]

A self-model is important in enabling a system to represent itself *to* itself as an agent. If this system possesses the physical resources to activate abstract, allocentric representations of actions and action goals, then it also possesses one of the most important building blocks for language acquisition and social cognition (see chapter 22 in this volume). However, it also faces new computational tasks: It now has to reliably differentiate between own and foreign actions. It has to find a reliable way of integrating only the right subset of currently active goal and action representations into its self-model. Cortical activity in the representation of own and foreign actions clearly overlaps and, interestingly, non-schizophrenic subjects are not able to phenomenally represent the relevant signals generated by their own limb movements (Georgieff and Jeannerod 1998).

Action-relative information seems to be coded in two pathways in systems like ourselves, because the action representation via the phenomenal self-model does not depend on the same information that is used in generating automatic actions. In other words, the capacity to differentiate between first-person and third-person actions utilizing proprioceptive, endogenous signals is itself not localized on the phenomenal level, is not being carried out through accessing phenomenally available information. What actually enters into phenomenal self-experience may just be the global state of a comparator module (Georgieff and Jeannerod 1998). Therefore, two major classes of hallucinations exist: perceptions without objects and actions (including cognitive actions) without subjects. We do not yet know anything about the detailed mech-

anisms generating the corresponding classes of phenomenal states (the medial prefrontal area may constitute a major component of their neural correlate; see Frith 1996). However, it is conceivable that a functional dedifferentiation of the mechanism which integrates action representations into the self-model as *intended* or as *imagined* actions, versus leaving them in a more abstract, allocentric status as elements of the external world model (and therefore only as *observed* actions), leads to the pathological phenomenology in question.

The neural correlates of this type of deviant representational dynamics are slowly beginning to emerge. They seem to be related to hyperactivational states in the right inferior parietal lobule (Brodmann area 40) and the cingulate gyrus (e.g., Spence et al. 1997). Interestingly, what in scientific practice leads us from the representational analysis of such uncommon classes of phenomenal states to the delineation of their physical correlates, is imaging their functional correlates. An important aspect of these functional correlates seems to consist in disordered ways of making the structure of external and internal bodily space available for the system and in deficits of the internal monitoring of ongoing motor acts (Spence et al. 1997).

• Alien hand syndrome (Goldstein 1908; Brion and Jedynak 1972) is characterized by a global experiential state in which the patient typically is well aware of complex, observable movements carried out by the nondominant hand, while at the same time experiencing no corresponding volitional acts. Subjectively (as well as functionally) the arm is "out of control," with a sense of intermanual conflict. On the other hand, many such arm movements clearly seem to be goal-directed actions, although no such goal representation is available either on the phenomenal level in general or on the level of conscious self-representation. Geschwind and his colleagues (1995) offer a case report of a 68-year-old woman suffering from a transient alien hand syndrome caused by a stroke limited only to the middle and posterior portions of the body of the corpus callosum:

> On postoperative day 11, she was noted by nursing staff to have left-sided weakness and difficulty walking. According to her family, she had complained of loss of control of her left hand for the previous three days, as if the hand were performing on its own. She awoke several times with her left hand choking her, and while she was awake, her left hand would unbutton her gown, crush cups on her tray, and fight with the right hand while she was answering the phone. To keep her left hand from doing mischief, she would subdue it with the right hand. She described this unpleasant situation as if someone "from the moon" were controlling her hand (Geschwind et al. 1995: 803).[11]

In this case the functional correlate of representational shift is likely to have been an inter-hemispheric motor disconnection, whereas the neural correlate of this functional deficit was a rather circumscribed lesion in the midbody of the corpus callosum. On the representational level we see that the triggering events leading to a certain subset of contradictory, but impressively complex and very obviously goal-directed, patterns of motor behavior, cannot be depicted as *my own* volitional acts anymore. In other words, the information about these events taking place within the system cannot be integrated into the phenomenal self-model. It is no longer globally available information for the system, either as a property of the world or as a property of the system itself. Therefore these action-generating events are—from the patient's perspective—not part of *her* phenomenal biography anymore. Only the visually and proprioceptively represented arm movements themselves are endowed with phenomenal subjectivity in the sense of ownership. They are, however, *not* subjective in the sense of phenomenal agenthood. Again, what is missing is a certain integrative capacity: the capacity to integrate a representation of the causal history of certain motor commands into the phenomenal self-model. (Note the implicit parallels to the discussions of schizophrenia in

Daprati et al. 1997; Georgieff and Jeannerod 1998). On the functional level this loss is possibly mirrored in the loss of interhemispheric integration of motor and supplementary motor areas (Geschwind et al. 1995: 807).

• Hemi-neglect and other attention disorders seem to present an especially interesting case: You have an active self-representational structure, parts of which cannot be "read out" by higher-order attentional processes. Therefore you do not have a phenomenal self-model of this region in state-space; information already contained in the system is not available under what the philosopher might want to call an internal context or an "ego-mode of presentation" (Newen 1997: 117).

Attention is important in constituting phenomenal content. Bernard Baars and David Chalmers have repeatedly pointed out that "global availability" may be one of the central functional criteria to mark out active phenomenal information. (see Baars 1988; Chalmers 1997). I think that given the material from psychophysics and neuropsychology, we need to differentiate this concept into at least three subcategories: *attentional* availability, *cognitive* availability, and *volitional* availability. In alien hand syndrome you seem to have a deficit that destroys volitional availability, but not attentional or cognitive availability. In hemi-neglect, however, attentional unavailability of information contained in an existing self-model can lead to a loss of cognitive availability (as in confabulatory activity and in anosognosia) and volitional availability (as in paralysis). There are of course generalized versions of this type of deviant phenomenal self-modeling.

One also has to do justice to situations in which certain layers of the self-model seem to be extended to the very border of the global model of reality.

• In some cases of mania or during certain religious experiences, the patient (or the mystic) is convinced that *all* events he experiences as taking place in the world are caused by his own volitional acts.

Philosophically speaking, the implicit ontology underlying these states is a Platonistic version of solipsism: All causation is mental causation, and there is only one causal agent in the world.[12] From a representationalist perspective we clearly seem to be confronted with a hypertrophy of self-representation: External events are endowed with phenomenal agenthood because their causal history is represented as an internal part of the system itself.[13] One may therefore speculate that the corresponding functional correlate must consist in a dedifferentiation of the integrational mechanism, which embeds some event representations into the currently active self-model while constantly excluding others. To my knowledge, nothing about the neural correlates realizing such a pathological function is known to date.

Let us take a look at the second target property.

The Property of Selfhood   Phenomenal selfhood is what makes us an experiential subject. In German the property in question has sometimes been called *präreflexive Selbstvertrautheit* (prereflexive self-intimacy; e.g., Frank 1991). It is a very basic and seemingly spontaneous, effortless way of inner acquaintance, of "being in touch with yourself," a fundamental form of nonconceptual self-knowledge that precedes any higher forms of cognitive self-consciousness. In fact, this basic form of primitive self-awareness is what makes quasi-propositional and conceptually mediated forms of self-consciousness possible, by preventing them from becoming circular and empty (Bermúdez 1995; Metzinger 1993). From a representationalist perspective it clearly must be the result of an ongoing subsymbolic dynamics: the existence of a single, coherent, and temporally extended self-representation forming the center of the global representational state. The resulting *centeredness* of the overall representational state, however, is a functional prop-

erty (to which I will come back later). If the representational module I just mentioned is damaged or disintegrates, or if multiple structures of this type alternate in the system or are simultaneously active, different neuropsychological syndromes or altered states result.

Here are some brief examples:

• Anosognosias and anosodiaphorias: loss of higher-order insight into an existing deficit, as in blindness denial (Anton's syndrome). This extensive and well-documented class of disorders is theoretically relevant, because it falsifies the "epistemic transparency" assumption, under which many classical theories of subjectivity have operated: There exist unnoticed and unnoticeable forms of mis(self-)representation, because large portions of the subsymbolic self-model seem to be cognitively and introspectively impenetrable (see also section "The Central Theoretical Problem on the Representational Level of Description," below).

• Dissociative identity disorder (DID; for diagnostic features, see *DSM-IV*: 300.14). The system uses different and alternating self-models to functionally adapt to extremely traumatizing or socially inconsistent situations. On the phenomenal level this results in the presence of two or more distinct "identities" or personality states, and sometimes in asymmetric amnesias.

Since I cannot enter an extended discussion of this specific class of phenomenal states here,[14] I only want to draw readers' attention to two important points that demonstrate the explanatory power of the naturalized representationalist approach as opposed to classical philosophical theories of subjectivity. First, it is of course well conceivable that a system generates a number of different self-models which are functionally incompatible, and therefore modularized. They nevertheless could be internally coherent, each endowed with its own characteristic phenomenal content and behavioral profile. Second, this does not have to be a pathological situation. Operating under different self-models in different situational contexts may be biologically as well as socially adaptive. Don't we all to some extent use multiple personalities to cope efficiently with different parts of our lives?

• *Ich-Störungen*[15] are a large class of psychiatric disorders accompanied by changes in the conscious experience of one's own identity. (For useful conceptual discussions and a number of case studies, see, e.g., Halligan and Marshall 1996.)

In these cases, the phenomenal self starts to disintegrate. Schizophrenia and DID are examples, as are depersonalization disorders. Self-models can lack information or become multiplied. They also can lose internal coherence. Phenomenological data from clinical neuropsychology and cognitive neuropsychiatry show that the internal correlation strength between the set of properties which is being depicted in the mode of phenomenal self-representation can vary greatly. If the phenomenal self-model, as I propose, at any given moment is a unified representation that can also dissolve or disintegrate, then there might of course be something like a *gradient of coherence* for this structure. In principle some metric for the internal coherence of a self-model should exist. Once the neural correlate of the phenomenal self-model in humans can be described in sufficient detail, this observation will constitute an interesting target for formal modeling.

The Property of Perspectivalness   The third and last phenomenal target property is "perspectivalness": the existence of a single, coherent, and temporally stable model of reality that is representationally centered on a single, coherent, and temporally extended phenomenal subject. A phenomenal subject is a model of the system *as experiencing*.[16] To analyze perspectivalness, a second theoretical entity has to be introduced: "the phenomenal model of the intentionality-relation," i.e., an ongoing, dynamical representation of the system *as currently interacting with an object-component* (see section "Step 5" and chapter 7, this volume). This structural feature of

the global representational space leads to the instantiation of a temporally extended, nonconceptual, first-person perspective. Again, if this global structural feature is lost, phenomenology changes and different neuropsychological disorders or classes of certain altered states emerge. Here are two last examples of situations in which conscious experience seems to remain while no longer being phenomenologically *subjective* experience. In these configurations the first-person perspective has been dissolved:

• Complete depersonalization (see *DSM-IV*: 300.6): loss of the phenomenal first-person perspective, accompanied by dysphoric states and functional deficits (*Angstvolle Ich-Auflösung*, "dreadful ego-dissolution"; see Dittrich 1985).

• Mystical states and religious experiences: self-less and noncentered global states that are later described and "autobiographically experienced" as nonpathological and nonthreatening (*Ozeanische Selbstentgrenzung*, "oceanic boundary loss"; see Dittrich 1985; "The Great View from Nowhere").

The interesting insight at this point seems to be that there is in fact something like phenomenologically nonsubjective consciousness (see Castaneda 1966; Chisholm 1981; Lewis 1979; Perry 1993; Shoemaker 1996). Obviously a full-blown theory of mind will have to do justice to the full spectrum of phenomenal states undergone by human beings. Mystical experiences as well as fully depersonalized pathological situations are important elements of this spectrum. The major epistemological obstacle in turning such states—be they pathological or spiritual—into explananda for neuroscientific research lies in the logical contradiction inherent in all reports from a purportedly *auto*biographical type of memory. The self-contradictory nature of such reports makes them a very doubtful source of information from a methodological perspective. I will now consider the two most important objections to the approach sketched in this paper.

The Central Theoretical Problem on the Functional Level of Description

The obvious criticism at this point is: This analysis does not do full justice to the phenomenology of self-consciousness, and it also cannot help us in understanding why a self-representation can be used as the immovable center of an egocentric world model in a purely functional sense. To take the phenomenology seriously means doing justice to the fact that the first-person perspective is always privileged among all other perspectives, which may be mentally represented in my conscious space as well.[17] In what way does the phenomenal self-model differ from all other currently active phenomenal models, be they models of objects or models of other persons? Which functional property marks out its special role in the informational architecture of the system, and exactly how does it become the stable *center*, not only of phenomenal but of behavioral space as well?

Here is my answer: The self-model is the only representational structure that is anchored in the brain by a continuous source of *internally* generated input. Whenever conscious experience (i.e., the activation of a stable, integrated model of reality) takes place at all, this continual source of internal, proprioceptive input exists as well. The body is always there, and although its relational properties in space and in movement constantly change, the body is the only coherent perceptual object that *constantly* generates input. If one treats the many different internal sources of information flowing from tactile, visceral, vestibular, and other proprioceptors within the body as one single sensory modality, one arrives at an interesting conclusion: Body perception is unique not only from an epistemological, but also from a functional perspective, in that it has only one singular object ever (see Martin 1995; Bermúdez 1998: chap. 6). And this elementary body percept will always contain a subvolume, which is unique in that it integrates a region

of maximal invariance into phenomenal state-space, a region which is generated from an information flow originating exclusively in internal transducers and which is strictly stimulus-correlated. I call this stimulus-correlated part of the self-model a self-*presentation* (see Metzinger 1993, 1997), because it makes fine-grained information available to the system that, according to my hypothesis, can be *presented*, but not *re*presented.[18] The self-model becomes the functional center of representational as well as of behavioral space, because its purely presentational basis contributes to the only perceptual object that is permanently stimulus-correlated. Within that object we have something like a "background 'buzz' of somatosensory input" (Kinsbourne 1995: 217), which on the subcognitive level of phenomenal experience enables us to *feel ourselves* as continuously embodied and as present within a subjective now.

This answer to the functionalist question posed above immediately leads to testable hypotheses, because it makes the step from functional to neural correlates possible. If, e.g., it is really true that the constant activity of that part of the neuromatrix of the spatial model of one's own body, which is independent of external input, becomes the center of experiential space by forming an invariant background of bodily awareness, then this constitutes an empirical hypothesis. Of course, as a philosopher I should now definitely step back and refrain from any dilettante, amateurish speculation. However, let me draw my readers' attention to the fact that new results concerning research on pain experience in phantom limbs may point to the existence of a genetically determined neuromatrix, the input-independent activation pattern of which could form the functional basis of the most invariant partitions in the phenomenal body image ("phylomatrix of the body-schema"; see Melzack 1989, 1990, 1992; Melzack et al. 1997; for a possibly more fundamental, but compatible approach see also Damasio 1994, 1999; Damasio and Damasio 1996a,b).

Of course, one might think that the elementary body percept is consolidated in social interactions only after birth, or during earlier motor behavior in the womb.[19] On the other hand, a persistent functional link between regions of primary somatosensory cortex and certain regions in the bodily self-model is proved by direct electrical stimulation during neurosurgical operations under local anesthesia (see Melzack et al. 1997). Of course, sensory body and motor maps are highly plastic and subject to the influence of experience even in the adult organism. And, of course, one has to see that there is probably no such thing as *absolute* invariance or functional rigidity. But there is good evidence for some kind of innate "body prototype," as can, for instance, be seen from the phantom sensations reported by some phocomelic children, who are born without one or more limbs. It seems that these data show that even people born without limbs develop complex bodily self-models which sometimes *include* limbs—even if there never has been a source of input.

Melzack's case studies provide convincing evidence that phantom limbs are experienced by at least 20 percent of congenitally limb-deficient subjects and by 50 percent of those who underwent amputations before the age of six years. If *all* of the congenital cases failed to have phantom experiences, it would be plausible that all self-modeling is only experientially based, but taken together with the fact that some of these patients do not lose the relevant parts of their phenomenal self-model even as adults, these cases seem to constitute plausible evidence that the neural correlate of the spatial model of the self is partly immune to local neuroplasticity in the somatosensory cortex. Melzack also points to numerous cases in which excision of the somatosensory cortex did not prevent the reappearance of a phantom limb at follow-up. Therefore the neural correlate of self-consciousness (NCSC) must be highly distributed.[20] In an earlier publication, Melzack writes:

In essence, I postulate that the brain contains a neuromatrix, or network of neurons, that, in addition to responding to sensory stimulation, continuously generates a characteristic pattern of impulses indicating that the body is intact and unequivocally one's own. I call this pattern a neurosignature. If such a matrix operated in the absence of sensory inputs from the periphery of the body, it would create the impression of having a limb even when that limb has been removed. (1992: 93)

Again, I do not want to indulge in any amateurish speculation at this point. On the level of conceptual analysis my answer to the first problem is that the self-model is the only active representational structure in the system which is functionally anchored in a continuous, internally generated source of input. If this is correct, there should be many empirical routes to successfully take the step from the functional to the neural correlates of preconceptual self-consciousness.

The Central Theoretical Problem on the Representational Level of Description

Step 3: Transparency and Naive Realism

The antireductionist reply to the theoretical model sketched in this essay is obvious and straightforward. There seems to be no necessary connection between the functional and representational basis properties and the phenomenal target properties of "mineness," "selfhood," and "perspectivalness." Everything described so far could, of course, happen without the instantiation of the phenomenal properties of "mineness," "selfhood," and "perspectivalness." It is conceivable, a property dualist might argue, that a biological information-processing system opens a centered representational space and then always embeds a model of itself into the model of reality active within this space *without* automatically generating a phenomenal self. An active, dynamical "self-model" still is just a representation of the system; it is a *system* model—

not an instance of genuine self-consciousness. In order for the functional property of centeredness to contribute to the phenomenal property of perspectivalness, the model of the system has to become a phenomenal self. From a philosophical point of view the cardinal question is What is needed—by conceptual necessity—to make a phenomenal first-person perspective emerge from a representational space that is already functionally centered? In short, how do you get from the functional property of "centeredness" and the representational property of "self-modeling" to the phenomenal property of "selfhood"?

The answer lies in what one might call the "semantic transparency" of the data structures used by the system. Terminological details[21] aside, the general idea is that the representational vehicles[22] employed by the system are transparent in the sense that they do not contain the information *that* they are models on the level of their content (see Metzinger 1993; Van Gulick 1988a, 1988b). In our present context "transparency" means that we are systems which are not able to recognize their own representational instruments *as* representational instruments. That is why we "look through" those representational structures, as if we were in direct and immediate contact with their content, with what they represent for us (see also row 2 of table 20.1).

Again, one may move downward and speculate about certain functional properties of the internal instruments the system uses to represent the world and itself *to* itself. A simple functional hypothesis might say that the respective data structures are activated in such a fast and reliable way that the system itself is not able to recognize them as such anymore (e.g., because of a lower temporal resolution of metarepresentational processes; see, e.g., Metzinger 1995c). This can then be supplemented by a plausible teleofunctionalist assumption: For biological systems like ourselves—who always had to minimize computational load and find simple but viable solutions—naive realism was a functionally adequate "back-

ground assumption" to achieve reproductive success. In short, there has been no evolutionary pressure on our representational architecture to overcome the naive realism inherent in semantic transparency. The decisive step of my argument consists in applying this point to the self-model.

Step 4: Autoepistemic Boundedness

Let us take stock. So far we have taken three steps in our investigation: First, the self-model was introduced as a theoretical entity. Second, we made a brief representationalist analysis of the target properties possible. Third, we then introduced an empirically highly plausible assumption regarding the nature of many phenomenal representations, the transparency assumption. We now have two more steps, both of which are decisive. The first consists in applying the transparency assumption to the self-model and thereby solving the homunculus problem.

We are systems that are not able to recognize their subsymbolic self-model *as* a model. For this reason we are permanently operating under the conditions of a "naive-realistic self-misunderstanding": We experience ourselves as constantly being in direct and immediate epistemic contact with ourselves. What we have in the past simply called a "self" is not a nonphysical individual, but only the content of an ongoing, dynamical process—the process of transparent self-modeling. Any system that, because of its functional architecture, is not able to recognize its self-generated subconceptual representation of itself *as* a representation, will inevitably fall into a naive-realistic relationship toward the content of this representation.[23] On the representationalist level of analysis, this clearly seems to be a conceptual necessity. And as an empirical assumption about the way our brain actually works, it is highly plausible. A prereflexive phenomenal self, therefore, emerges if a system operates under a model of reality centered by a transparent self-model.

Step 5:   The Phenomenal Model of the Intentionality Relation

The last step consists in applying the transparency constraint to the internal representation of the relation between subject and perceptual object, to the relation between agent and goal. If, for instance, the phenomenal model of one's own perceptual states contains a transparent representation of their causal history, then inevitably convolved global states will result, the content of which can only be truthfully described by the system itself as (e.g.) "I *myself* [= the content of a transparent self-model] am now seeing *this object* [= the content of a transparent object representation], and I am seeing it *with my own eyes*" [= the simple story about immediate sensory perception, which sufficed for the brain's evolutionary purposes]. The phenomenal self is a virtual agent perceiving virtual objects in a virtual world. This agent doesn't know that it possesses a visual cortex, and it does not know what electromagnetic radiation is: It just sees "with its own eyes"—by, as it were, effortlessly directing its visual attention. This virtual agent does not know that it possesses a motor system which, for instance, needs an internal emulator for fast, goal-driven reaching movements. It just acts "with its own hands." It doesn't know what a sensorimotor loop is—it just effortlessly enjoys what researchers in the field of virtual reality design call "full immersion," which for them is still a distant goal. To achieve this global effect, what is needed is a dynamic and transparent subject-object relation that episodically integrates the self-model and those perceptual objects which cause the changes in its content by telling an internal story about how these changes came about. This story does not have to be the true story; it may well be a greatly simplified internal confabulation that has proved to be functionally adequate.

Based on the arguments given above, I claim that phenomenal subjectivity emerges precisely at this stage: As soon as the system transparently models itself as an epistemic or causal agent, you have a transparent representation of episodic subject-object relations. For philosophers, of course, the new distinction of *phenomenal* intentionality as opposed to unconscious processes bearing intentional content will not be too surprising a move. It certainly is exciting that we presently witness this notion surfacing at the frontier of neuroscientific theory formation as well (see, e.g., Damasio 1994, 1999; Damasio and Damasio 1996a: 172, 1996b: 24; chapter 7, this volume; Delacour 1997: 138; LaBerge 1997: 150, 172).

Why would a concise research program for the neural correlate of self-consciousness (the NCSC) be of highest relevance for understanding phenomenal experience? If all the above is true (or if it at least points in the right direction), then it should prove to be more than heuristically fruitful. The vast majority of phenomenal states are *subjective* states in the way I have just analyzed: Not only are they elements of a coherent internal model of reality used by the system; not only are they activated within a window of presence; not only does their phenomenal content supervene entirely on internal functional and physical properties; but they are bound into a transparently centered representational space. The maximally salient focus of conscious experience will always be constituted by the object-component of the phenomenal model of the intentionality-relation, with the subject-component, the self-model, providing a source of invariance and stability. If I am correct —and that is what it actually means when one says that such states are subjective states—then a straightforward empirical prediction will follow: Under standard conditions a very large class of phenomenal states should become episodically integrated with the current self-model on a very small time scale, as attention, as volition, as cognition wander around in representational space, selecting ever new object-components for the conscious first-person perspective. Global availability of information means availability for transient, dynamical integration into the currently active self-model, generating a "self in the act of knowing." In other words, the self-model theory of subjectivity can serve to mark out a specific and highly interesting class of neural correlates of consciousness.

And that is why the NCSC is important: Only if we find the neural and functional correlates of the phenomenal self will we be able to discover a more *general* theoretical framework into which all data can fit. Only then will we have a chance to understand what we are actually talking about when we say that phenomenal experience is a *subjective* phenomenon. It is for this reason that I have introduced two new theoretical entities in this chapter, the notion of a "transparent self-model" and the concept of the "phenomenal model of the intentionality-relation." Two predictions are associated with them. First, if—all other constraints held constant—the self-model of a conscious system would become fully *opaque*, then the phenomenal target property of experiential "selfhood" would disappear. Second, if the phenomenal model of the intentionality-relation collapses or cannot be sustained in a given conscious system, phenomenal states may exist, but will not be experientially *subjective* states any more, because the phenomenal first-person perspective has disappeared in this system. Intentionality-modeling is a necessary condition for perspectivalness.

In conclusion, let me once again illustrate the central thought of the argument by a metaphor. Interestingly, the point of this metaphor is that it contains a logical mistake: We are systems which were configured by evolution in such a way that they constantly *confuse* themselves with the content of their phenomenal self-model. In other words, we are physical systems that *on the level of phenomenal representation* are not able to differentiate between themselves and the content of their currently active self-model. We know ourselves only under a representation, and we are not able to *subjectively* represent this very fact. The evolutionary advantage of the underlying

dynamical process of constantly confusing yourself with your own self-model is obvious: It makes a selfless biological system *egotistic* by generating a very robust self-illusion. Now here is the logical mistake: *Whose* illusion could that be? It makes sense to speak of truth and falsity, of knowledge and illusion, only if you already have an epistemic agent in the sense of a system possessing conceptualized knowledge in a strong propositional sense. But this is not the case: We have just solved the homunculus problem; there is nobody in there who could be wrong about anything. All you have is a functionally grounded self-modeling system under the condition of a naive-realistic self-misunderstanding. So, if you would really want to carry this metaphor even further, what I have been saying in this paper is that the conscious self is an illusion which is *no one's* illusion.

Acknowledgments

I wish to thank William Banks, Patricia Churchland, Christof Koch, Francis Crick, Antonio Damasio, and Mirko von Elstermann for helpful comments and critical discussions of earlier versions of this paper.

Notes

1. This, of course, is a point Paul Churchland has often made: "I suggest, then, that those of us who prize the flux and content of our subjective phenomenological experience need not view the advance of materialist neuroscience with fear and foreboding. Quite the contrary. The genuine arrival of a materialist kinematics and dynamics for psychological states and cognitive processes will constitute not a gloom in which our inner life is suppressed or eclipsed, but rather a dawning, in which its marvellous intricacies are finally revealed—most notably, if we apply [it] ourselves, in direct self-conscious introspection." See Churchland 1989: 66.

2. Although this structure may already contain primitive, self-specifying information. See especially Bermúdez 1998: chap. 5.

3. Higher-order, conceptually mediated forms of self-consciousness are always anchored in more primitive forms of noncategorizable, cognitively unavailabe forms of content (from which they very likely have developed: see Bermúdez 1998; Metzinger 1993). It is exciting to see how currently the best philosophical theorists working on analytical theories of self-representation and self-consciousness are starting to do justice to the importance of bodily awareness in the constitution of higher-level forms of subjectivity (see, e.g., Bermúdez 1998 or Cassam 1997). However, one should be careful as not to introduce a principled distinction (and hence a new dualism between reified conceptual and nonconceptual forms of content) at this point. Content is not a mysterious type of *thing*, but an abstract property of a highly fluid and complex cognitive dynamics, and the best empirically plausible models of representational content we have at this point clearly suggest the existence of a *continuum* reaching from simple sensory content to more abstract, conceptlike forms (see Churchland 1998: 32). I would like to suggest that we will find exactly such a continuum in the case of self-representation as well.

4. This, of course, is just another way of describing what happens when you wake up in the morning. There is a formal proof that every regulator of a complex system will automatically become a *model* of that system. See Conant and Ashby 1970.

5. In table 20.1 I have tried to give an overview of what I think are the seven most important phenomenological characteristics of subjective states. For each case, a convincing representationalist analysis could constitute another necessary, but not sufficient, ascription criterion for conscious experience in standard cases. However, consciousness is such a rich and complex phenomenon that counter examples can always be found if our domain is sufficiently wide (e.g., considering case studies from clinical neuropsychology, see Metzinger 2002). Therefore, my goal in this paper is rather modest: I am not claiming that even if we had all seven criteria (let's call them weak subjectivity 1–7) clearly defined in a conceptually convincing and empirically contentful manner, the conjunction of these criteria would already constitute a *necessary* condition. I am not even claiming that the criterion investigated here is a necessary criterion in a strict analytical sense (see note 6).

The reasons for concentrating on perspectivalness and self-representation are in part philosophical and in part methodological (see the section "Step 5"). From a philosophical perspective, for many reasons the subjectivity of our target phenomenon is arguably the most interesting aspect of the problem. If one is interested in generating empirical research programs, then the neural correlates of phenomenal self-modeling are especially interesting, because under standard conditions, they will constitute the most *invariant* aspect of state-space.

6. Note that in certain contexts this condition may not even be a *necessary* condition for the ascription of phenomenal experience in general: If we allow for noncentered, selfless states of phenomenal experience (e.g., in psychiatric cases like full depersonalization or during some classes of mystical or religious experiences), then we will have to conceptually describe these state classes as aperspectival or *nonsubjective* varieties of conscious experience. As exclusively *internal* representations, such states may still be "subjective" from an epistemological perspective (and in a quite weak sense), but they are nonsubjective on a phenomenological level of description.

7. I think that "virtual reality" is the best technological metaphor which is currently available as a source for generating new theoretical intuitions. In the context of this paper, heuristically the most interesting concept may be that of "full immersion." Here, my own ideas converge strongly with those of Antti Revonsuo. See Revonsuo 1995; and chapter 4 in this volume.

8. See Ramachandran and Blakeslee 1998: 47. For clinical and experimental details, see Ramachandran and Rogers-Ramachandran 1996.

9. Depersonalization is here understood as the loss of phenomenal agenthood, namely, the specific form of phenomenal content that Karl Jaspers called "Vollzugsbewußtsein" (executive consciousness).

10. Frith (1996: 1509) points out that attributions of heard voices to external *agents* are more strongly correlated to current delusions than to actually occurring hallucinations, and therefore are in some sense independent from the tendency to phenomenally represent self-generated events as external. McKay, McKenna, and Laws (1986) offer a case study and a number of considerations concerning the clinical concept of schizophrenia that may be helpful for philosophers.

11. I am indebted to Andreas Kleinschmidt for useful advice with regard to relevant literature and possible interpretations of data.

12. This way of analyzing phenomenal state classes, according to the brain's implicit ontology or functionally active "existence assumptions," also opens a new hermeneutic research program for the history of ideas. It is the mirror image of the approach sketched here: What kinds of neuropsychiatric diagnoses would correspond to which types of classical philosophical models of reality, if their ontology were interpreted as an actual, individual *phenomenal* representation of reality?

13. Such overattributions could, for instance, be interpreted as a dysfunction of the hypothetical comparator module postulated in Georgieff and Jeannerod 1998.

14. But see Metzinger 1993, 1996, 2002. For an early philosophical discussion and a striking case study, see Dennett and Humphrey 1989; for further references and some critical remarks, see Miller and Triggiano 1992; David et al. 1996.

15. There is no canonical and taxonomically established translation for the German category of an *Ich-Störung* (ego disorder). What in English is often termed "passivity phenomena" and "delusions of control" are prototypical examples of this disorder. Henrik Walter points out that this may be due to the influence of German idealism on theoretical psychiatry (see Walter 2000).

16. To speak about a model of self *as experiencing* does not necessary lead to circularity. The phenomenal content of the self-model includes dynamical relations to the world—for instance, to perceived objects. I will say more about this feature of self-representation *as phenomenal subject* in the section "Step 5." Closely related considerations of course apply to the model of self *as acting*.

17. For a recent antireductionist description of the problem of the experiential *individuality* of self-consciousness, see e.g., Nagel 1986: chap. 4. For criticisms, see Lycan 1996; Malcolm 1988; Metzinger 1995a.

18. Concerning the notion of "presentational content," see Metzinger 1997, 2002, chapter 2. Presentational content is subconceptual, nondoxastic, stimulus-correlated, and homogeneous sensory content, given within a subjective window of presence. The information given by presentational content is attentionally and volitionally, but not cognitively, available for the system.

19. I am greatly indebted to Toemme Nösselt for a number of helpful discussions on this issue.

20. This has consequences for a philosophical theory of self-representation because it sets a major constraint with regard to the possible *formats* of mental content. Connectionist theories of representation meet this constraint.

21. See Van Gulick 1988a, 1988b; Metzinger 1993; see also Harman 1990; McGinn 1982; Shoemaker 1990; Tye 1991, 1995. In the Anglo-Saxon world the first occurrence of the related concept of "diaphanousness" may have been Moore 1903: 450. Note that not all phenomenal representations are characterized by this feature: Pseudohallucinations or contents of lucid dreams are examples in which the information that these states are *representational* states is experientially available to the phenomenal subject. The most important *opaque* layer of the human self-model is arguably formed by conscious, self-directed thought; see note 23.

22. I call these vehicles "phenomenal mental models," assuming that we will eventually be able to describe them as a definite subclass of connectionist representations, the content of which can very likely analyzed through some sort of state-space semantics. See Metzinger 1995b; Churchland 1986, 1989, 1998.

23. It is interesting to note that there are of course layers within the human self-model that are *not* characterized by the transparency mentioned above. As *cognitive agents*, as thinkers of thoughts in a quasi-linguistic format, we generate intended simulations of certain states of affairs that may or may not hold in the world. On the level of phenomenal experience we clearly recognize these cognitive processes *as* self-initiated representational activities; and, interestingly, it is only through the use of precisely these representational instruments—through theory formation—that we can in effect transcend our naive-realistic self-misunderstanding—if only by intellectual insight, and not on the level of subjective experience itself. What we often call the "cognitive subject," the thinking self, actually is a rather small partition of the human self-model, presumably also one that is phylogenetically very young. Maybe the fact that it is this partition which holds the capacity for epistemically transcending the situation I have described above, is responsible for the obvious fact of philosophers traditionally being most interested in this part of the human self. Cognitive activities in a narrower sense are processes that internally simulate compositionality and syntactical operations on quasi-linguistic symbol-tokens to a suffi-

cient degree of approximation. And it is precisely for linguistic entities that we can make a distinction between form and content, between syntax and semantics.

References

Baars, B. J. (1988). *A Cognitive Theory of Consciousness*. Cambridge: Cambridge University Press.

Bermúdez, J. L. (1995). Ecological perception and the notion of a nonconceptual point of view. In Bermúdez et al. 1995.

Bermúdez, J. L. (1998). *The Paradox of Self-Consciousness*. Cambridge, MA: MIT Press.

Bermúdez, J. L., Marcel, A., and Eilan, N., eds. (1995). *The Body and the Self*. Cambridge, MA: MIT Press.

Block, N., Flanagan, O., and Güzeldere, G., eds. (1997). *Consciousness: Philosophical Debates*. Cambridge, MA: MIT Press.

Brentano, F. (1973) [1874]. *Psychologie vom empirischen Standpunkt. Erster Band*. Hamburg: Meiner.

Brion, S., and Jedynak, C.-P. (1972). Troubles du transfert interhémisphérique (callosal disconnection). A propos de trois observations de tumeurs du corps calleux. Le signe de lamain étrangère. *Revue neurologique* (Paris) 126: 257–266.

Cassam, Q. (1997). *Self and World*. Oxford: Clarendon Press.

Castañeda, H. N. (1966). >He<: A study on the logic of self-consciousness. *Ratio* 8: 130–157.

Chalmers, D. J. (1997). Availability: The cognitive basis of experience? In Block et al. 1997.

Chisholm, R. M. (1981). *The First Person. An Essay on Reference and Intentionality*. Minneapolis: University of Minnesota Press.

Churchland, P. M. (1986). Some reductive strategies in cognitive neurobiology. *Mind* 95: 279–309. Reprinted in Churchland 1989.

Churchland, P. M. (1989). *A Neurocomputational Perspective*. Cambridge, MA: MIT Press.

Churchland, P. M. (1998). Conceptual similarity across sensory and neural diversity: The Fodor/Lepore challenge answered. *Journal of Philosophy* 65: 5–32.

Clark, A. (1989). *Microcognition: Philosophy, Cognitive Science, and Parallel Distributed Processing*. Cambridge, MA: MIT Press.

Conant, R. C., and Ashby, W. R. (1970). Every good regulator of a system must be a model of that system. *International Journal of Systems Science* 2: 89–97.

Damasio, A. (1994). *Descartes' Error*. New York: Putnam/Grosset.

Damasio, A. (1999). *The Feeling of What Happens: Body and Emotion in the Making of Consciousness*. New York: Harcourt Brace and Company.

Damasio, A., and Damasio, H. (1996a). Images and subjectivity: Neurobiological trials and tribulations. In R. N. McCauley, ed., *The Churchlands and Their Critics*. Cambridge, MA: Blackwell.

Damasio, A., and Damasio, H. (1996b). Making images and creating subjectivity. In R. Llinás and S. Churchland, eds., *The Mind–Brain Continuum*. Cambridge, MA: MIT Press.

Daprati, E., Franck, N., Georgieff, N., Proust, J., Pacherie, E., Dalery, J., and Jeannerod, M. (1997). Looking for the agent: An investigation into consciousness of action and self-consciousness in schizophrenic patients. *Cognition* 65: 71–86.

David, A., Kemp, R., Smith, L., and Fahy, T. (1996). Split minds: Multiple personality and schizophrenia. In Halligan and Marshall 1996.

Delacour, J. (1997). Neurobiology of consciousness: An overview. *Behavioural Brain Research* 85: 127–141.

Dennett, D. C. (1987). *The Intentional Stance*. Cambridge, MA: MIT Press.

Dennett, D. C., and Humphrey, N. (1989). Speaking for ourselves: An assessment of multiple personality disorder. *Raritan: A Quarterly Review* 9, no. 1: 68–98.

Diagnostic and Statistical Manual of Mental Disorders: DSM-IV. 4th ed. (1994). Prepared by the Task Force on DSM-IV and other committees and work groups of the American Psychiatric Association Washington, DC: American Psychiatric Association.

Dittrich, A. (1985). *Ätiologie-unabhängige Strukturen veränderter Wachbewußtseinszustände*. Stuttgart: Enke.

Dretske, F. (1995). *Naturalizing the Mind*. Cambridge, MA: MIT Press.

Frank, M. (1991). *Selbstbewußtsein und Selbsterkenntnis*. Stuttgart: Reclam.

Frith, C. (1996). The role of prefrontal cortex in self-consciousness: The case of auditory hallucinations. *Philosophical Transactions of the Royal Society of London* B351: 1505–1512.

Georgieff, N., and Jeannerod, M. (1998). Beyond consciousness of external reality: A "Who" system for consciousness and action and self-consciousness. *Consciousness and Cognition* 7: 465–487.

Geschwind, D. H., Iacoboni, M., Mega, M. S., Zaidel, D. W., Clughesy, T., and Zaidel, E. (1995). Alien hand syndrome: Interhemispheric disconnection due to lesion in the midbody of the corpus callosum. *Neurology* 45: 802–808.

Goldstein, K. (1908). Zur Lehre der motorischen Apraxie. *Journal für Psychologie und Neurologie* 11: 169–187.

Grush, R. (1997). The architecture of representation. *Philosophical Psychology* 10: 5–25.

Grush, R. (1998). Wahrnehmung, Vorstellung, und die sensomotorische Schleife. In H.-D. Heckmann and F. Esken, eds., *Bewußtsein und Repräsentation*. Paderborn: mentis.

Halligan, P. W., and Marshall, J. J., eds. (1996). *Method in Madness: Case Studies in Cognitive Neuropsychiatry*. Hove, UK: Psychology Press.

Harman, G. (1990). The intrinsic quality of experience. In J. Tomberlin, ed., *Philosophical Perspectives*, vol. 4, *Action Theory and Philosophy of Mind*. Atascadero, CA: Ridgeview. Reprinted in Block et al. 1997.

Kinsbourne, M. (1995). Awareness of one's own body: An attentional theory of its nature, development, and brain basis. In Bermúdez et al. 1995.

Koch, C., and Davis, J. L., eds. (1994). *Large-Scale Neuronal Theories of the Brain*. Cambridge, MA: MIT Press.

LaBerge, D. (1997). Attention, awareness, and the triangular circuit. *Consciousness and Cognition* 6: 149–181.

Lewis, D. K. (1979). Attitudes de dicto and de se. *Philosophical Review* 88: 513–542.

Lycan, W. G. (1996). *Consciousness and Experience*. Cambridge, MA: MIT Press.

Malcolm, N. (1988). Subjectivity. *Philosophy* 63: 147–160.

Marcel, A., and Bisiach, E., eds. (1988). *Consciousness in Contemporary Science*. Oxford: Oxford University Press.

Martin, M. G. F. (1995). Bodily awareness: A sense of ownership. In Bermúdez et al. 1995.

McGinn, C. (1982). *The Character of Mind*. Oxford: Oxford University Press.

McKay, A. P., McKenna, P. J., and Laws, K. (1996). Severe schizophrenia: What is it like? In Halligan and Marshall 1996.

Melzack, R. (1989). Phantom limbs, the self and the brain: The D. O. Hebb memorial lecture. *Canadian Psychology* 30: 1–16.

Melzack, R. (1990). Phantom limbs and the concept of a neuromatrix. *Trends in Neurosciences* 13: 88–92.

Melzack, R. (1992). Phantom limbs. *Scientific American* 266: 90–96.

Melzack, R., Israel, R., Lacroix, R., and Schultz, G. (1997). Phantom limbs in people with congenital limb deficiency or amputation in early childhood. *Brain* 120, pt. 9: 1603–1620.

Metzinger, T. (1993). *Subjekt und Selbstmodell: Die Perspektivität phänomenalen Bewußtseins vor dem Hintergrund einer naturalistischen Theorie mentaler Repräsentation*. Paderborn: mentis.

Metzinger, T. (1995a). Perspektivische Fakten? Die Naturalisierung des "Blick von nirgendwo." In G. Meggle and J. Nida-Rümelin, eds. (1997). *ANALYOMEN 2—Perspektiven der Analytischen Philosophie*. Berlin: De Gruyter.

Metzinger, T. (1995b). Phänomenale mentale Modelle. In K. Sachs-Hombach, ed., *Bilder im Geiste: Zur kognitiven und erkenntnistheoretischen Funktion piktorialer Repräsentationen*. Amsterdam: Rodopi.

Metzinger, T. (1995c). Faster than thought: Holism, homogeneity and temporal coding. In Metzinger 1995d.

Metzinger, T., ed. (1995d). *Conscious Experience*. Thorverton, UK: Imprint Academic; Paderborn: mentis.

Metzinger, T. (1997). *Präsentationaler Gehalt*. In H.-D. Heckmann and F. Esken, eds., *Bewußtsein und Repräsentation*. Paderborn: mentis.

Metzinger, T. (2002). *Being No One: The Self-Model Theory of Subjectivity*. Cambridge, MA: MIT Press.

Miller, S. D., and Triggiano, P. J. (1992). The psychophysiological investigation of multiple personality disorder: Review and update. *American Journal of Clinical Hypnosis* 35: 47–61.

Moore, G. E. (1903). The refutation of idealism. *Mind* 12: 433–453.

Nagel, T. (1986). *The View from Nowhere*. New York: Oxford University Press.

Newen, A. (1997). The logic of indexical thoughts and the metaphysics of the "self." In W. Künne, A. Newen, and M. Anduschus, (eds.), *Direct Reference, Indexicality and Propositional Attitudes.* Stanford: CSLI.

O'Shaughnessy, B. (1995). Proprioception and the body image. In Bermúdez et al. 1995.

Perry, J. (1993). *The Problem of the Essential Indexical and Other Essays.* Oxford: Oxford University Press.

Ramachandran, V. S., and Blakeslee, S. (1998). *Phantoms in the Brain.* New York: William Morrow.

Raffman, D. (1995). On the persistence of phenomenology. In Metzinger 1995b.

Ramachandran, V. S., and Rogers-Ramachandran, D. (1996). Synaesthesia in phantom limbs induced with mirrors. *Proceedings of the Royal Society London* B 263: 377–386.

Revonsuo, A. (1995). Consciousness, dreams, and virtual realities. *Philosophical Psychology* 8: 35–58.

Shoemaker, S. (1990). Qualities and qualia: What's in the mind? *Philosophy and Phenomenological Research Supplement* 50: 109–131.

Shoemaker, S. (1996). *The First-Person Perspective and Other Essays.* Cambridge, UK: Cambridge University Press.

Singer, W. (1993). Synchronization of cortical activity and its putative role in information processing and learning. *Annual Review of Physiology* 55: 349–384.

Singer, W. (1994). Putative functions of temporal correlations in neocortical processing. In Koch and Davis 1994.

Spence, S. A., Brooks, D. J., Hirsch, S. R., Liddle, P. F., Meehan, J., and Grasby, P. M. (1997). A PET study of voluntary movement in schizophrenic patients experiencing passivity phenomena (delusions of alien control). *Brain* 120: 1997–2011.

Tye, M. (1991). *The Imagery Debate.* Cambridge, MA: MIT Press.

Tye, M. (1995). *Ten Problems of Consciousness.* Cambridge, MA: MIT Press.

Van Gulick, R. (1988a). Consciousness, intrinsic intentionality, and self-understanding machines. In Marcel and Bisiach 1988.

Van Gulick, R. (1988b). A functionalist plea for self-consciousness. *Philosophical Review* 97: 149–188.

Walter, H. (1998). Emergence and the cognitive neuroscience approach to psychiatry. *Zeitschrift für Naturforschung* 53c: 723–737.

Walter, H. (2000). Emotionales Denken statt kalter Vernunft: Das Konzept des Selbst in der Neurophilosophie der Willensfreiheit. In A. Newen and K. Vogeley, eds., *Das Selbst und seine neurobiologischen Grundlagen.* Paderborn: mentis.

Yates, J. (1975). The content of awareness is a model of the world. *Psychological Review* 92: 249–284.

21

Awareness of Agency: Three Levels of Analysis

Joëlle Proust

Exploring the neural correlates of consciousness presents three kinds of challenges. The first has to do with the difficult notion of a neural—or of a cerebral—realization of a function. Although everyone agrees that every mental function supervenes on the activity of some part of the brain, some indeterminacy may arise regarding the kind of supervenience basis that is to be looked for. A common view is that every mental function, even highly modular ones, operates only on the background of other mental functions or cerebral systems. Therefore, when one looks for neural correlates of any particular function, one has to differentiate those neural or brain properties which are identifiable as directly correlated to that function from those which are only indirectly correlated to it. In other words, there are two ways of understanding the neural correlation of a mental state to a cerebral state. In the stronger sense, such a correlation should be both necessary and sufficient. The causal entanglement of cerebral functions makes such a demand implausible. What can be looked for is at most a weaker kind of correlation: only against the background of a normally functioning brain can some particular neural states be associated with particular mental properties. In the case of interest here, the effort to locate the supervenience basis of consciousness in one definite, well-circumscribed center is at odds with the notion that conscious states are information-processing states using widely distributed data analyses and retrieval.

The second challenge consists in specifying what the term "consciousness" is supposed to refer to. As Block (1995) shows convincingly, several different concepts are often confused under this word. Phenomenal consciousness refers to experiential states, like seeing green or feeling a pain. Access consciousness has to do with the rational control of speech and behavior. Whereas phenomenal states have a nonconceptual content, access consciousness involves inference, and thus conceptual content.

This second challenge is made still more difficult when one realizes that conscious states of both categories (phenomenal and inferential) might be related to a specific function which itself depends both on implicit (unconscious) and on explicit learning (i.e., attention). Attention cannot itself be identified with some conscious state, because if it helps to determine which kinds of contents will be made phenomenally salient and inferentially promiscuous, it cannot without circularity be itself triggered by phenomenally and inferentially salient features of incoming or stored data (see Proust 1998).

The third challenge consists in a well-known, venerable set of worries linked to the fact that after all, there is nothing we can tell about the causal connection between some neural activation—more generally, some physical structure—and a particular phenomenal quality. Shepard (1995) gives an interesting twist to the problem. Given that nonhuman animals cannot report on their internal states, how are we to establish in any principled way what kind of organism can enjoy conscious states? Neither would the ability to report subjective feelings and experiences, as displayed by humans, suffice to establish that consciousness emerges at the agent level. Does, then, the ability to have conscious experiences depend on complexity in the underlying system? Is this a holistic capacity? Is the property of being conscious a quality emerging, say, at the level of the neuron or of the neuron assembly?

However laden which conceptual difficulties, these problems cannot be articulated and solved without relying on scientific inquiry. Folk psychology is a dubious adviser in such a task, which consists partly in understanding the possibility of folk psychology. One way to circumvent suggestions from folk psychology is to concentrate on the data of mental pathology. This domain, poorly described and understood by ordinary psychology, offers interesting correlations between functional alterations and perturbations of consciousness.

We will concentrate here on the subjective impression associated with the notion that one is the actor of one's own acts. Taking the subjective lead, we will try to look for a functional basis and for a neural correlate for this "feeling in charge." Although it is a platitude to say that one did something on the basis of one's own intention to act, it is not all that clear how an action is actually planned and executed; how a subject becomes conscious of intending, acting, and having completed the action; and how far prior or current conscious states are necessary for the whole process to develop. Studying a pathological case, where a patient may either misattribute some action as being his own or, on the contrary, disavow being the actor of a particular action—claiming that a foreign influence had him move—should shed some light on the relationships between functional data, subjective reports of agency or loss thereof, and neural correlates. Schizophrenia offers such cases.

The clinical symptoms of schizophrenia include disturbances in visual experience, blocking phenomena, and specific problems in speech production, speech understanding, and thought control. The patients often have delusions of control (they see themselves as endowed with specific, more or less extensive powers over other people) or delusions of reference (other people in the street are perceived as having something particular to communicate to them). A significant proportion of patients experience hallucinations, in general (verbal-) auditory, haptic, or olfactory. They also experience a number of difficulties related to action, also called "executive" difficulties. These perturbations are manifest both in the subjective reports issued by the patients and in their results on executive tests such as the Tower of London and the Wisconsin Card Sorting Test (WCST). Being requested to tell how it all started, a patient gives the follow-ing account: "I get shaky in the knees and my chest is like a mountain in front of me, and my body actions are different. The arms and legs are apart and away from me, and they go on their own. That's when I feel I am the other person and copy their movements, or else stop and stand like a statue. I have to stop to find out whether my hand is in my pocket or not.... Sometimes the legs walk on by themselves or sometimes I let my arms roll to see where they will land" (Chapman 1966, 232).

From the mosaic of reported perturbations in the domain of action there emerges a sense of imposed actions, of being subject to a foreign will or, conversely, of exerting influence on others; a disposition to copy others without pre-established intention of doing so; and a relative difficulty in resisting impulses triggered by contextual cues.

If we want to contrast the levels of analysis of the awareness of agency in these disorders, it is important to insist that this way of summarizing the clinical evidence is shaped by covert functional hypotheses, which will be made explicit below. A patient normally couches his own experience in qualitative, holistic terms involving not only a change in his own mind but also a severe change both in the external world and in several of his bodily functions. Delusions can be seen as normal inferences from puzzling new experiences, against the background of an existing system of beliefs. Any systematic change in the quality of perception can receive a subjective explanation in epistemic and motivational terms with a considerable impact on the subject's apprehension of his world and of his role in it.

The description just given of the schizophrenic syndrome is compatible with a functional hypothesis according to which the disease would be in part constituted by a perturbed monitoring of action. By "action monitoring" is understood a set of complementary operations such as instigating an action in the correct time and place, exerting a feedback control on the movement toward the goal or target event, or stopping the movement when the goal is reached or when crucial preconditions fail to be met.

Before we examine various ways of articulating this hypothesis, we need to define an action. According to neuroscientists as well as philosophers sensitive to the issue of animal psychology (Jeannerod 1995; Frankfurt 1988), an action should be defined not on the basis of its source (in terms of relevant beliefs and desires) but as a process that develops from an internal model toward a goal with an appropriately monitored execution. In other words, feedback is the central notion for an action: A movement has to be guided in an internally controlled way up to goal attainment in order to be called an action. In this view of action, the source of the action (i.e., the actual cause that triggers it) may be external as well as internal. The fact that an action can be carried out consciously or not, in an automatic or in a deliberate way, is also an extrinsic property of action that does not need to enter its definition. As a consequence, one can also, at least as a matter of conceptual distinction, separate control of an action from conscious access to control mechanisms. On the other hand, an essential ingredient is a comparator, through which a system can modify the current steps toward the goal as a function of the difference between observed and predicted output.

According to an influential theory (Frith 1992), many of the clinical data reported above, besides the openly executive symptoms, result from impairments in processes related to the monitoring of action. Within this general framework, Christopher Frith has an interesting strategy for explaining schizophrenic symptoms. The first step consists in broadening the executive hypothesis in such a way that it encompasses action proper as well as the mental activity related to action. The second step consists in extending the hypothesis still further, by considering the previous perturbations as special cases of an overarching metarepresentational capacity. Let us examine these two steps in turn.

From Monitoring Actions to Monitoring Intentions and Self

In schizophrenia, both the monitoring of action and the monitoring of the intentions to act would be disturbed (Frith 1992: 81). Positive symptoms, such as delusion of control or verbal-auditory hallucinations, would be explained by an inability to distinguish changes due to our own actions from changes due to external events. The patient who hallucinates is seen as failing to recognize an internal speech production as his own. Similarly, in thought insertion, a patient is taken to be unable to recognize a thought as his own.

Why would these failures occur? Normally, any mental or physical activity is perceived as originating in self or in some external event thanks to the information carried by a dedicated signal, telling whether a movement was effected by the individual; when the signal is absent, the system interprets a movement as unwilled, as when the body is passively subjected to some external force. The relevant signal is supposed to help compare reafferent signals with the signals that are expected on the basis of the current willed action. It has been suggested that such a signal would be delivered by a mechanism underlying active perceptual activities called corollary discharge (Sperry 1950) or efferent copy (von Holst and Mittelstaedt 1950). Although it is only hypothetical at this stage of our knowledge of brain functions, such a mechanism is required to explain, for example, how ocular saccades can be taken into account and neutralized in interpreting visual input. When no such efferent copy signal is produced (e.g, one is sitting in a moving train), it is much more difficult to say whether one is moving or whether the perceived scene is. In our conscious sense of agency, a major component would thus consist in the sense of effort that is the subjective correlate of the corollary discharge of any action.

Granted that a sense of effort is responsible for being aware that one acts, why not suppose that a similar subjective sense allows knowing that one thinks? To give his hypothesis a wider scope, Frith suggests that the same "sense of effort" could be present when a thought is produced. A loss of such a (thought- or action-related) sense of effort would issue in an experience of either thought insertion or externally controlled action. In the case of ordinary thoughts, it is plausible that thoughts one does not identify as one's own are taken to be alien, inserted thoughts. Being a particular kind of thought, an intention to act could thus be misattributed as somebody else's intention to act.

These intriguing hypotheses have received partial support from clinical and experimental data. In particular, the difficulty in monitoring one's own actions is experimentally testable through standard executive tests such as WCST, or through specific tasks such as the ability to correct videogame motor responses used by Frith and Done (1989; see also Malenka et al. 1982). Schizophrenic patients with passivity experiences (delusions of control and thought insertion) are shown to be abnormally impaired in a motor correction task when they are not provided with visual feedback on their own actions. Using the theoretical apparatus summarized above, the idea is that while normal subjects can use central "efference copy" signals to compare the actual with the expected output of their actions, schizophrenics seem not to be able to produce, or at least to use, these signals. Being unaware of their own intentions, they will experience their actions as having an external agent. This inference is based on an incorrect memory of the type of action effected. The delusion of control thus expresses a defect in self-monitoring.

Problems of Monitoring and Metarepresentational Deficits

Frith (1992, 1994) suggests that the disorders described above, affecting both self-monitoring

and the monitoring of intentions, could after all express deeper-rooted problems having to do with the structure of conscious experience. His argument develops on both conceptual and empirical grounds. Conceptually, Frith relies on what philosophers call a "higher-order theory of conscious states" (see Rosenthal 1993). To be consciously looking at a tree, for example, you must form the thought representing the fact that you look at a tree, and hence you must form a metarepresentation of your looking at a tree. If metarepresentation is crucial for self-awareness, then people having problems with metarepresenting states (their own or others' states) should have problems with self-consciousness as well as with interpreting other people's mental states.

Empirically, Frith proposes that what is disturbed is not only some kind of low-level mechanism (such as the efferent copy mechanism evoked above) but also the ability to recognize that one is in a certain mental state (intention or belief). This ability could depend on a high-level, general-purpose mechanism responsible for a large part of metarepresentational performances. This system, called the supervisory attentional system (SAS), was first described by Shallice (1988). It is the set of control functions involved in nonroutine, willed operations. In this model, pursuing a goal may be a matter of a routine that is performed by "contention scheduling." But representing this goal, that is, making it the content of a conscious intention, is the duty of SAS. Thus, in the reading that Frith offers of Shallice's SAS, operation of the will is indeed dependent on self-consciousness. In this view, to be efficacious in guiding behavior, a state of affairs has to be represented as the content of an intention. All willed action therefore has a metarepresentational structure. Deliberate intentional action implies that a connection between two representations is established: one for a primary condition (like "do X") and one for the function that is allocated to the primary representation (like intending, believing, knowing) (Frith 1992: 130).

To understand how metarepresentation could be instantiated in the brain, one should therefore, according to Frith, concentrate on the relationship between contention schedule and SAS: The first gives primary information—"do X"—about a movement to be performed. Such information can be understood as a first-order proposition, or as some representation activated in motor cortex. SAS then specifies what the function of the proposition will be; an additional brain representation interacting with the proposition will thus allow forming of the metarepresentation "I intend to do X." This additional structure could be different according to the kind of connection between the metarepresentation and its primary content. Looking at the relevant brain areas, it is found that tasks which require inhibition of prepotent responses involve the orbito-frontal lobe, whereas tasks requiring delayed reponses activate dorsolateral frontal areas. Prefrontal cortex, supplementary motor area (SMA), and the basal ganglia would be in charge of the proper control of the use to which the primary content (represented in the relevant part of motor or temporal cortex) should be put (Frith 1992: 130).

Let us summarize. For Frith, monitoring one's actions presupposes monitoring one's intentions, which in turn presupposes being conscious of having those intentions. For example, the fact that rats can monitor their own actions ipso facto indicates that these animals "have some kind of self-awareness" (Frith 1992: 131). In this metarepresentational framework, schizophrenic symptoms result from the underlying disorder in the ability to metarepresent mental states, both in the self and in other people. In auditory hallucination, a patient hears a voice and does not recognize it as his own for lack of a self-attribution; in reference delusion the patient makes incorrect inferences about the intentions of other people, misattributing a mental state to someone who does not have it. A patient with a delusion of influence does not recognize his own intentions and takes them to be somebody else's.

Frith's model thus sees schizophrenia as lying on a continuum with a developmental disorder such as autism. Autistic children present a perturbation in understanding mental states in themselves and others, as is shown by their specific difficulty in solving the false belief task. To succeed at such a task, one must take someone else's point of view on a situation even though the corresponding belief is false (outdated). Let us suppose that an autistic child watches the following scene: A toy is removed from where child A has put it when A is out of the room. Now let us ask the following question to the autistic child: Where will A look for his toy? An autistic child—as well as a normal child under the age of three or four—will attribute to A a piece of knowledge that he acquired himself, but that A fails to have. According to the "theory theory" of mind, favored by Frith, autistic children fail the false belief task because they are unable to metarepresent states, which in turn expresses the impairment of a specialized module, the theory of mind module. In contradistinction with autistic patients, schizophrenic patients, according to Frith, had access to this module during their earlier life but become unable to use it. Such a disorder would affect their present performance in representing various kinds of mental states: their own goals (grandiosity, unrealistic goal attribution), their own intentions (delusions of control, thought insertion), and the goals and intentions of others (persecution, verbal-auditory hallucination) (Frith 1994: 156).

Discussion

Several methodological objections can be addressed to this type of theory, understood as a common explanation for autism and schizophrenia. Before such an innate theory of mind module is postulated—or, in general, before one tries to understand a symptom in terms of some higher-level functional hypothesis—one should first investigate which lower-level processes might jointly result in the ability to understand mental facts. In autism, it may be that affects fail to be perceived and recognized by the baby, which would prevent him/her from extracting the relevant information for categorizing internal states (see Hobson 1993). Another possibility would be a specific deficit in memorizing motor imagery or in imitating (see Meltzoff and Gopnik 1993; Pacherie 1997), or in inhibiting prepotent stimuli (see Russell 1997). In schizophrenia, disorders in metarepresentation may also be derived from an executive disorder, or be linked to a deficit in working memory or to an attentional disorder.

Another objection has to do with the notion of explanation in psychiatry. When a pathological symptom is to be explained, it is not informative to invoke a hypothetical corresponding function whose alleged disorder causes the symptom. What is needed is an independent proof of the existence of the "new" function, in particular of the information used and of the processor using it (see David 1994; 295). In all cases, it must be shown that the disturbances in the known functions cannot account for the symptom. It must also be demonstrated that the symptom as described forms a "natural class," that is, that its defining properties help in determining a common causal structure. In the particular case of Frith's theory, it is unclear why two different kinds of explanation are offered for the same class of symptoms. One is, as we saw, that a patient does not have a proper corollary discharge mechanism allowing him to know what action he has performed. He therefore has not a conceptual problem with his own intentions but a content-identification problem. The other is, according to the modular view, that a schizophrenic patient fails to master intentional concepts; his module for a theory of mind is impaired. In this case the patient does not know what belief is, and commits mistakes on contents in a derivative way (i.e., because he has an inadequate understanding of what a belief, a desire, an intention should be). Each explanation—the

lower-level theory of efference copy and the higher-level modular theory of mentalization—seems to preempt the other.

Claiming that a particular module has the effect of performing some particular cognitive task clearly does not suffice to establish that this module in fact exists independently of other functions, in particular that it uses specific inputs and delivers specific outputs in the fast, automatic, and informationally encapsulated way associated with the concept of module (see Fodor 1983; Russell 1997). Now how can the existence of a module be established? Developmental data suggest constraints on functional links, but do not by themselves speak in favor of a particular mental architecture. By contrast, neurological data may support modular claims because they allow for the possibility of identifying various cerebral areas functionally through the method of double dissociation (see Shallice 1988).

From a philosophical point of view, Frith's approach exemplifies a theory in which consciousness is taken to be a mental function alongside other functions such as language, perception, and action planning. Whether self-awareness is explained through the SAS model or through a modular mechanism such as the theory of mind module, in both cases it is suggested that the brain has specialized mechanisms for becoming aware of mental facts allowing the subject to know not only what he believes but also that he has beliefs. Mental pathology would thus reflect the fact that mental information failed to be processed.

Also, although this point is often left implicit, it is presupposed in this view that the mechanisms for self-awareness are also those responsible for self-identity. There are several arguments against such an assimilation. If consciousness of one's own states is distributed at many different levels—such as memory, perception, action—it may be more questionable to identify the acquisition of a concept of a self with the various types of conscious states emerging from monitoring the various kinds of internal information. Data from animal psychology prevent an assimilation between elementary reflexive states such as these and the building blocks of the concept of a self. Research in the corollary discharge in the fruit fly never tackled the concept of an emergent fly selfhood. To detect who did the action requests a restricted answer, in terms of a GO-NOGO type of switch. No decision on personal identity is involved in agency attribution, although conversely there can be no personal identity without a capacity for answering "who" questions.

Self-awareness may therefore alternatively be understood as emerging from underlying functional processes that in specific cases mediate consciously accessible or reportable outputs. In this perspective, conscious states may occur in a variety of mental functions without having to be dealt with separately, in the sense that their being conscious makes them functionally special. As Rizzolatti (1994, 220) emphasizes, "Motor preparation is not a category of neural operations ("unconscious") opposed to another category of neural operations ("conscious"), but rather a term which describes the effect that some neural operations may have on motor responses regardless of whether or not they are conscious." This view on consciousness is of a radically different kind than the view described above, where self-awareness and awareness of others are entirely realized at the theory-of-mind level and seem to emerge at a very late stage in phylogeny.

It is worth exploring a theory that purports to explain the symptoms of schizophrenia listed above in a more parsimonious way, that is, in terms of lower-level mechanisms that may indeed have far-reaching effects on the system of beliefs and of motivations of the disturbed patient. This theory, developed by Marc Jeannerod and his collaborators, tries, as Frith's theory does, to understand the altered conscious states in deluded patients in terms of a monitoring of action deficit. Interestingly, this theory also is relevant to explaining part of the autistic syndrome, without having to hypothesize a disturbed

module for the theory-of-mind mechanism. I will present this theory in my own terms, hoping that, in its core, it is faithful to Jeannerod's general intentions.

Jeannerod's Concept of Action Awareness

Frith's theory paved the way for distinguishing various ways in which attributing a mental state may go wrong. Although he did make some of the crucial distinctions, he failed to provide a description of what the normal individual is able to perceive and of what he has to infer. Let us then start by distinguishing at a conceptual level several types of attribution that may contribute to action awareness. I will contrast agency awareness, goal awareness, and sensorimotor awareness. Agency awareness is typically a conscious realization that I—or someone else—did or did not perform an action. It is the state in which an organism finds itself when detecting its being active or passive in a particular situation. In particular, it is a state that is activated when interpreting input signals (afferences or reafferences) that in turn allow achieving a veridical perception of the environment. Goal awareness individuates the action through its intentional content. This dimension of action awareness allows categorizing actions according to their adaptive meaning. It focuses on the motive that drives the execution of the corresponding action. Sensorimotor awareness is related to the motor content of an action. It is the form of awareness that identifies an action through its dynamics, that is, via the spatial and temporal properties of the bodily movement involved in the action.

Common sense has it that in a normal subject, these three forms of action awareness are present in most types of action. Here is the folk story: An agent forms the conscious intention to do X. He does X by moving in a Q way. He knows that he Qs to reach X (sensorimotor awareness). He knows that he wants to have X done (goal awareness). He knows that he and no one else did X (agency awareness).

Schizophrenic patients' difficulties with the monitoring of action may disturb this picture. As we said earlier, a patient may do X without acknowledging that he was the agent of the action X ("someone else made me act"); he may also do X without having a particular conscious goal in doing X (this is a case of automatic or stimulus-driven behavior, such as psychotic roaming or stripping clothes off in public; but this latter class of dissociations is problematic, for we saw earlier that a subject in such a case always finds a way to rationalize his action by making up a goal). Even folk psychologists have to admit that sensorimotor content offers a perplexing case. Although one usually believes one is conscious of one's own motor activity, there are many cases in which one is unable not only to explain verbally how one does X but also to do it "in the abstract," in the absence of the relevant contextual cues and motivational pressures.

To provide a low-level theory of the schizophrenic symptoms listed above, it is necessary to explain how the three components of action awareness can be dissociated. Whereas Frith offers an explanation in terms of a metarepresentational disorder (what goes wrong is that the patient cannot form a mental representation of his own states), Jeannerod (1999) suggests that the problem stems from the representational structure of action: the possibility of a pathological dissociation suggests that several subfunctions work in a more or less independent way. In its broad lines, the hypothesis advanced by Jeannerod is that, in the normal subject, a goal representation is in itself agent-neutral and coded in allocentric coordinates. Sensorimotor representations are egocentrically coded but short-lived; activated mainly at a nonconscious level, they are often not—or only poorly—memorized when the action is completed. Agency representation is effected separately, through an inference based on both internal and external cues.

In this perspective, the schizophrenic symptoms have nothing to do with a specific disorder in metarepresentation. The altered conscious states may appear at each functional level where signals are received and used to monitor action. If the signals used for controlling motor execution are not the same as those used for generating a conscious judgment on the action, then subjects engaged in an action may have a poor conscious model of what they do, at least at the sensorimotor level. If the signals used in identifying a goal representation are different from those used in attributing the action to oneself, then patients may have a conscious representation of the goal of an action while rejecting their role in executing it.

As Jeannerod's target article shows in detail (Jeannerod 1994), various sources of data indicate that the same representational format is used to imagine, plan, memorize, prepare the action, and guide its execution. In the definition of action proposed earlier, to which Jeannerod subscribes, an action implies the existence of an internal model of the goal that guides the execution until completion. The internal, dynamical model for a particular action can be run beforehand to test the viability of the action, in a simulatory way, or run on-line to guide the action. It can also be activated by the perception of some external performance of this very same action. This format can be called semantic, if one understands under this term that the conditions of satisfaction of the action are couched in external, allocentric terms: The target event of an action normally includes both the object on which the action is exerted and the final state of the organism in relation to this object. Therefore the representation of the goal of an action must also code the dynamics of the action as a function of the properties of the target object. This aspect of goal representation should be called pragmatic (see Jeannerod 1994: 198) because it draws on the pragmatic information in visual cortex, devoted to the properties of objects relevant for action. The latter are represented in the dorsal stream as "affordances," not as cues for symbolic categorization (represented in the ventral stream).[1]

Consciousness of action is, in this view, intrinsically related to the representational format for action. The very awareness of an action being performed by the self (i.e., motor imagery) is the subjective, felt correlate of the representation on which the execution relies, and is "functionally equivalent" to the representation used in preparing the action. A number of studies indeed show that mental imagery shares several key physiological correlates with the corresponding real action. For example, heart rate, respiration rate, and end-tidal PCO_2 are increased in imagery because they are in the corresponding preparations of actions (Decety et al. 1991). Deliberate mental simulation of an action also activates motor pathways (Bonnet et al. 1997) as well as the corresponding areas of the sensorimotor cortex and supplementary motor area (Roth et al. 1996). The wealth of data gathered about the neural correlates of action indicate that a common network of neurons is activated for all conditions involving action: intending, imitating, observing, preparing—the inferior parietal lobule (Brodmann area 40), the ventral premotor area (ventral area 6), and part of SMA. This network could constitute a general vocabulary of actions for all kinds of uses. In addition, an overlap in dedicated areas can be observed between performing and simulating, simulating and observing, and performing and observing a particular action, which suggests close functional links between these activities.

Goal Representations Are Agent-Neutral

Of particular interest for schizophrenic symptoms is that one and the same representation can normally be used to produce a goal-oriented behavior or to recognize a behavior in someone else as being goal-oriented. It has been known for some time that neural assemblies in the su-

perior temporal sulcus are involved in the recognition of specific movements in other organisms (Perrett et al. 1989). More recently, it was shown that neurons from the macaque brain in F5, called "mirror-neurons," are able to respond both to visual stimuli of an action and to the production of movement by the self. A series of neural cell recordings in the macaque shows that groups of neurons in the premotor cortex are activated both by a particular movement effected by another individual—animal or human—and by the active performance of the same movement (Di Pellegrino et al. 1992; Rizzolatti et al. 1996; Gallese et al. 1996). These mirror neurons respond only when the observed agent acts on an object; they do not fire when the agent mimes an action in the absence of an object, or when only the object is presented. Transcranial magnetic stimulation of the motor cortex (Fadiga et al. 1995) and PET studies on normal human subjects observing someone grasping objects (Rizzolatti et al. 1996) suggest that the same kinds of neurons are present in homologous areas of the human brain (Broca's area). The presence of mirror neurons in this cerebral area might give an additional plausibility to the motor theory of speech defended by Liberman (1996).

According to Jeannerod, the discovery of mirror neurons suggests that goal representations may at some level be agent-independent. Becoming conscious of an action such as grasping or walking does not involve first identifying an agent, then specifying its current activity. It relies on the activation of a representation that is neutral as to the agent. Before we get to the question of how to proceed from goal identification to agent identification, let us examine the sensorimotor content of an action more closely.

Recognizing the Sensorimotor Content of an Action

To what extent is a normal subject conscious of the dynamics of his own actions? One way of ascribing an action to oneself could consist in relying on the internal model activated in the course of the execution. A decisive argument for such a claim would be that subjects have access to accurate internal information on what kind of movement they have done. "Internal" here means the central or proprioceptive dynamics of the action, also called "internal feedback," as contrasted with the external feedback provided by visual reafferences.

Recent work by Fourneret and Jeannerod (1998; Jeannerod 1999) indicates that normal subjects, as well as schizophrenic patients, have a poor access to the internal model of the movement they have effected. When they are deprived of accurate visual feedback, and are instead given spurious visual reafferences in the course of their actions, they are quite unable to identify the actual movement they have produced. Their conscious sense of their own movement in space seems to be overwhelmed by the visual cues that are provided, even though these cues grossly depart from the actual direction of the movement. This result is coherent with experimental evidence concerning the lack of awareness of subjects having to adjust their movements for grasping an object to a sudden jump of the target (Goodale et al. 1986). Again, the signals used in generating or correcting an action seem to depart from the signals used in forming a conscious judgment on which sensorimotor sequence occurred. It seems that subjects use external cues to consciously identify the sensorimotor content of their own actions, whereas they essentially rely on internal cues to make the necessary adjustments in an unconscious and automatic way.

Let us pause to observe the contrast between rehearsing the sensorimotor content of a past action and planning to act according to a particular sensorimotor content. While a subject can memorize quite well, and produce mental imagery, for sensorimotor contents that he plans to execute, he is quite unable to reactivate the mental imagery of a sensorimotor content for a past action when the latter has been produced as a response to contextual cues. I know how to cut a piece of cake or how to press an orange. But how did I grasp this object while it was falling? How did I manage not to slide on the icy pavement? These constrasts suggest that conscious access to the sensorimotor content of one's action requires two types of additional conditions relative to simple use of that content in ordinary learning tasks. First, there must be public, allocentric features to ground the sensorimotor judgment. As we will see below, this could indicate that conscious experience of verbally reportable experiences is functionally dependent on coding public, shared features of the environment. Second, the action features need to be controlled on-line. Mental imagery does occur in cases of careful motor preparation or execution. It does not need to occur in routine tasks. Once an action is executed, its sensorimotor content is rapidly erased from consciously accessible memory.

Judging Who

One of the misleading intuitions about agency attribution consists in taking mental imagery to provide a complete picture of an action, including the agent, the target event, and the instrumental behavior. According to this intuition, everyone would have a direct impression of who does what in the content of his own mental imagery. "This action feels like mine," in this view, means that "I have the current experience of moving this particular way, and I see it happening in my own sphere, that is, within my reach." "That action does not feel like mine" would mean, conversely, that "It happens outside my sphere, outside my reach, and with no associated phenomenal awareness."

This intuition is challenged by the dissociations, articulated above, between the three levels of action representation: The goal content, the sensorimotor content, and the agency content are three different kinds of information that require different procedures to be correctly extracted and used, and that provide different (if any) conscious experiences. Let us suppose that you are watching a soccer game on TV: You may well share a large part of the phenomenology of the active player. As you work at identifying particular goal contents, you form various mental images of the smart moves to perform, and may even feel "I can make it." This empathy does not help in locating the true agent; it makes the solution more difficult to find. Although there is obviously a difference in neuronal activation when one looks at an action and when one performs it (in the latter case only, your brain launches the action, and receives feedback of both the internal and the external varieties), there is no exact mapping, as we saw, between our representational states, on the one hand, and our conscious phenomenology and agency attributions, on the other hand.

One practical, although by no means infallible, way of finding out who the agent is, seems to be to identify where the action took place. If something happens within your reach in the right temporal sequence, then you may safely infer that you are the agent for the action you have individuated. You are at home sitting in your armchair and not on a soccer field, and there is no ball around. This is (partly) how you know that you did not score a goal.

If this is true, then one way of testing the ability of a subject to determine whether or not he is the agent of a particular action consists in providing him with an ambiguous visual feedback about the spatial and temporal properties of his actions, in a context where agency attributions cannot be easily inferred. This can be done using an experimental paradigm in which the subject looks at his own gloved hand behind a transparent screen. What he considers as his hand can also be the video image of a similar but alien hand. He must carefully compare his own internal representation of the action with the available visual feedback in order to detect possible mismatches (Nielsen 1963). This paradigm was used to investigate the performance of schizophrenic patients in attributing to themselves a token of action on the basis of a visual feedback that can be either veridical (what they see is their own hand) or spurious (they see a similar alien hand) (Daprati et al. 1997). This experiment included three conditions: The seen hand could be the subject's (condition I) or the experimenter's; in the latter case, the movement of the alien hand could be identical to the subject's response (condition II) or not (condition III).

It was found that normal subjects misjudged the alien hand as theirs in condition II only, in roughly 30 percent of the cases, and never misattributed their own hand movement to the experimenter. Schizophrenic patients had a performance similar to normal subjects in conditions I and III, but their error rate was 77 percent for patients with hallucinations and 80 percent for patients with delusions in condition II.

These results raise a set of new questions. First, how can one explain the contrasting results in conditions I and II? When a subject does a simple action, such as raising one finger when hearing a tone, and watches a simultaneous action by the gloved hand, he must compare fine central or proprioceptive details of timing and kinematics in the internal model of the movement effected with the visual cues to detect who the agent is. Normal subjects fail occasionally, when the mismatch between cues lies below a certain threshold. This failure is consistent with the data gathered by Fourneret and Jeannerod reported above. Vision may win over proprioception and convince the subject that what he did was what he saw. Let us note, however, that the present task is explicitly one of detection, whereas the explicit task in Fourneret and Jeannerod was a motor performance with visual feedback (drawing a straight line). This difference in goal could account for the better performance of subjects engaged in detection. Not having to use the visual feedback for pursuing the task may help the subjects to focus on their own sensorimotor experience, however impoverished it may be.

It is interesting to note that failure in normal subjects always consists in overattributing to themselves visual tokens of movements of the alien hand, never in denying that a movement was theirs. This asymmetry in the pattern of failures may be explained by claiming that the subjects are indeed conscious of having done the same type of movement as the one observed, have learned to identify their movement in their peripheral space, and therefore are driven to adapt (within limits) their visual experience to their motor experience by neglecting the possible mismatches. (Still, subjects with delusion of control do have a slightly stronger tendency in this experiment to incorrectly identify a gesture of theirs as the experimenter's.)

The degraded performance of schizophrenic patients relative to controls in condition II needs to be accounted for. Why would patients with hallucinations and delusions make 77 percent and 80 percent, respectively, of agency misattributions to self, while other patients have a 50 percent rate of errors? Several hypotheses come to mind, some of them explored in Daprati et al. (1997). The simplest and most venerable is that the system fails to produce or to use a sufficiently strong copy of the efferent signal. In this view, the system fails to keep track of its own representation of the action as effected. For lack of such a signal, the organism fails to correctly anticipate the feedback that should occur as a consequence of the executed movement. What this hypothesis does not explain, though, is the asymmetry between the patients' performances in conditions I and II. The learning bias postulated above could again account for it. Also, this hypothesis fails to account for the fact that schizophrenics do not have problems automatically correcting their own intentional movements in simple tasks.

A second general type of hypothesis, compatible with the first, consists in examining the relationship between sensorimotor representation and agency representation. Granted that a corollary discharge regulates the execution of an action and the extraction of the relevant feedback, one sees that this mechanism is purely "private," in the sense that it has to use egocentric coding: Only in this way can a comparison be made between efference copy and reafferences. On the other hand, determining who did an action is a perceptual judgment made on the basis of public cues represented in allocentric coding. To know that I am the agent of my actions, I need to represent the goal, as well as the relevant visual features of a current action, and determine whether these correspond to any internal model. Although, as we saw, the sensorimotor representation of the action is not consciously driving every step of the action, still some salient parts of the sensorimotor control of the action may be represented explicitly, in terms of the physical changes that occur in the world. The main evidence that I am the agent in a particular action is that the relevant aspects of the environment and of my body are successively felt to be affected in the planned way. If for some reason the world around me was changing successively in exactly the way it would if I acted on it intentionally, while I am only forming intentions to act, I would have a hard time, in the absence of a plausible explanation, resisting the idea that I am acting on it. Thus it may not be so much internal as external cues—as predicted by an action plan—that have the main burden in agency judgments.

Thus it is plausible that schizophrenic patients have a specific difficulty either in comparing egocentric with allocentric representations, or in using the sequence of environmental cues to produce a conscious and verbally reportable agency judgment. Let us briefly explore these two routes.

It is a well established fact that schizophrenics have a specific deficit in integrating multiple sources of information. In particular, they have a specific difficulty in integrating proprioceptive and sensorimotor representations with visual inputs. Clinical reports on schizophrenics frequently describe an egocentric perception of the outside world: Patients tend to see people as similar to themselves in their physical appearance; in verbal hallucinations they hear voices directed to themselves. In delusion of reference, they have the impression that unknown passersby wish to communicate with them. In a few cases, patients have distorted impressions concerning the boundaries of their own body (Cutting 1994). This perturbation in the egocentric-allocentric representation of states of affair may express a dramatically reduced ability to utilize contextual information in a task-relevant way (Cohen and Servan-Schreiber 1993; Silverstein et al. 1996). In this hypothesis, whatever the present task is, reception of familiar or egocentric information is facilitated, while features of the environment that are novel or foreign tend to be ignored. (Cohen and Servan-Schreiber suggest that variations of dopamine in the brain are responsible for these changes.)

Such an explanation could account for the clinical cases in which patients with delusion misattribute to themselves actions of other people, as well as for Daprati et al.'s results. In this view, agency attribution is taken to be a cognitive task that involves selecting relevant cues and balancing egocentric and allocentric sources of evidence. One difficulty is again to explain how these same patients may have normal performance in integrating proprioception and visual data in other tasks and in daily routines. As we saw earlier, Malenka et al. (1982) had shown that patients do indeed use visual feedback to correct their errors in motor performance, and seem unable to make the adequate corrections when they lack such visual feedback.

A way out of the difficulty, explored by Jeannerod (1999), consists in denying that the various agency tasks under consideration present the same cognitive demands. Some are automatic: The adequate responses are either innate or overlearned. The common feature in these automatic tasks is that they do not involve any specific control. They are stimulus-driven, and do not require any attentional resources. Some are controlled: In other words, they are either new or still to be learned; they cannot be executed without exerting a deliberate selection of inputs; to succeed in these tasks, subjects have to keep in working memory the goal and subgoals of the action. Now it seems obvious that the agency attribution task in Daprati et al.'s experiment belongs to the latter category. Subjects cannot rely on familiar routines to respond correctly. They have to find by themselves a strategy for detecting who the agent is.

An important finding in this perspective is that, in schizophrenics, automatic processes (such as the inhibition of a blink reflex through presentation of a weak prestimulus) resist interference better, while voluntary processes (such as pressing a key as soon as a checkerboard seen on a screen disappears) are more subject to interference than in normal subjects (Callaway and Naghdi 1982). Dominey and Georgieff (1997) show that schizophrenics do better, in a sequence learning paradigm, in learning the surface structure of sequences than in learning the abstract structure, which again indicates that their implicit learning is spared while their controlled, explicit processing may be impaired. This contrast between automatic and controlled processing could account for the impaired agency attribution in situations demanding a high level of explicit processing. Agency judgments happen in a variety of contexts, the less natural being the experimental ones. Ordinarily, a subject does not have to ask himself explicitly whether he was the agent of an act. Still, the information on who did what is critical for the success of any active perception, as well as for any action. This contrast between agency information and agency conscious attribution appears also in clinical data, where the schizophrenic patients seem to be considerably more disturbed in their conscious sense of agency than in their actual interaction with the world.

In this view, altered conscious states in patients would not result from a general consciousness-related deficit, but from local difficulties with processing cues relevant for identifying an action and retaining them in working memory. Thus they would not be primarily impaired in the processing of first-person information, but in context-sensitivity, that is, the way in which the context is taken to be relevant and is used for controlling one's actions.

Self-Consciousness, Simulation, and the Theory of Mind: Concluding Remarks

In the present state of research on conscious agency attribution, there are still many questions to be answered, concerning in particular the cerebral mechanisms for agency attribution that are impaired in schizophrenic patients, and the difference between the impairments underlying, respectively, the delusion of influence (where the subject is not conscious of acting, but of being acted upon) and the delusion of control (where the subject believes that he can cause other people to act). One question raised earlier in this chapter needs to be explored again in the light of the preceding discussion: Is there any uniform notion of self-consciousness? Is such a notion a product of metarepresentational abilities?

Let us note that even in those cases where patients attribute their own acts to some external force, they experience agency deprivation in a first-person way. Similarly, a depersonalized patient reports having a feeling of depersonalization, or a patient with Cotard syndrome reports that he does not exist anymore. It seems paradoxical that a subject could retain a first-person experience of episodes that seem associated with no feeling at all. One could submit that these states lie on a continuum with extreme cases where no first-person experience is present and for that very reason is not reported ("negative" symptoms such as catatonia could raise this kind of problem). But this line of response fails to acknowledge what has been the main theme in this chapter. If there is a functional disconnection between conscious representation and unconscious information processing, then it is perfectly possible for someone to report abnormal qualia while not being impaired in automatically processing the corresponding stimuli.

The preceding discussion leads us to resist the view that reflexive conscious states would depend on the operation of some central mechanism generally responsible for metarepresentation. Clearly, many different types of information are used in the course of an action to know who did what (corollary discharge, parameters of movement velocity, body vs target orientation, etc.). Among these, few can be directly made the content of a conscious experience. You don't feel in charge in the same direct way that you see a certain shade of green or that you feel a prick in your finger. An agent does not have access to his own central efferent signals. Agent-related conscious representations may be, with respect to their informational basis, distributed on several distinct functions, such as visual perception, proprioceptive and haptic processing, inferential capacities, and verbal representations. When an agent becomes conscious of acting, it may be, as we saw, on the basis of third-person accessible information.

A second important fact that emerged is that goal representation is self-other neutral. If goal representations are essentially sharable, then we do not understand other people by projecting a piece of internal knowledge onto them, as is often assumed. The problem that our brain has to solve is the converse problem: determining who the agent is, once a goal is identified. This fact does not imply that we become conscious of "detached" goal representations. What it does imply is that it is certainly possible to identify the goal of an action without specifying who the agent is. A corresponding intuition of this phenomenon is offered by a type of mental imagery in which a pattern of movement is both visualized and effected mentally. This kind of simulation does not seem to call for an explicit representation of the agent. Mentally simulating an action in a first-person way, and looking at someone with the intention of imitating his movement, share important cerebral as well as phenomenological properties. (Decety et al. 1994, 1997; see Jeannerod 1999 for a review). Simulation would in both cases appeal to the memory of a goal-directed action, and possibly carry with it part of the sensorimotor representation typical of the action. Control of such an ability, which seems denied to nonhuman animals, is the basis for craftsmanship and for artistic and sport practices.

This view has interesting consequences for the theory of mentalization, that is, for the explanation of what makes a human being able to attribute to others and to himself mental states such as believing and desiring. Here, too, it must be decided whether this ability develops as a whole, as a module coming to maturity around four years of age, or whether it results from the interaction of other independent subcapacities. Whereas, as we saw, Frith's theory of schizophrenia invokes the impairment of a metarepresentational module, a view that Jeannerod seems to have adopted in some of his writings, the discussion above is compatible with another picture of the conscious attribution of mental states. The concept of simulation has been used by philosophers (see Goldman 1993; Heal 1986; Gordon 1996a, 1996b; Gallese and Goldman 1998; Proust 1999a) to show that a theory of mind is not needed to attribute intentional states to others. According to this view, one can predict and explain another's behavior by simulating the decision processes in the other as well as in oneself. Mental concepts such as belief, desire, and agency would in this analysis not precede, but result from, actively simulating others entertaining goals and motivational states. Autistic children would accordingly lack a theory of mind because they would have a primary trouble appropriately simulating the situation in which another is involved.

The preceding discussion brings important additions to the simulation theory of mind, with the notion of the shared character of goal representations. One can plausibly speculate that observed action and the simulatory component of action memory form a major building block for understanding other minds. Metarepresenting, in this perspective, would depend on additional executive capacities for maintaining distinct the inferences from diverse simulated contexts of action. Simulating aspects of action and perception could thus give us a key to context processing and its disorders, that is, those which seem to be instrumental in schizophrenia and in autism.

Acknowledgments

I thank Elisabeth Pacherie for her comments on a previous version, and Marc Jeannerod, Jean Decety, and Jacques Paillard for helpful discussions.

Note

1. On the functional distribution of cortical pathways for vision, see Ungerleider and Mishkin (1982) and Jeannerod (1997). My use of the contrast between "semantic" and "pragmatic" modes of representation differs slightly from Jeannerod's.

References

American Psychiatric Association. (1987). *Diagnostic and Statistical Manual of Mental Disorders*, 3rd ed., rev. (*DSM IIIR*). Washington D.C.: American Psychiatric Association.

Block, N. (1995). On a confusion of a function of consciousness. *Behavioral and Brain Sciences* 18, no. 2: 227–287.

Bonnet, M., Decety, J., Requin, J., and Jeannerod, M. (1997). Mental simulation of an action modulates the excitability of spinal reflex pathways in man. *Cognitive Brain Research* 5: 221–228.

Callaway, E., and Naghdi, S. (1982). An information processing model for schizophrenia. *Archives of General Psychiatry* 39: 339–347.

Chapman, J. (1966). The early symptoms of schizophrenia. *British Journal of Psychiatry* 112: 225–251.

Cohen, J. D., and Servan-Schreiber, D. (1992). Context, cortex and dopamine: A connectionist approach to behavior and biology in schizophrenia. *Psychological Review* 99, no. 1: 45–87.

Cohen, J. D., and Servan-Schreiber, D. (1993). A theory of dopamine function and its role in cognitive deficits in schizophrenia. *Schizophrenia Bulletin* 19: 85–104.

Cutting, J. C. (1994). Evidence for right hemisphere dysfunction in schizophrenia. In A. S. David and J. C. Cutting, eds., *The Neuropsychology of Schizophrenia*, pp. 231–242. Hillsdale, NJ: Lawrence Erlbaum.

Daprati, E., Franck, N., Georgieff, N., Proust, J., Pacherie, E., Dalery, J., and Jeannerod, M. (1997). Looking for the agent: An investigation into self-consciousness and consciousness of the action in schizophrenic patients. *Cognition* 65: 71–86.

David, A. S. (1994). The neuropsychological origin of auditory hallucinations. In A. S. David and J. C. Cutting eds., *The Neuropsychology of Schizophrenia*, 269–313. Hillsdale, NJ: Lawrence Erlbaum.

Decety, J., Grezes, J., Costes, N., Perani, D., Jeannerod, M., Procyk, E., Grassi, F., and Fazio, F. (1997). Brain activity during observation of action: Influence of action content and subject's strategy. *Brain* 120: 1763–1777.

Decety, J., Jeannerod, M., Germain, M., and Pastene, J. (1991). Vegetative response during imagined movement is proportional to mental effort. *Behavioral and Brain Research* 42: 1–5.

Decety, J., Perani, D., Jeannerod, M., Bettinardi, V., Tadary, B., Woods, R., Mazziotta, J. C., and Fazio, F. (1994). Mapping motor representations with PET. *Nature* 371: 600–602.

Di Pellegrino, G., Fadiga, L., Fogassi, L., Gallese, V., and Rizzolatti, G. (1992). Understanding motor events: A neurophysiological study. *Experimental Brain Research* 91: 176–180.

Dominey, P. F., and Georgieff, N. (1997). Schizophrenics learn surface but not abstract structure in a serial reaction time task. *NeuroReport* 8: 2877–2882.

Fadiga, L., Fogassi, L., Pavesi, G., and Rizzolatti, G. (1995). Motor facilitation during action observation: A magnetic stimulation study. *Journal of Neurophysiology* 73: 2608–2611.

Feinberg, I. (1978). Efference copy and corollary discharge: Implications for thinking and its disorders. *Schizophrenia Bulletin* 4: 636–640.

Fodor, J. (1983). *The Modularity of Mind*. Cambridge, MA: MIT Press.

Fourneret. P., and Jeannerod, M. (1998). Limited conscious monitoring of motor performance in normal subjects. *Neuropsychologia* 36: 1133–1140.

Frankfurt, H. (1988). *The Importance of What We Care About*. Cambridge: Cambridge University Press.

Freedman, B. J., and Chapman, L. J. (1973). Early subjective experience in schizophrenic episodes. *Journal of Abnormal Psychology* 82: 46–54.

Frith, C. D. (1979). Consciousness, information processing and schizophrenia. *British Journal of Psychiatry* 134: 225–235.

Frith, C. D. (1992). *The Cognitive Neuropsychology of Schizophrenia*. Hillsdale, NJ: Lawrence Erlbaum.

Frith, C. D. (1994). Theory of mind in schizophrenia. In A. S. David and J. C. Cutting, eds., *The Neuropsychology of Schizophrenia*, 147–161. Hillsdale, NJ: Lawrence Erlbaum.

Frith, C. D. (1995). Consciousness is for other people. *Behavioral and Brain Sciences* 18, no. 4: 682–683.

Frith, C. D., and Done, D. J. (1989). Experiences of alien control in schizophrenia reflect a disorder in the central monitoring of action. *Psychological Medicine* 19: 359–363.

Gallese, V., Fadiga, L., Fogassi, L., and Rizzolatti, G. (1996). Action recognition in the premotor cortex. *Brain* 119: 593–609.

Gallese, V., and Goldman, A. (1998). Mirror neurons and the simulation theory of mind-reading. *Trends in Neuroscience* 2, no. 12: 493–501.

Georgieff, N., and Jeannerod, M. (1998). Beyond consciousness of external reality: A "who" system for consciousness of action and self-consciousness. *Consciousness and Cognition* 7: 465–477.

Goldman, A. (1993). The psychology of folk psychology. *Behavioral and Brain Sciences* 16: 15–28.

Goodale, M. A., Pélisson, D., and Prablanc, C. (1986). Large adjustments in visually guided reaching do not depend on vision of the hand or perception of target displacement. *Nature* 320: 748–750.

Gordon, R. M. (1996a). Simulation without introspection or inference from me to you. In M. Davies, and T. Stone, eds., *Mental Simulation*, 53–67. Oxford: Blackwell.

Gordon, R. M. (1996b). "Radical" simulationism. In P. Carruthers and P. K. Smith, eds., *Theories of Theories of Mind*, 11–21. Cambridge: Cambridge University Press.

Gray J. A., Feldon, J., Rawlins, J. N. P., Hemsley, D. R., and Smith, A. D. (1991). The neuropsychology of schizophrenia. *Behavioral and Brain Sciences* 14: 1–84.

Heal, J. (1986). Replication and functionalism. In J. Butterfield, ed., *Language, Mind and Logic*, 135–150. Cambridge: Cambridge University Press.

Hobson, P. (1993). *Autism and the Development of Mind*. Hove, UK: Lawrence Erlbaum Associates.

Jahanshahi, M., and Frith, C. D. (1998). Willed action and its impairments. *Cognitive Neuropsychology* 15: 483–533.

Jeannerod, M. (1990). Traitement conscient et inconscient de l'information perceptive. *Revue internationale de psychopathologie* 1: 13–34.

Jeannerod, M. (1993). Intention, représentation, action. *Revue internationale de psychopathologie* 10: 167–191.

Jeannerod, M. (1994). The representing brain: Neural correlates of motor intention and imagery. *Behavioral and Brain Sciences* 17: 187–245.

Jeannerod, M. (1997). *The Cognitive Neuroscience of Action*. Oxford: Basil Blackwell.

Jeannerod, M. (1999). To act or not to act: Perspectives on the representation of actions. *Quarterly Journal of Experimental Psychology* 52A: 1–29.

Jeannerod, M., and Biguer, B. (1982). Visuomotor mechanisms in reaching within extrapersonal space. In D. Ingle, M. A. Goodale, and R. Mansfield, eds., *Advances in the Analysis of Visual Behavior*, 387–409. Cambridge, MA: MIT Press.

Jeannerod, M., and Fourneret, P. (1998). Etre agent ou être agi? Sur les critères d'auto-attribution d'une action. In H. Grivois and J. Proust, eds., *Subjectivité et conscience d'agir dans la schizophrénie et dans l'autisme*. Paris: Presses Universitaires de France.

Liberman, A. (1996). *Speech: A Special Code*. Cambridge, MA: MIT Press.

Malenka, R. C., Angel, R. W., Hampton, B., and Berger, P. A. (1982). Impaired central error-correcting behavior in schizophrenia. *Archives of General Psychiatry* 39: 101–107.

McGhie, A., and Chapman, J. (1961). Disorders of attention and perception in early schizophrenia. *British Journal of Psychiatry* 34: 103–116.

Meltzoff, A. N., and Gopnik, A. (1993). The role of imitation in understanding persons and developing a theory of mind. in S. Baron-Cohen, H. Tager-Flusberg, and D. J. Cohen, eds., *Understanding Other Minds*, 335–366. Oxford: Oxford University Press.

Nielsen, T. I. (1963). Volition: A new experimental approach. Scandinavian Journal of Psychology 4: 225–230.

Pacherie, E. (1997). Motor-images, self-consciousness, and autism. In J. Russell, ed., *Autism as an Executive Disorder*, 215–255. Oxford: Oxford University Press.

Perrett, D. I., Harries, M. H., Bevan, M. R., Thomas, S., Benson, P. J., Mistlin, A. J., Chitty, A. J., Hietanen, J. K., and Ortega, J. E. (1989). Frameworks of analysis for the neural representation of animate objects and actions. *Journal of Experimental Biology* 146: 87–113.

Proust, J. (1998). *A Plea for Mental Acts*. CREA report no. 9901. Paris: Ecole Polytechnique.

Proust, J. (1999a). Indexes for action. *Revue internationale de philosophie* 3: 321–345.

Proust, J. (1999b). Mind-reading in non-human primates. *Philosophical Topics*, in press.

Rizzolatti, G. (1994). Nonconscious motor images. *Behavioral and Brain Sciences* 17, no. 2: 220.

Rizzolatti, G., Camarda, R., Fogassi, L., Gentilucci, M., Luppino, G., and Matelli, M. (1988). Functional organization of area 6 in the macaque monkey. II, Area F5 and the control of distal movements. *Experimental Brain Research* 71: 491–507.

Rosenthal, D. (1993). Thinking that one thinks. In M. Davies and G. W. Humphreys, ed., Consciousness: Psychological and Philosophical Essays, 197–223. Oxford: Blackwell.

Roth, M., Decety, J., Raybaudi, M., Massarelli, R., Delon-Martin, C., Segebarth, C., Morand, S., Gemignani, A., Décorps, M., and Jeannerod, M. (1996). Possible involvement of primary motor cortex in mentally simulated movement. A functional magnetic-resonance imaging study. *NeuroReport* 7: 1280–1284.

Russell, J. (1996). *Agency: Its Role in Mental Development*. Hove: Erlbaum (UK), Taylor and Francis.

Russell, J. (1997). Les racines exécutives (non modulaires) des perturbations de la mentalisation dans l'autisme. In H. Grivois and J. Proust, eds., *Subjectivité et conscience d'agir: Approches clinique et cognitive de la psychose*, 139–206. Paris: Presses Universitaires de France.

Schwartz-Place, E. J. S., and Gillmore, G. C. (1980). Perceptual organization in schizophrenia. *Journal of Abnormal Psychology* 89: 408–418.

Shallice, T. (1988). *From Neuropsychology to Mental Structure*. Cambridge: Cambridge University Press.

Shepard, A. (1995). What is an agent that it experiences P-consciousness? And what is P-consciousness that it moves an agent? *Behavioral and Brain Sciences* 18, no. 2: 267–268.

Silverstein, S. M., Matteson, S., and Knight, R. A. (1996). Reduced top-down influence in auditory perceptual organization in schizophrenia. *Journal of Abnormal Psychology* 105: 663–667.

Sperry, R. W. (1950). Neural basis of the spontaneous optokinetic response produced by visual inversion. *Journal of Comparative and Physiological Psychology* 43: 482–489.

Swerdlow, N. R., and Koob, G. F. (1987). Dopamine, schizophrenia, mania and depression: Toward a unified hypothesis of cortico-striato-pallido-thalamic function. *Behavioral and Brain Sciences* 10: 197–245.

Ungerleider, L., and Mishkin, M. (1982). Two cortical visual systems. In D. J. Ingle, M. A. Goodale, and R. J. W. Mansfield, eds., *Analysis of Visual Behavior*, 549–586. Cambridge, MA: MIT Press.

Venables, P. H. (1964). Input dysfunction in schizophrenia. In B. A. Maher, ed., *Progress in Experimental Personality Research*, vol. 1. New York: Academic Press.

von Holst, E., and Mittaelstaedt, H. (1950). Das Reafferenzprinzip: Wechselwirkung zwischen Zentralnervensystem und Peripherie. *Naturwissenschaften* 37: 464–476.

Widlöcher, D., and Hardy-Bayle, M.-C. (1989). Cognition and control of action in psychopathology. *Cahiers de psychologie cognitive* 9, no. 6: 583–615.

Vittorio Gallese

Neurophysiology, the discipline that investigates the functional organization of the brain and its relation to behavior, has traditionally privileged a strictly reductionist approach. Thus, in most cases neurophysiologists addressed "simple" problems such as the organization of sensory systems or the way in which movements of effectors are programmed and controlled. Since the 1980s, however, issues such as attention, intention, intentionality, and ultimately even consciousness, traditionally fields of investigation in the cognitive sciences, have progressively become the challenging target of more and more neuroscientists. This fact certainly represents a major turn in the history of the scientific study of brain functions.

From a neurophysiological perspective, the brain's functions can be investigated only by considering the dynamic interplay between the biological agent, who possesses the brain, and the external world. A scientific account of the way in which our brain "represents" the world cannot neglect the reciprocal connection between the two. So we must study the brain, trying as much as possible to bring the "world" into the laboratory, by using a "naturalistic" approach. A naturalistic approach, when applied to neurophysiology, consists in choosing the most appropriate way of testing neurons' activity, by figuring out what stimuli or behavioral situation would more closely approximate what the animal from which we are recording would experience in its natural environment. Single-neuron recording then becomes an exciting investigation by which significant correlations between neural activity and behavior can be established only after having falsified, and therefore discarded, the various possible alternative explanations for a given pattern of neural discharge.

The brain is the anatomical and the functional site of a broad range of multilevel processes.

Neurophysiology investigates the neuronal level. The complexity into which the billions of neurons composing the brain are organized implies, in addition, the potential combinatorial explosion of the ways in which information can be processed. These considerations may induce one to postulate that brain functions are completely distributed, discarding as useless the heuristical value of the single-neuron recording approach. The findings reported in the present article suggest that this is not necessarily true. By means of a naturalistic approach it is possible to reliably correlate a given function or behavior with the properties of a given cortical neural circuit. Furthermore, by using this approach to study apparently simple processes, such as the integration of visual and motor information required to program purposeful acts like grasping, I believe that it is possible to provide an explanatory frame which also can be applied to cognitive functions.

In the first part of the article the functional properties of a premotor area of the monkey, area F5, will be described. In the second, more speculative, part of the article, it will be argued that the visuomotor processes occurring in the macaque monkey premotor cortex may provide new insights on issues such as action understanding, intersubjectivity, and theory of mind. I will conclude that these new findings may help in reshaping some of our ideas about the way in which the human brain "represents" the reality it is enmeshed in.

A New Perspective on the Motor System: The Ventral Premotor Area F5 of the Monkey

Convergent anatomical evidence (see Matelli and Luppino 1997) shows that the ventral premotor cortex (also referred to as inferior area 6) is composed of two distinct areas, designated as F4 and F5 (Matelli et al. 1985). Area F5 occupies the rostralmost part of inferior area 6, extending rostrally within the posterior bank of the inferior limb of the arcuate sulcus. Area F5 is connected with the hand field of the primary motor cortex (Matelli et al. 1986) and has direct, although limited, projections to the upper cervical segments of the spinal cord (He et al. 1993). Intracortical microstimulation in F5 evokes hand and mouth movements at thresholds generally higher than in the primary motor cortex (Gentilucci et al. 1988; Hepp-Reymond et al. 1994). The functional properties of F5 neurons were assessed in a series of single-unit recording experiments (Rizzolatti et al. 1981; Okano and Tanji 1987; Rizzolatti et al. 1988). These experiments showed that the activity of F5 neurons is correlated with specific distal motor acts and not with the execution of individual movements.

An important distinction is that between movement and motor act: What makes a movement a motor act is the presence of a goal. Using the effective motor act as the classification criterion, the following classes of neurons were described: "grasping neurons," "holding neurons," "tearing neurons," and "manipulation neurons." Grasping neurons discharge when the monkey performs movements aimed to take possession of objects with the hand ("grasping-with the-hand neurons"), with the mouth ("grasping-with-the-mouth neurons"), or with both ("grasping-with-the-hand-and-the-mouth neurons").

Grasping-with-the-hand neurons form the largest class of F5 neurons. Most neurons of this class are selective for different types of grip. The majority of F5 grasping neurons are selective for precision grip (opposition of the pulpar surface of the index finger and thumb, normally used to grasp small objects).

The most interesting aspect of F5 neurons is that they code movement in quite abstract terms. What is coded is not simply a parameter such as force or movement direction, but rather the relationship, in motor terms, between the agent and the object of the action. F5 neurons become active only if a particular type of action (e.g., grasp, hold, etc.) is executed to achieve a particular type of goal (e.g., to take possession of a piece of food, to throw away an object, etc.).

The metaphor of a "motor vocabulary" was introduced (Gentilucci and Rizzolatti 1990; Rizzolatti et al. 1988) in order to conceptualize the function of these neurons. This vocabulary collects various "words," each constituted by groups of neurons related to different motor acts. The hierarchical value of these "words" can be different: Some of them indicate the general goal of the action (e.g., grasp, hold, tear). Some others concern the way in which a particular action has to be executed, such as to grasp with the index finger and the thumb (precision grip). Another group of "words" deals with the temporal phases into which the action to be performed can be segmented (e.g., hand aperture phase).

The presence in the motor system of a "vocabulary" of motor acts allows a much simpler selection of a particular action within a given context. When the action is either self-generated or externally generated, only a few "words" need to be selected. Let us imagine that a monkey is presented with a small object, say a raisin, within its reaching distance. If the motivational value of the stimulus is powerful enough to trigger an appetitive behavior, it will evoke a command for a grasping action; then the command will address a specific finger configuration suitable to grasp the raisin in that particular situation. Within the context of a motor "vocabulary," motor action can be conceived as a simple assembly of words instead of being described in the less economical terms of the control of individual movements. This radically new way to conceive the function of the motor system opened the possibility, which will become clearer below, to tackle cognitive aspects of behavior such as intersubjectivity from a neurobiological perspective.

Canonical Neurons

Since most grasping actions are executed under visual guidance, it is extremely interesting to elucidate the relationship between the features of 3D visual objects and the specific "words" of the motor vocabulary. In this logic the appearance of a graspable object in the visual space will immediately retrieve the appropriate ensemble of "words." This process, in neurophysiological terms, implies that the same neuron must be able not only to code motor acts but also to respond to the visual features triggering them.

A considerable percentage of F5 grasping neurons, "canonical neurons," responds to the visual presentation of objects of different sizes and shapes in the absence of any detectable movement (Rizzolatti et al. 1988; Jeannerod et al. 1995; Murata et al. 1997). Very often a strict congruence has been observed between the type of grip coded by a given neuron and the size or the shape of the object effective in triggering its visual response. The most interesting aspect, however, is the fact that in a considerable percentage of neurons the congruence is observed between the high selectivity for a given type of executed grip and the selectivity for the visual presentation of a group of objects that, although differing in shape, nevertheless all "afford" the same type of grip, which is identical to the motorically coded one.

A first conclusion that can be drawn from these data is that it is extremely difficult to conceptualize the function of F5 canonical grasping neurons in purely sensory or motor terms. At this stage objects seem to be processed in *relational terms*. In other words, by means of a neural network a series of physical entities, 3D objects, is identified and differentiated not in relation to mere physical appearance, but in

relation to the effect of the interaction with an acting agent.

Mirror Neurons

A second class of grasping-related neurons, mirror neurons, has been described in area F5 of the macaque monkey (Gallese et al. 1996; Rizzolatti et al. 1996). These neurons, although having the same motor properties as canonical neurons, differ sharply in the nature of their visual properties. Mirror neurons are not activated during the observation of objects but only during the observation of an agent (a human being or a monkey) acting in a purposeful way upon objects with his hand or his mouth. Neither the sight of the object alone nor of the agent alone is effective in driving these neurons. Mimicking the action in the absence of the target object or using a tool to execute the object-related action is similarly ineffective in driving mirror neurons' activity.

In a relevant percentage of mirror neurons a strict congruence between the observed action effective in triggering the neural visual response and the executed action effective in driving the motor response has been observed. In other words, the observed action performed by another individual evokes in the observer the same neural pattern that occurs during the active execution of that action. Grasping, holding, manipulating, and tearing objects are the actions that, both when observed and when executed, most frequently activate these neurons.

On the basis of their functional properties, mirror neurons can be considered as constituting an action observation/execution matching system. What is the link between acting and observing someone else acting? This link is constituted by the presence in both instances of a goal. This goal is recognized and "understood" by the observer by mapping it on a shared motor representation. Again, as in the case of canonical neurons, the motor system exhibits a double function. On one side it supervises action execution, and on the other it "validates" what is perceived in motor terms.

The Nature of Motor Representations and Their Pertinence to Intersubjectivity

What Is a Motor Representation?

In this second part of the article the neuroscientific evidence will be used as a starting point for developing a more speculative approach.

So far we have seen that two distinct classes of premotor neurons (F5 canonical and mirror neurons) are endowed with the property of coding goal-directed movements. Both canonical and mirror neurons become motorically active only when a given movement pattern of the hand is aimed to a certain target in a certain way to achieve a certain goal. Within this context, a goal could be conceptually defined as the explanation in teleological terms of a willed relational attitude. I posit that this relational attitude is also used to give, at a preconceptual level (well before the development of the linguistic competence), preliminary "intentional" coherence to the array of visual stimuli we are exposed to. An object, as coded by canonical neurons, is transformed from a physical textured pattern of given shape, size, and color into something that acquires its meaning in virtue of being constituted as the target of an action. The physical object becomes an *intentional object*.

At this stage, the nervous system elaborates a code that "classifies" the objects of the external world according to their relational value for the acting subject. The object ceases to exist by itself but acquires a meaning in virtue of its relation to the acting subject. There is undoubtedly a similarity between this "intentional" model of object coding and the "pragmatic" type of coding considered as the distinctive hallmark of the visual processing occurring in the dorsal stream (see Jeannerod 1994). Within the "pragmatic" model, however, the emphasis is placed on the

physical properties of a given object that can "afford" a given pragmatic relation with the acting agent, whereas the "intentional" model places more stress on the relevant role of the acting subject in determining the meaning of the physical world (see also Bermudez 1995).

The same relational attitude is applied when observing other behaving individuals. The observer begins to "understand" the observed behavior of a second party when this process of "motor equivalence" between action observation and action execution is established by means of a shared motor representation.

We can do something, see someone doing something, or imagine someone doing something. These conditions all share the same system of "implementation": the motor system. What is shared by "grasping a glass," "seeing someone grasping a glass," and "imagining someone grasping a glass" is the presence of a moving hand aimed to a target. Evidence from brain imaging studies in humans (Decety et al. 1994; Stephan et al. 1995; Grafton et al. 1996) and the neurophysiological data reported here both show that the motor system is mastering not only the actual expression of its domain feature, movement; the motor system also masters its own representation. The contribution of Marc Jeannerod is seminal in this respect. According to Jeannerod (1994, 1997), all different aspects of action, from its intention to its execution or observation, are part of a single representation-execution continuum.

This notion of motor representation configures a preconceptual level of analysis of information that is deeply rooted in the intrinsically relational nature of the motor system. From this perspective, agency constitutes the key for understanding, in both phylogenetic and ontogenetic terms, how our knowledge of the world is built. Piaget (1955) stressed the importance of agency for the development of the capacity to discriminate between an objective world and our experience of being subjects representing a physically independent "world outside." This perspective has been revitalized by Russell (1995). According to Russell, an essential characteristic of agency is the capacity to determine the sequence of one's perceptual inputs. We are always able to discriminate between displacements within our visual field originated by movements in the external world and those originated by our own movements. This ability is the consequence of the process of action monitoring, by which we can tell real movements (those happening independently of us) from apparent movements (those occurring as a consequence of our own movements). The neurophysiological mechanism of "efference copying," elucidated by von Holst and Mittelstaedt (1973), explains how the nervous system is able to record when a movement (e.g., a head turn) is being performed, thus compensating for the visual changes that this movement produces. A similar mechanism may give account of the fact that executed and observed actions, despite their sharing of the same neural representation, usually do not, when attributing the role of agent, engender any ambiguity in the normal subject.

In Russell's analysis, another aspect of agency that is relevant for the development of the self/world distinction is reversibility. By means of movement we can direct the focus of our attention in one direction and then reverse it at will: "The order of perceptions is irreversible, and its possible repetition is something over which we have no power." In contrast, when acting, we have a relative freedom to determine what we experience at a given time and in the order we choose" (Russell 1995, 133). What is self-determined is delimited from what is totally independent from our power, and therefore intrinsically irreversible. The "world outside," by resisting us, sets the limits of our experience of being a distinct entity, a subject. By relentlessly acting, subjects develop the capacity to carve out their sense of identity by putting themselves in a relational attitude to the world. Acting on the world becomes progressively distinct from being acted upon by the world. But this is only one side

of the coin. The subject of experience is constituted in relation to a twofold "world outside": the world of objects, inanimate things, and the social world, the world of other beings.

Agency and Intersubjectivity

Mammals are usually in mutual relationship with conspecifics. This social attitude is particularly developed among primates. Macaque monkeys live in groups characterized by several sophisticated social interactions, such as grooming (see Dunbar 1993), that are usually disciplined by a well delineated hierarchical organization. It is therefore very important for each member of a given social group to be able to recognize the presence of another individual performing an action, to identify his social rank, to discriminate the observed action from others, and to "understand" the meaning of the observed action in order to react to it appropriately.

The data reported here help to clarify some of the neurophysiological mechanisms that might be at the basis of the sophisticated social competence displayed by nonhuman primates. Whenever an individual emits an action, it is able to predict its consequences. This knowledge is likely built by associating, through learning, the goal of the action, coded in the motor centers, with its consequences, as monitored by the sensory systems. The matching system represented by mirror neurons could provide the neuronal basis for such a process of "action understanding." Meaning would be assigned to the observed actions by matching them on the same neuronal machinery that generates them.

As human beings, we are constantly trying to find a balance between our need to express our individuality and the need to follow the social "rules" dictated by our highly structured society. All our social activities depend on mutual understanding. Mutual understanding requires the capacity to attribute, both to the self and to others, intentions, desires, and beliefs, by implying that both the self and others are endowed with mental states. This capacity has been explained as the ability to build a conceptual system, commonly designated as "theory of mind" (see Premack and Woodruff 1978). Theory of mind offers the possibility to investigate the mechanisms of social cognition, and it has been proposed as a suitable common framework for interpreting psychopathological states such as autism and schizophrenia (Frith 1992).

How this endowment of humans is structured, how it is functionally organized, is matter of debate. Even more debated is the problem of determining whether theory of mind, or whatever else is at the basis of "mentalism" (defined here as our capacity to attribute beliefs, desires, intentions to others), is an innate capacity of our species or whether it has been achieved over an evolutionary continuum, during which pre-adapted functional mechanisms have "developed" a new functional meaning, subserving newly acquired skills, "mentalism" included. Although such a dilemma would require a thorough treatment for which there is not room here, what I wish to say is that the results of neuroscientific research point to the second, evolutionary answer as the more likely account of the origin of "mentalism." Whether "mentalism" is synonymous with theory of mind remains to be ascertained.

It is undeniable that, as human beings, we are capable not only to "represent" the world but also to represent ourselves representing the world. It has been argued that this second-order representation, or metarepresentation (see Leslie 1987), is subserved by a modular system. According to Baron-Cohen (1995), humans evolved a neurocognitive system (mind-reading system) allowing them to attribute mental states to other individuals. This system is modular, composed of four components: intentionality detector, eye direction detector, shared attention mechanism, theory of mind mechanism. The intentionality detector recognizes stimuli as volitional by detecting their goal.

Setting the problem of modularity aside, Baron-Cohen's model is very stimulating because it provides a functional architecture that can easily be matched with the mechanisms discovered by neuroscience at the neural level. Mirror neurons, for example, could provide the neuronal basis for the proposed intentionality detector. It is also possible that the eye direction detector, supposed to recognize eye behavior as an index of another volitional entity, could be subserved by a set of neurons matching gaze direction of both the agent and the observer. Brain imaging studies (Puce et al. 1998) and neurophysiological data (for review, see Carey et al. 1997) seem to suggest that this is more than a speculative hypothesis.

I referred to Baron-Cohen's model not to support the theory-theory version of "mentalism" (I would rather endorse the simulationist version; see Gallese and Goldman 1998), but to show that even the models heralded by the supporters of a strictly cognitivist account of "mentalism" are composed of elementary units that happen to be pretheoretical, and can easily be "embodied" in known neural circuits.

If we analyze what is at the basis of intersubjectivity, what it is that allows individuals to "see" the social world as meaningful, we discover that agency plays a major role in all these phenomena. Agency allows one to define the problems of both subjectivity and intersubjectivity within the same framework (see Proust 1998). At the same time, agency allows one to give a prelinguistic, preconceptual account of what is at the basis of mentalism (see Bermudez 1995; Pacherie 1998).

Developmental psychology has provided evidence demonstrating that the capacity to understand causal relations and the goals of actions develops well before conceptualization and language competence have been achieved. Most directly relevant is the work of Meltzoff (1995), who describes eighteen-month-old children re-enacting the *intended* behavior they observe in adults, not their *actual* behavior. It appears, then, that children as young as eighteen months do not simply imitate observed behavior. They track the (mental) *intentions* of people they observe.

The long path started by our primate ancestors with the development of manual skills and tool use has led in the course of time to the sophisticated epistemological attitude of human beings. The cognitive development that we experience in the course of our personal lives epitomizes the same path, leading from the construction of a sharp demarcation between the acting self and the world to the magic ability of the developing child to unravel the ever less mysterious social world that surrounds him/her. The new perspective on the motor system and on its fundamental role in constituting the intentionality of our approach to the "world outside," briefly presented here, provides, I think, few solid steps toward a neurobiological explanation of social cognition.

Conclusions

Our capacity to put ourselves in relation to a world inhabited by inanimate things and by living persons whom we recognize as similar to ourselves, resides in the functional properties of an intricate network of neural cells. The perspective that I have tried to sketch in the present article suggests that today it is concretely possible to address the problems of intersubjectivity and social cognition from a neuroscientific perspective. After positing that, we are left with the need to accommodate the "personal level" description of our mental attitudes with the "subpersonal level" description of the cortico-cortical circuits that allow these attitudes to be expressed. One way to solve this problem may be to adopt a multilevel analysis/description of the explananda. By doing this we are released from the temptation to use the same type of analysis, the same conceptual linguistic framework, to

describe levels that are different although correlated. This difference, however, is not ontological but epistemological. A spike train of a given population of neurons occurring while we are trying to understand someone's behavior is, in turn, occurring while a certain number of Na^+ ions are massively entering the very same neurons' cellular bodies. We have described the situation by choosing three different and, at the same time, coherent levels of instantiation. Why are we talking about the "neural correlate" and not about the "Na^+ correlate" of social cognition? We use a higher-level description because its complexity is more apt to capture our inherently complex experience of the world. Our complex experience of the world, nevertheless, is made out of simpler behavioral mechanisms, very much as our cortical circuits are made of neurons whose activity is in turn made out of the ions' flow. In other words, among all these different levels of description there is no ontological gap to be crossed, just a continuum of increasing organizational complexity. Neurophysiology, in this view, represents a sort of "cognitive archaeology," a lantern projecting its light onto the ever less obscure remnants of our long animal past.

Acknowledgments

The author wishes to thank Luciano Fadiga, Leonardo Fogassi, and Giacomo Rizzolatti for their valuable comments and criticisms of an earlier version of this article. The preparation of this article was supported by the Human Frontier Scientific Program.

References

Baron-Cohen, S. (1995). *Mindblindness. An Essay on Autism and Theory of Mind*. Cambridge, MA: MIT Press.

Bermudez, J. L. (1995). Ecological perception and the notion of a nonconceptual point of view. In J. L.

Bermudez, A. Marcel, and N. Eilan, eds., *The Body and the Self*, 153–173. Cambridge, MA: MIT Press.

Carey, D. P., Perrett, D. I., and Oram, M. W. (1997). Recognizing, understanding and reproducing actions. In M. Jeannerod and J. Grafman, eds., In Action and cognition, *Handbook of Neuropsychology*, vol. 11, sec. 16, 111–130. Amsterdam: Elsevier Science.

Decety, J., Perani, D., Jeannerod, M., Bettinardi, V., Tadary, B., Woods, R., Mazziotta, J. C., and Fazio, F. (1994). Mapping motor representations with positron emission tomography. *Nature* 371: 600–602.

Dunbar, R. I. M. (1993). Coevolution of neocortical size, group size and language in humans. *Behavioral Brain Sciences* 16: 681–694.

Fadiga, L., Fogassi, L., Pavesi, G., and Rizzolatti, G. (1995). Motor facilitation during action observation: A magnetic stimulation study. *Journal of Neurophysiology* 73: 2608–2611.

Frith, C. D. (1992). *The Cognitive Neuropsychology of Schizophrenia*. Hillsdale, NJ: Lawrence Erlbaum.

Gallese, V., Fadiga, L., Fogassi, L., and Rizzolatti, G. (1996). Action recognition in the premotor cortex. *Brain* 119: 593–609.

Gallese, V., and Goldman, A. (1998). Mirror neurons and the simulation theory of mind-reading. *Trends in Cognitive Sciences* 12: 493–501.

Gentilucci, M., Fogassi, L., Luppino, G., Matelli, M., Camarda, R., and Rizzolatti, G. (1988). Functional organization of inferior area 6 in the macaque monkey: I. Somatotopy and the control of proximal movements. *Experimental Brain Research* 71: 475–490.

Gentilucci, M., and Rizzolatti, G. (1990). Motor and visual-motor functions of the premotor cortex. In P. Rakic and W. Singer, eds., *Neurobiology of Neocortex*, 269–284. Chichester, UK: Wiley.

Grafton, S. T., Arbib, M. A., Fadiga, L., and Rizzolatti, G. (1996). Localization of grasp representations in humans by PET: 2. Observation compared with imagination. *Experimental Brain Research*, 112: 103–111.

He, S. Q., Dum, R. P., and Strick, P. L. (1993). Topographic organization of corticospinal projections from the frontal lobe—motor areas on the lateral surface of the hemisphere. *Journal of Neuroscience* 13: 952–980.

Hepp-Reymond, M.-C., Husler, E. J., Maier, M. A., and Qi, H.-X. (1994). Force-related neuronal activity in two regions of the primate ventral premotor cortex.

Canadian Journal of Physiology and Pharmacology 72: 571–579.

Jeannerod, M. (1994). The representing brain: Neural correlates of motor intention and imagery. *Behavioral Brain Sciences* 17: 187–245.

Jeannerod, M. (1997). *The Cognitive Neuroscience of Action*. Oxford: Blackwell.

Jeannerod, J., Arbib, M. A., Rizzolatti, G., and Sakata, H. (1995). Grasping objects: The cortical mechanisms of visuomotor transformation. *Trends in Neurosciences* 18: 314–320.

Leslie, A. M. (1987). Pretence and representation. The origins of "theory of mind." *Psychol. Rev.* 94: 412–426.

Matelli, M., Camarda, M., Glickstein, M., and Rizzolatti, G. (1986). Afferent and efferent projections of the inferior area 6 in the macaque monkey. *J. Comp. Neurol.* 251: 281–298.

Matelli, M., and Luppino, G. (1997). Functional anatomy of human motor cortical areas. In F. Boller, and J. Grafman, eds., *Handbook of Neuropsychology*, vol. 11. Elsevier Science.

Matelli, M., Luppino, G., and Rizzolatti, G. (1985). Patterns of cytochrome oxidase activity in the frontal agranular cortex of macaque monkey. *Behav. Brain Res.* 18: 125–137.

Meltzoff, A. (1995). Understanding the intentions of others: Re-enactment of intended acts by 18-month-old children. *Developmental Psychology* 31: 838–850.

Murata, A., Fadiga, L., Fogassi, L., Gallese, V., Raos, V., and Rizzolatti, G. (1997). Object representation in the ventral premotor cortex (area F5) of the monkey. *Journal of Neurophysiology* 78: 2226–2230.

Okano, K., and Tanji, J. (1987). Neuronal activities in the primate motor fields of the agranular frontal cortex preceding visually triggered and self-paced movement. *Exp. Brain Res.* 66: 155–166.

Pacherie, E. (1998). Représentations motrices, imitation et théorie de l'esprit: Le Cas de l'autisme. In H. Grivois and J. Proust, eds., *Subjectivité et conscience d'agir*, 207–248. Paris: Presses Universitaires de France.

Piaget, J. (1955). *The Child's Construction of Reality*. London: Routledge and Kegan Paul.

Premack, D., and Woodruff, G. (1978). Does the chimpanzee have a theory of mind? *Behavioral Brain Sciences* 4: 515–526.

Proust, J. (1998). Présentation. In H. Grivois and J. Proust, eds., *Subjectivité et conscience d'agir*, 1–33. Paris: Presses Universitaires de France.

Puce, A., Allison, T., Bentin, S., Gore, J. C., and McCarthy, G. (1998). Temporal cortex activation in humans viewing eye and mouth movements. *Journal of Neuroscience* 18: 2188–2199.

Rizzolatti, G., Camarda, R., Fogassi, L., Gentilucci, M., Luppino, G., and Matelli, M. (1988). Functional organization of inferior area 6 in the macaque monkey: II. Area F5 and the control of distal movements. *Experimental Brain Research* 71: 491–507.

Rizzolatti G., Fadiga, L., Gallese, V., and Fogassi L. (1996). Premotor cortex and the recognition of motor actions. *Cogn. Brain Res.* 3: 131–141.

Rizzolatti G., Scandolara, C., Matelli, M., and Gentilucci, M. (1981). Afferent properties of periarcuate neurons in macaque monkey. II. Visual responses. *Behavioral Brain Research*, 2: 147–163.

Russell, J. (1995). At two with nature: Agency and the development of self-world dualism. In J. L. Bermudez, A. Marcel, and N. Eilan, eds., *The Body and the Self*, 127–151. Cambridge, MA: MIT Press.

Stephan, K. M., Fink, G., Passingham, R. E., Silberzweig, D., Ceballos-Baumann, A. O., Frith, C. D., and Frackowiak, R. S. J. (1995). Functional anatomy of the mental representation of upper extremity movements in healthy subjects. *Journal of Neurophysiology* 73: 373–386.

von Holst, E., and Mittelstaedt, H. (1973). Das Reafferenzprinzip: Wechselwirkung zwischen Zentralnervensystem und Peripherie. Trans. R. D. Martin. In *The Behavioral Physiology of Animals and Man: Selected Papers of E. von Holst*, vol. 1. Coral Gables, FL: University of Miami Press.

Contributors

Jackie Andrade
Department of Psychology
University of Sheffield
Sheffield, United Kingdom

Ansgar Beckermann
Department of Philosophy
University of Bielefeld
Bielefeld, Germany

David J. Chalmers
Department of Philosophy
University of Arizona
Tucson, Arizona

Francis Crick
The Salk Institute for Biological Studies
San Diego, California

Antonio R. Damasio
M. W. Van Allen Professor and
Head, Department of Neurology
University of Iowa Hospitals and Clinics
Iowa City, Iowa

Gerald M. Edelman
The Neurosciences Institute
San Diego, California

Dominic ffytche
Institute of Psychiatry
London, United Kingdom

Hans Flohr
Brain Research Institute
University of Bremen
Bremen, Germany

Nicholas P. Franks
Biophysics Section, The Blackett Laboratory
Imperial College of Science, Technology and Medicine
London, United Kingdom

Vittorio Gallese
Institute of Human Physiology
University of Parma
Parma, Italy

Melvyn A. Goodale
Department of Psychology
University of Western Ontario, London
Ontario, Canada

Valerie Gray Hardcastle
Department of Philosophy
Virginia Polytechnic Institute
Blacksburg, Virginia

Beena Khurana
Computation and Neural Systems Program
California Institute of Technology
Pasadena, California

Christof Koch
Computation and Neural Systems Program
California Institute of Technology
Pasadena, California

William R. Lieb
Biophysics Section, The Blackett Laboratory
Imperial College of Science, Technology and Medicine
London, United Kingdom

Erik D. Lumer
Wellcome Department of Cognitive Neurology
Institute of Neurology
University College London
London, United Kingdom

Thomas Metzinger
Department of Philosophy
International Programme in Cognitive Science
University of Osnabrück
Osnabrück, Germany

Kelly J. Murphy
The Rotman Research Institute of Baycrest Centre
The University of Toronto
Ontario, Canada

Romi Nijhawan
Computation and Neural Systems
Division of Biology
California Institute of Technology
Pasadena, California

Joëlle Proust
Centre de Recherche en Epistemologie Appliquée
Ecole Polytechnique
Paris, France

Antti Revonsuo
Department of Philosophy
Center for Cognitive Neuroscience
University of Turku
Turku, Finland

Gerhard Roth
Brain Research Institute, University of Bremen,
and Hanse Institute for Advanced Study
Delmenhorst, Germany

Thomas Schmidt
Institute of Psychology
University of Göttingen
Göttingen, Germany

Wolf Singer
Department of Neurophysiology
Max-Planck Institute of Neuroscience
Frankfurt am Main, Germany

Giulio Tononi
The Neurosciences Institute
San Diego, California

The Association for the Scientific Study of
Consciousness
http://assc.caltech.edu

Index